BIOLOGICAL MARKERS IN EPIDEMIOLOGY

BIOLOGICAL MARKERS IN EPIDEMIOLOGY

BARBARA S. HULKA
M.D., M.P.H.

TIMOTHY C. WILCOSKY
Ph.D.

JACK D. GRIFFITH
Ph.D.

New York   Oxford
OXFORD UNIVERSITY PRESS
1990

Oxford University Press

Oxford   New York   Toronto
Delhi   Bombay   Calcutta   Madras   Karachi
Petaling Jaya   Singapore   Hong Kong   Tokyo
Nairobi   Dar es Salaam   Cape Town
Melbourne   Auckland

and associated companies in
Berlin   Ibadan

Library of Congress Cataloging-in-Publication Data
Biological markers in epidemiology / Barbara S. Hulka, Jack D. Griffith,
and Timothy C. Wilcosky.
p.   cm.
Bibliography: p.   Includes index.
ISBN 0-19-505984-0
1. Epidemiology.   2. Pathology, Molecular.   I. Hulka, Barbara S.
II. Griffith, Jack D.   III. Wilcosky, Timothy C.
RA652.B56 1990
614.4—dc20   89-16049   CIP

9 8 7 6 5 4 3 2 1

Printed in the United States of America
on acid-free paper

FOREWORD

F.P. PERERA

Prevention of environmentally related diseases such as cancer and reproductive illness hinges on identifying causative factors and mechanisms. However, the role of environmental exposures to toxic chemicals has proved especially elusive to epidemiologists who are usually forced to rely on insensitive and nonspecific exposure measures and on clinical disease as the outcome. Both formulation of research questions and interpretation of epidemiologic data suffer from a lack of understanding of mechanisms. These problems are exacerbated in studies of populations exposed to low levels of toxic chemicals, such as pesticides in the diet and emissions from hazardous waste sites or industrial operations. Here the possibility of exposure misclassification, the low frequency of disease outcomes, the multiplicity of causal factors and (in the case of cancer) the long latency of disease, all conspire against identification of causal associations. As noted in the book, associations of the magnitude of cigarette smoking and lung cancer, which are invulnerable to possible flaws in study design and analysis, are fortunately rare. Therefore, epidemiologic research strategies must be appreciably strengthened.

Enter biological markers. Although markers such as serum cholesterol and antibodies to bacterial and viral agents have been used by epidemiologists for generations, "biomarkers" have taken on a new importance as a result of dramatic advances in the fields of molecular biology and toxicology. For the first time, exquisitely sensitive laboratory techniques can detect subtle alterations in molecular processes that reflect events known or believed to occur along the continuum between exposure and disease. In theory, these mechanistically relevant biomarkers can provide information on the molecular dose of a toxic chemical, the resultant preclinical biological effect, and even specific genetic and acquired factors that modify the effect of exposure in the study population. With these tools in hand, the "molecular epidemiologist" could not only achieve greater resolution of exposure–disease relationships, but could also enhance our understanding of disease pathogenesis, including the nature of individual variation in sensitivity.

During the past 7 years, the field of biomonitoring and molecular epidemiology has seen a surge of activity in the development and characterization (validation) of methods. Numerous pilot-type studies have been undertaken in small populations with "model" exposure to genotoxic or carcinogenic compounds: cigarette smoke, the diet, the workplace, the community, and the clinical setting. These small-scale field studies have demonstrated that the "molecular epidemiologic" approach is feasible and that a number of methods are adequately sensitive and reproducible for human studies. However, considerable groundwork is needed to relate biomarkers in tissues readily available for human monitoring (e.g., peripheral blood) to those in target tissue (e.g., lung). In most cases, it would also be premature to deploy biomarkers in full-scale epidemiologic studies without additional information regarding the mechanisms they reflect. The extent to which individuals vary over time despite constant exposure must also be understood. In laying this groundwork, epidemiologists, environmental toxicologists, and laboratory scientists must work together.

As noted in the conclusion of this excellent review, "Biologic markers will play a prominent role in epidemiologic research of the 1990s. Growth in the use of biomarkers may be as important to epidemiologic research as the development of quantitative methods was during the 1970s and 1980s. Although these developments are taking place outside of epidemiology, the opportunities that they provide are causing them to be drawn inexorably into the fabric of epidemiologic research." *Biological Markers in Epidemiology* provides epidemiologists with a valuable road map into this new area. It gives a thoughtful and detailed discussion of biomarkers (urine mutagenicity, DNA and protein adducts, sister chromatid exchanges, micronuclei, chromosome aberrations, oncogenes, and indicators of susceptibility). It is more than a primer, however. The review is set firmly within the context of methodologic issues facing epidemiologists in the selection of biomarkers, study design, and interpretation of results. As such, it makes a real contribution to this interdisciplinary field and hopefully will wind up on the shelves of both laboratory investigators, and epidemiologists, who will become better collaborators as a result.

PREFACE

This book is the result of a cooperative agreement between the U.S. Environmental Protection Agency and the Department of Epidemiology at the University of North Carolina at Chapel Hill. It includes authors from these and other organizations in the Research Triangle area of North Carolina. The book has evolved over several years of study and learning on our part, and represents our effort to communicate the current status and future potential of molecular epidemiology as a field of scientific inquiry. Several things were learned quickly; the actual contributions of this field to cancer and reproductive epidemiology are less extensive than would be inferred from the amount of discussion that the topic has generated. In other words, much of the field is still a promise, to be consummated in the future. The other point that immediately came to the fore was that there was very little epidemiology, and few epidemiologists actually doing research in the field. Articles and book titles bore the label but the contributors and authors were consistently laboratory scientists, with a sprinkling of policy makers and occupational physicians/epidemiologists. The mainstream of epidemiology was rarely represented. Because of our frustration with the laboratory sciences literature, finding it difficult reading and not of primary relevance to epidemiologists, and because of our belief that molecular epidemiology is a major current and future direction for epidemiology, we decided that there should be an introductory book written by epidemiologists, primarily for epidemiologists. This is the background for this book.

There are many participants in this book in addition to those who are noted as authors or editors. These include molecular biologists, biochemists, toxicologists, geneticists, statisticians, and physicians in different specialties. All have contributed; some on defined topics within individual chapters while others have reviewed full chapters. These reviews have been particularly important to this effort in order to keep the laboratory components of the science accurate. We have tried to simplify difficult concepts, avoid unnecessary detail and still be accurate and reasonably current. This was not an easy task. The one individual to whom we are most indebted for this continuing guidance is David G. Kaufman, M.D., Ph.D., professor of pathology at the

University of North Carolina School of Medicine. He reviewed every chapter of the book, using his keen mind and red pencil liberally, to assure the integrity of the laboratory science concepts and assays.

We also want to thank the many other reviewers of individual chapters. These include Dr. Kaufman's colleagues in the UNC Department of Pathology and other scientists from the U.S. Environmental Protection Agency and the UNC School of Public Health, Department of Environmental Sciences and Engineering and Department of Biostatistics.

A number of individuals have served on advisory committees, which were particularly influential in guiding the directions for this book in its formative stages. These advisors include:

Philip G. Archer, Sc.D., University of Colorado Medical School
Arthur D. Bloom, M.D., Columbia University
Robert C. Duncan, Ph.D., University of Miami
John R. Fowle, III, Ph.D., U.S. Environmental Protection Agency
Brian P. Leaderer, Ph.D., Yale University
Frederica P. Perera, Dr.P.H., Columbia University
Cheryl Siegal-Scott, M.S.P.H., U.S. Environmental Protection Agency

It was during early meetings and discussions with these consultants that the direction for the book, emphasizing genotoxicity and carcinogenesis, evolved. This was a fortunate decision from my perspective since it coincided with my own interests and research experience; however, reasonable arguments can be made for alternate pathways. Most cogent of these is the relative lack of reviews of biological markers for neurobehavioral or respiratory health effects, as examples. This deficiency should certainly be corrected, and offers an opportunity for other authors and future volumes.

Most thanks is due to the chapters' authors, who have submitted gracefully to Dr. Kaufman's red pencil and my own entreaties about clarity, brevity, and simplicity. For those who find this book too unsophisticated and introductory, I accept responsibility. All material pertaining to laboratory assays and modern biology had to be readily understandable by the book's editors, who served as the representative epidemiologic audience. Those who are extensively trained in the laboratory sciences will find the descriptions of concepts and assays elementary. It is our judgment, however, that most epidemiologists will find the material helpful; for some it will integrate and highlight previously gained knowledge, whereas others will be reading new material.

We extend our appreciation to several other individuals; to Ms. Barbara Scott-Murdock who provided a scientifically knowledgeable editorial review, improving our flow of language and written presentation. Ms. Carol D. Morton persisted with professional competency on the word processing of numerous manuscript versions and revisions. Finally, we want to recognize Richard B. Everson, M.D., M.P.H. of the Environmental Protection Agency, whose intellectual vitality and scientific knowledge have invigorated the research activities and elevated the level of scientific inquiry within the EPA Cooperative Agreement.

Chapel Hill, N.C.   B.S.H
May 1989

CONTENTS

CONTRIBUTORS

Jay M. Goldring, M.S.P.H.
MD C3-03
National Institute of Environmental Health Sciences
Box 12233
Research Triangle Park, NC 27709

Jack Griffith, Ph.D.
U.S. Environmental Protection Agency
Health Effects Research Laboratory
MD-55A
Research Triangle Park, NC 27711

Barbara S. Hulka, M.D., M.P.H.
Kenan Professor and Chair
Department of Epidemiology
The University of North Carolina
Chapel Hill, NC 27599-7400

George W. Lucier, Ph.D.
National Institute of Environmental Health Sciences
Box 12233
Research Triangle Park, NC 27709

Lisa T. McFarland, M.S.P.H.
SRA Technologies
Research Triangle Park Offices
2515 Hwy 54, Building 2200
Durham, NC 27713

Susan M. Rynard, M.S.P.H.
Chief, Chronic Disease Section
Indiana State Board of Health
1330 West Michigan
P.O. Box 1964
Indianapolis, IN 46206-1964

Gary G. Schwartz, Ph.D., M.P.H.
Postdoctoral Fellow
Department of Epidemiology
The University of North Carolina
Chapel Hill, NC 27599-7400

Marilyn F. Vine, Ph.D.
Research Assistant Professor
Department of Epidemiology
The University of North Carolina
Chapel Hill, NC 27599-7400

Timothy C. Wilcosky, Ph.D.
Research Assistant Professor
Department of Epidemiology
The University of North Carolina
Chapel Hill, NC 27599-7400

BIOLOGICAL MARKERS IN EPIDEMIOLOGY

1

OVERVIEW OF BIOLOGICAL MARKERS

BARBARA S. HULKA

INTRODUCTION
Defining the Field

Molecular epidemiology is a research domain of significant promise but only modest current fulfillment. As first defined by Higginson (1977), molecular epidemiology referred to "the application of sophisticated techniques to the epidemiologic study of biologic material." Perera and Weinstein (1982) used the term *molecular cancer epidemiology* "to describe an approach in which advanced laboratory methods are used in combination with analytical epidemiology to identify at the biochemical or molecular level specific exogenous agents and/or host factors that play a role in human cancer causation." Although this definition gives a fuller flavor of the topic, it concentrates on elements of the exposure variable, "exogenous agents and/or host factors," without emphasizing the role of molecular epidemiology in identifying markers of subclinical disease. In fact, molecular epidemiology can be used to advantage in studying numerous health effects or diseases, not just cancer.

From the perspective of epidemiologists, "biochemical or molecular epidemiology" is the incorporation of biological markers (biomarkers) into analytic epidemiologic research. Biomarkers, defined as cellular, biochemical, or molecular alterations that are measurable in biological media, such as human tissues, cells, or fluids, have been used by generations of epidemiologists in their research. Cardiovascular disease epidemiologists have focused on serum cholesterol, lipids, and lipoprotein fractions with great success. This approach has increased knowledge of the causes of atherosclerosis and myocardial infarction, and has been used to further the goals of prevention. In infectious disease epidemiology, the identification of antibodies to bacterial and viral agents, as well as direct culture of these organisms from body fluids and tissues, has been a mainstay of the field. The term *seroepidemiology* was coined by those who studied immunologic responses to various organisms and then related these responses to patterns of disease occurrence. Even in the field of cancer epidemiology, as applied to screening, we have successfully identified cervical cancer precursors through cervical cytology, by characterizing cellular alterations that can be observed under simple light microscopy.

What is new, then, about biomarkers in epidemiologic research? It is mostly the extent to which these markers can identify molecular or biochemical alterations, which were not recognized or observed before the molecular biology revolution and its concomitant development of sophisticated laboratory technology. Today, biomarkers can be identified down to a level of less than one alteration in 10^6 DNA bases. Such precision allows the development of a mechanistic understanding of disease causation. It has the potential to draw the exposure variables and their disease outcomes closer together.

The last decade has witnessed an exponential growth in molecular biology and in the laboratory technology that made this growth possible. The human genome is being mapped to specific regions on each chromosome and the protein products of genes are being characterized with great rapidity. These areas of scientific advance are important to epidemiology. The reasons are many, including the most global: to remain scientifically relevant, epidemiologic research must evolve within the entire body of scientific knowledge. In addition, these advances have the potential to improve the capability of epidemiologic research in understanding and quantifying the spectrum of exposure to disease relationships, and in increasing opportunities for intervention research, including prevention trials.

Biomarkers may be internal indicators of exposure to external xenobiotics, they may reflect early, subclinical adverse health effects, or they may define the innate susceptibility of the human host. Furthermore, a given biomarker may serve one or more of these functions depending on how it is used in the context of the objectives and design of a study. For example, DNA adducts to benzo(a)pyrene might be the dependent variables in a study of occupational exposure to polycyclic aromatic hydrocarbons, independent variables in a study of lung cancer, or indicators of cigarette smoking, a confounding variable in many studies. Adducts could even be surrogates for susceptibility, depending on the extent to which cigarette smoke constituents stimulated aryl hydrocarbon hydroxylase activity and thereby affected the level of adduct formation. Thus, there are multiple roles for any particular biomarker in epidemiologic studies.

Although we categorize biomarkers in later sections of this book, some of these categories actually reflect a continuum of events from external exposure through internal interactions with host susceptibility factors to eventual disease outcomes. Any classification scheme we choose, whether categorical or continuous, will undoubtedly change as our understanding of disease processes and the markers we use to identify them are better understood.

Audience for Book

A review of the recent literature on biomarkers found several books and review articles that addressed biomarkers in environmental health, occupational monitoring, epidemiology, or risk assessment (Perera and Weinstein, 1982; Board of Scientific Counselors, 1984; IARC, 1984; Third Task Force, 1984; Harris, 1986; Sorsa and Norppa,

1986; Alavanja et al., 1987; Draggan et al., 1987; Higginson, 1977; NRC, 1987; Perera, 1987). With few exceptions, these publications were authored by researchers in the laboratory sciences. Thus, the topics and language of these publications are more understandable to laboratory scientists than to epidemiologists. Training in clinical epidemiology, to whatever extent it differs from traditional epidemiology, carries no advantage; it contains no elements of the molecular epidemiology perspective. Perhaps the most compatible literature for epidemiologists appears in the occupational health literature from Europe, and particularly Scandinavia (Sorsa and Norppa, 1986) where biomonitoring of occupational groups has been accepted for over two decades. Papers by Perera (1987), Gann et al. (1985), Everson (1987), and Hulka and Wilcosky (1988) also provide a framework amenable to epidemiologic thinking.

Because the collaborative nature of molecular epidemiology is self-evident, we hope that laboratory scientists, who foresee the application of their assays to large groups of people in field settings, will find this book informative. Chapter 3, which points out the criteria for selecting and evaluating potential biomarkers for an epidemiologic study, may be of particular interest to laboratory scientists. Our intent is to introduce the field of molecular epidemiology to epidemiologists and laboratory scientists from the perspective of research-oriented epidemiologists.

Focus of Book

Although biomarkers generally are not new to epidemiologic research, certain types, such as those related to genotoxicity, are relative newcomers. Chapters 5 through 10 concentrate on markers related to genetic mutational events. Because mutational events are thought to be an initial step in carcinogenesis, these markers may be suspect for the development of subsequent cancers (somatic cell mutations) or reproductive adverse effects (germinal cell mutations). We want to emphasize the word *suspect* because there are few, if any, empirical observations in humans to substantiate these associations.

We selected the particular markers described in Chapters 4 through 10 with attention to both their availability and their potential usefulness for epidemiologic research. Although human studies can be cited for each of these markers, studies that could be classified as epidemiologic, in terms of population selection and adherence to standards of design, data collection, and analysis, are few. In general, these limitations reflect the developmental state of both the laboratory capability and the markers themselves.

We made another choice concerning which type of exogenous exposure to emphasize. Although the full spectrum of xenobiotics includes chemical, physical (e.g., ionizing radiation), and biological (e.g., viruses), we chose to concentrate on chemical exposures. The reason for this choice was that chemical exposures appeared to have received the least attention in the epidemiologic literature on biomarkers. Chemicals are also a timely choice in view of the current interest in environmental chemical exposures (e.g., toxic waste dumps) and risk assessment strategies. We should note, however, that the molecular or biochemical derangement proximate to the clinical manifestations of cancer may be similar, whether the insult is viral genetic material integrated into the genome or genotoxicity caused by ionizing radiation or chemicals.

RATIONALE FOR USE OF BIOMARKERS

Using biomarkers in epidemiologic research has potential for both improving validity and reducing bias. Consider the problems encountered in studies of disease occurrence in relation to environmental exposure, where accurate information on amount and duration of exposure to a particular agent may be nearly impossible to obtain. In occupational studies, the main sources of exposure information are job classification and estimates of chemical exposures reported to be associated with these jobs. More direct information is sometimes available from sporadic monitoring of the ambient environment and occasionally from personal monitors attached to individual workers. All but the latter strategy represent ecologic measurements of a variable for which precise individual data are needed. In epidemiologic terms, an ecologic measurement indicates that the group value of some variable is assigned to the individual, under the assumption that the group value is a reasonable surrogate for the individual. The ecologic approach carries the potential for significant misclassification of individual exposure (Brunekreef et al., 1987). Such misclassification reduces the power of studies to detect health effects and can produce erroneous and misleading results. Biomarkers have the potential to improve the sensitivity and specificity of our exposure measures and thus increase the validity of results.

Second, biological markers should enhance our understanding of disease pathogenesis and allow for earlier disease detection. Although our current disease classification systems, based on histologic diagnoses or standardized criteria for disease signs and symptoms, are quite accurate, there are earlier stages of disease before clinical manifestations. If we can use biological markers to accurately identify these, the study of preclinical disease will be enhanced, providing greater opportunities for preventive intervention.

Third, biological markers may assist in providing more homogeneous classifications of disease. To the extent that particular chromosomal aberrations are found in some adult acute leukemia patients and not in others, two case groups could be formed with respect to a particular exposure (Sandler and Collman, 1987). The exposure may be related to one group of cases but not to the other. Thus, biological markers could allow for more etiologically relevant disease classification.

Another relatively unexplored, but potentially very large domain in epidemiologic research, is the study of individual susceptibility and the markers that could identify such susceptibility. Epidemiologists usually classify people as exposed or unexposed and compare disease risk between groups. This is an artificial and biologically uninformed strategy, when within the most highly exposed group we know that only a small proportion will develop the disease. Even among cigarette smokers, the cumulative lifetime risk of clinically manifest lung cancer is only about 10 percent. Why do the other 90 percent not develop lung cancer? Very little attention has been paid to interindividual differences in susceptibility. Genetic epidemiology can help to increase our understanding of genetic variability, which alters individual responses to exogenous exposures. To the extent that biomarkers of genetic or acquired susceptibility are known and that laboratory assays for these markers are available, epidemiologic research can be strengthened. Susceptibility markers, which may be extremely potent effect modifiers, should make it possible to demonstrate high disease risks for exposed susceptibles and lower risks for nonsusceptible exposed and unexposed groups.

Prevention trials using intervention strategies illustrate a methodologic contribution of biomarkers. For example, trials of smoking cessation strategies (Abrams et al., 1987) have found that salivary cotinine is a more accurate measure of current smoking status than responses to questionnaires. In this example, smoking cessation is the outcome variable of interest. In other trials, biomarkers may be used to measure compliance with the intervention. In the Lipid Research Clinics Coronary Primary Prevention Trial (Lipid Research, 1984), which was designed to measure effects of a serum lipid-lowering agent (cholestyramine) on cardiovascular disease mortality and morbidity, serum cholesterol was used as a marker for adherence to the cholestyramine regimen.

Last, knowledge of biological markers can improve our understanding of the mechanisms of disease occurrence. To the extent that markers are themselves part of the causal link between exposure and disease, they help to elucidate the pathogenesis of disease. Surrogate markers are useful, if they accurately represent the true marker in target tissue. The examples of DNA and protein adducts illustrate mechanistic and surrogate markers, respectively. Information on mechanisms, derived from an array of scientific disciplines, strengthens the interpretation of epidemiologic data and the theoretical framework from which we identify gaps in knowledge and formulate research questions.

TYPES OF BIOMARKERS
Classification, Definitions, and Illustrations

Biological markers can be classified according to a variety of schemes, most of which are variations of the classification introduced by Perera and Weinstein (1982). In their terminology, markers were classified into categories of susceptibility, internal dose, biologically effective dose (BED), and biological response (BR). This approach suggests a sequence of events from exposure to disease. The sequence starts with an external exposure, defined as the concentration of a chemical substance in an individual's immediate environment. Estimates of external concentrations are based on ambient monitoring for the amount of the chemical in air, water, soil, or food. Personal monitoring, questionnaires, and mathematical modeling techniques have also been used to estimate exposures.

Figure 1-1 illustrates sites of uptake and target tissue for exogenous chemicals, and the media potentially available for studying biomarkers in humans. Circulating blood occupies a central position both as a means of distributing exogenous agents throughout the body and as a target for their action. Biological media available for identifying markers may be peripheral to the target tissue of importance for disease occurrence. For example, blood, including its constituent white and red blood cells, is readily available for study, whereas the true target organ might be epithelial cells in the lower respiratory tract or urinary bladder. Feasibility considerations may dictate the use of surrogate, rather than target tissues. For example, bone marrow stem cells may be the target tissue for exogenous chemicals such as benzene. Micronuclei in these cells would be a suitable biomarker, except that the invasiveness of specimen collection poses an obvious constraint to their use. Identifying biological markers from available media rather than the target tissue assumes that the surrogate is a true reflection of the target site. The extent to which this assumption is valid varies with the marker type, the

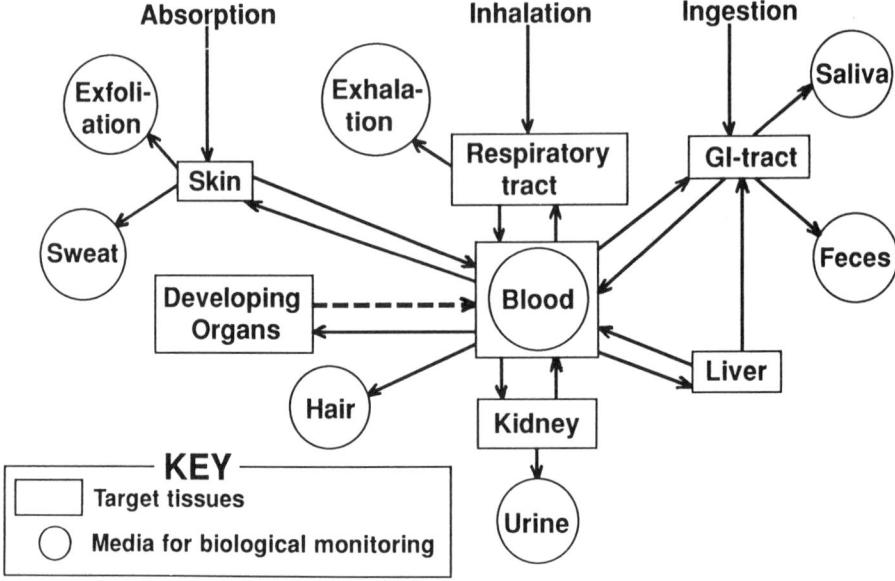

Figure 1-1. Sites of uptake, target tissue, and media for monitoring for xenobiotic compounds. (Adapted from Committee on Biological Markers, National Research Council. Biological Markers in Environmental Health Research. *Environ Health Perspect* 1987;77:3–9.)

particular chemical exposure, and the biological characteristics, including longevity of the surrogate tissue.

If an exogenous chemical is identified in body tissues or fluids through one of a variety of laboratory assays, it becomes a marker of internal dose. An internal dose marker indicates the amount of exogenous chemical, either unchanged or metabolically altered, absorbed by the human organism. Pharmacokinetic data, such as half-life, circulating peak dose, or cumulative dose, are frequently useful in quantifying internal dose. Chemicals, such as halogenated hydrocarbons that are stored in adipose tissue to form an accumulated body burden, represent an interesting subset of these markers. Other examples of internal dose markers appear in Table 1-1. Some of these are chemical specific, either metabolically altered (e.g., cotinine in urine) or chemically unchanged (e.g., urinary lead). Urinary alkyl phosphate residues, identified in farm workers after exposure to organic phosphate pesticides (Duncan and Griffith, 1985), are another example. Mutagenesis assays are chemically nonspecific but indicate exposure to chemicals that the host has activated to mutagenic, potentially carcinogenic, substances.

The next markers in sequence are those for BED, noted in Table 1-2. A BED marker indicates the amount of absorbed chemical that has interacted with critical subcellular targets, measured either in a target or surrogate tissue. Chemical addition products, unscheduled DNA synthesis, and DNA strand breaks may be included in this category, although it is primarily for adducts that laboratory assays applicable to human studies have been developed (Everson, 1987). DNA adducts are of particular interest

Table 1-1 Internal Dose Markers

Marker	Exposure	Biological Media
Cotinine	Nicotine in cigarette smoke	Body fluids
Lead	Lead in environment	Body fluids and tissues (hair, nails, teeth)
DDE	DDT	Adipose tissue
Aflatoxin	Aflatoxin in food stuff	Body fluids
Mutagenesis assays	Chemical mutagens	Body fluids

DDE, dichlorodiphenyldichloroethylene.

Hulka BS, Wilcosky TC: Biological markers in epidemiologic research. *Arch Environ Health* 1988;43:83–89.

because they are thought to initiate mutational events. But even when identified, their interpretation is not obvious. Although benzo(a)pyrene produces a specific adduct with DNA, the chemical's ubiquity in the environment hinders studies that purport to show adduct formation in relation to a specific source of exposure. On the other hand, methyl bromide produces a nonspecific methyl adduct with hemoglobin (Djalali-Behzad et al., 1981). Yet these can be informative, since background levels of methyl adducts should be modest relative to adducts from an occupational exposure. Furthermore, the methyl adducts formed with hemoglobin are thought to be reasonable proxies for DNA adducts.

Biological response (BR) markers are biological or biochemical changes in target cells or tissues that result from the action of the chemical and are thought to be a step in the pathologic process toward disease. We stress the word *thought* because empirical data in humans to link BR markers to clinically overt disease are for the most part lacking. The definition, however, is consistent with data obtained from animal models and with current concepts of carcinogenesis and other disease processes in humans. Table 1-3 lists some BR markers. The literature on chromosomal alterations is extensive and is well illustrated by the report from Stolley and colleagues (1984). They showed an association between frequency of sister chromatid exchanges (SCEs) in lymphocytes and level of exposure to ethylene oxide at the worksite. Chromosomal alterations presumably affect genetic material adjacent to the site of chromosomal breakage or reattachment, causing changes in the genes themselves or their products.

The BR markers differ from the BED markers by representing a more stable

Table 1-2 Biologically Effective Dose Markers

Marker	Exposure	Biological Media
DNA adducts	Benzo(a)pyrene	WBC
Protein adducts (hemoglobin)	Ethylene oxide	RBC

WBC, white blood cell; RBC, red blood cell.

Hulka BS, Wilcosky TC: Biological markers in epidemiologic research. *Arch Environ Health* 1988;432:83–89.

Table 1-3 Biological Response Markers

Markers	Exposure	Biological Media
Chromosomal	Mutagenic chemicals	
Aberrations		WBC
Sister chromatid exchange		WBC
Micronuclei		Epithelia
Point mutations	Mutagenic chemicals	
HGPRT		WBC
Thymidine-kinase		WBC
Oncogene activation	Chemical carcinogens (benzo(a)pyrene)	Tissue
Elevated protoporphyrin	Lead	RBC
Decreased acetylcholines- terase	Organic phosphate pesticides	Plasma

HGPRT, hypoxanthine–guanine phosphoribosyl transferase; RBC, red blood cell; WBC, white blood cell.
Hulka, BS, Wilcosky TC: Biological markers in epidemiologic research. *Arch Environ Health* 1988;43:83–89.

alteration in cells and tissues, with greater persistence over time. They are also likely to represent a more advanced mechanistic process in the continuum toward overt disease. Cytogenetic markers are prominent in this category. Theoretically, both BED and BR markers should have a quantitative relationship with a marker of internal dose.

Disease markers form the last group in the spectrum. Markers in this category are frequently proposed for disease screening purposes. A disease marker is a measurable indicator of a biological or biochemical event that either represents a subclinical stage of disease or is a manifestation of the disease itself. This indicator can be used as a dependent variable in a study of exposure and disease associations. Disease markers (Table 1-4) are frequently characterized by altered gene expression with inappropriate synthesis of fetal proteins or isoenzymes. Alpha-fetoprotein (AFP), carcinoembryonic antigen (CEA), and a variety of tumor-specific antigens have been proposed as markers for the early diagnosis of cancers at various sites. Unfortunately, because of their lack of specificity, these markers have not proved useful in screening for preclinical disease. For example, CEA may be present in patients with benign gastrointestinal disorders as well as in patients with cancer. Many tumor-specific antigens are useful in monitoring cancer recurrence and providing information on the extent of tumor burden. Tumor-specific antigens are helpful for prognostication in patients with diagnosed cancer.

Table 1-4 Markers of Subclinical Disease

Marker	Disease
Altered gene expression	
Serum alpha-fetoprotein	Liver cancer
	GI diseases
	Fetal neural tube defect
Carcinoembryonic antigen	GI cancers
	Other GI diseases
Tumor specific antigens	Various cancers
SGOT	Myocardial infarction

GI, gastrointestinal; SGOT, serum glutamic-oxaloacetic transaminase.
Hulka BS, Wilcosky TC: Biological markers in epidemiologic research. *Arch Environ Health* 1988;43:83–89.

A different kind of marker, which does not lie on the spectrum from exposure to disease but is of great importance in every step along the way and a major determinant of whether or not disease occurs, is the susceptibility marker. These markers are measurable indicators of the genetic or acquired factors, existing before and independent of exposure, that influence the probability that disease will result from external exposures. Although the examples listed in Table 1-5 are genetic markers, acquired diseases (including infections), physiologic changes and nutritional status can also alter individual susceptibility to carcinogens.

Differences in susceptibility are thought to account for much of the interindividual variability in some markers. For example, benzo(a)pyrene–DNA binding levels have been noted to vary 12–100-fold among individuals who smoke similar amounts of tobacco (Harris et al., 1978). Genetic differences, perhaps in aryl hydrocarbon hydroxylase activity, are likely to account for a significant amount of this variability but extraneous environmental exposures and lifestyle behaviors also contribute.

Individuals with rare autosomal recessive inherited diseases involving defects in DNA replication or repair (Bloom's syndrome and xeroderma pigmentosum) offer additional examples of differences in susceptibility. These people are at markedly increased risk of developing certain cancers. To the extent that persons heterozygous for these disease traits have an increased cancer risk, the genetic alteration could have a quantitatively important effect on population-based rates of cancer occurrence. A study of the blood relatives of patients with ataxia–telangiectasia, an autosomal recessive syndrome which infers very high cancer risk, illustrates this point (Swift et al., 1987). Among white patients with breast cancer in the United States, 8.8 percent were estimated to be heterozygous for ataxia–telangiectasia.

The effect of susceptibility markers can also be observed for some ingested medications. Genetically determined interindividual variability in the metabolism of drugs, which can influence their pharmacologic effects, has been clearly established. For example, some people are "slow" and others "fast" acetylators of hydralazine. Slow acetylators are subject to a longer duration of drug activity than are fast acetylators, a phenomenon that may influence the drug's effectiveness in the treatment of hypertension (Meyer, 1978). Although ingested medications may seem remote from the topic of environmental chemical exposures, the model of medication use is highly relevant. Precise external dose concentrations can be quantified and related to the internal dose level modified by individual susceptibility. Response in terms of altered signs and symptoms of disease can be measured accurately with standardized protocols. Thus,

Table 1-5 Susceptibility Markers

Markers[a]	Exposure	Disease
Alpha$_1$-antitrypsin	Smoking	Emphysema
N-acetyltransferase	Aromatic amines	Bladder cancer
Aryl hydrocarbon hydroxylase	Smoking	Lung cancer

[a]Marker affects relationship between exposure and disease.
Hulka BS, Wilcosky TC: Biological markers in epidemiologic research. *Arch Environ Health* 1988;43:83–89.

the model of human drug exposures in clinical settings should have important applicability to less precisely measured chemical exposure in environmental settings.

Relationship Among Biomarkers

Figure 1-2 is a schematic presentation of the relationship among markers (National Research Council, 1987). The scheme illustrates the distinctive role of susceptibility, which can affect each step in the process between exposure and disease. In epidemiologic terms, susceptibility markers would be considered effect modifiers. Effect modifiers are operative when uniformly exposed persons exhibit markedly different risks of disease. For example, postmenopausal women using exogenous estrogens exhibit different risks of developing endometrial carcinoma depending on whether or not they are obese (Hulka et al., 1980). Obesity is the effect modifier and estrogens the exposure, analogous to susceptibility markers and chemical exposures, respectively. The diagram omits a whole set of other potential effect modifiers and confounders that relate to extraneous environmental influences: chemical, physical, biological, and cultural. It is these factors that have influenced the development of epidemiologic methods. The goal has been to "control for" effects of these extraneous factors, through both design and analytic techniques, so that etiologic inferences between "exposure" and "disease" can be made.

CONSTRAINTS OF BIOMARKERS IN EPIDEMIOLOGIC RESEARCH

Quality research can only be achieved through collaborative efforts. Collaboration among scientists who are not familiar with each other's discipline, methods, or language requires tolerance and willingness to learn.

Most of the markers we know have been examined only to a limited extent in humans and some have been studied only in experimental systems (in vitro and in vivo). The research requirements for markers in epidemiologic studies include considerations of feasibility and applicability to large numbers of people in nonexperimental settings. A laboratory assay that appears highly developed to the molecular biologist may be only in a preliminary stage of development for epidemiologic studies.

In our enthusiam for this blossoming new field of research, it is important that we do not overextend the inferences and interpretations made from the observed data. Findings become credible only after replication in multiple studies, conducted among different groups of people, in various settings, over different points in time.

Even for common markers, data on marker frequency in general populations, including persons of different ages and gender, rarely exist. Although it may not be feasible to obtain baseline information for any but the most common markers and assays, appropriately designated and sampled control subjects can be used to help accumulate this store of information.

Researchers must address the issue of intraindividual and interindividual variability, although it is the between-group differences that are usually of interest. Epidemiologists who focus on groups rather than on individuals may not feel comfortable with this shift in emphasis. When considered within the framework of effect modification, however, interindividual variability becomes more compatible with epidemiologic concepts.

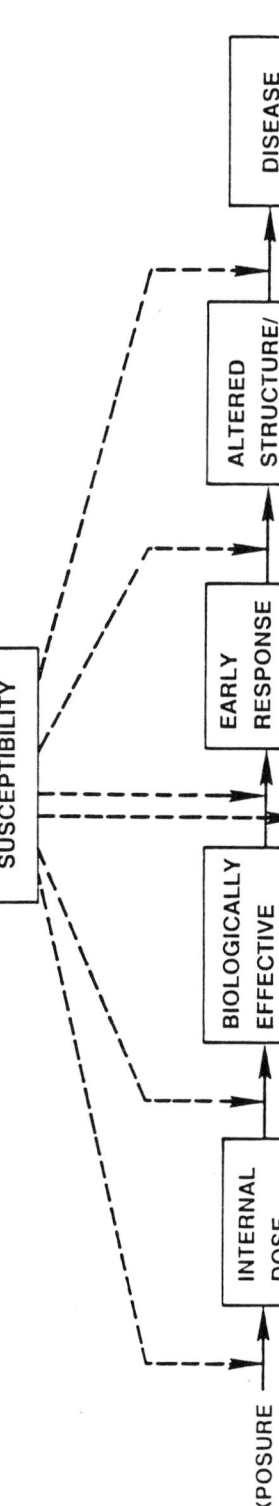

Figure 1-2. The relationship of biological markers to exposure and disease. (Adapted from Committee on Biological Markers, National Research Council. Biological Markers in Environmental Health Research. *Environ Health Perspect* 1987;77:3–9.)

In concluding this overview, we emphasize the uses of biomarkers in epidemiologic research. These include improvement in the accuracy of exposure measurement, identification of subclinical disease, provision of more homogeneous classifications of disease, identification of individuals susceptible to disease in the presence of adverse exposures, improvement in methodology for preventive and therapeutic trials, and an increase in knowledge of disease pathogenesis.

Existing constraints in the use of biomarkers in epidemiologic research indicate important avenues for future research. Much of the needed research is developmental: in the laboratory, in populations, and among individuals. First, many of the laboratory assays that the epidemiologist would like to employ require further development both to improve accuracy, reliability, and interpretability, and to reduce costs. Second, data on various markers, and assays, are needed for normal populations to identify marker distributions within different age and sex groupings. Third, we need more information on the extent of intraindividual variation in markers with respect to tissue localization and persistence, and interindividual variability due to genetic and acquired susceptibility factors. Developmental research should precede, or at least take place, concurrently with more classic epidemiologic research that is designed to increase substantive knowledge of disease etiology.

REFERENCES

Abrams DB, Follick MJ, Biener L, Carey KB, Hitti J: Saliva cotinine as a measure of smoking status in field settings. *AJPH* 1987;77:846–848.

Alavanja M, Aron J, Brown C, et al.: Cancer risk-assessment models: Anticipated contributions from biochemical epidemiology. *JNCI* 1987;78:633–643.

Board of Scientific Counselors: *Report of the NTP Ad Hoc Panel on Chemical Carcinogenesis Testing and Evaluation of the National Tox. Prog.* Unpublished, 1984.

Brunekoef B, Noy D, Clausing P: Variability of exposure measurements in environmental epidemiology. *Am J Epidemiol* 1987;125:892–898.

Djalali-Behzad G, Hussain S, Osterman-Golkar S, Segerbäck D: Estimation of genetic risks of alkylating agents. VI. Exposure of mice and bacteria to methyl bromide. *Mutat Res* 1981; 84:1–9.

Draggan S, Cohrssen JJ, Morrison RE, eds.: *Environmental Impacts on Human Health—The Agenda for Long-Term Research and Development.* New York, Praeger Publishers, 1987.

Duncan RC, Griffith J: Monitoring study of urinary metabolites and selected symptomatology among Flordia citrus workers. *J Toxicol Environ Health* 1985;16:509–521.

Everson RB: A review of approaches to the detection of genetic damage in the human fetus. *Environ Health Perspect* 1987;74:109–117.

Gann PH, Davis DL, Perera F: Biological Markers in Environmental Epidemiology: Constraints and Opportunities. Presented at the Fifth Workshop of the Scientific Group on Methodologies for the Safety Evaluation of Chemicals (SGOMSEC), Mexico City, 12–16 August 1985.

Harris CC, ed.: *Biochemical and Molecular Epidemiology of Cancer.* New York, Alan R. Liss, Inc., 1986.

Harris CC, Autrup H, Stoner G: Metabolism of benzo(a)pyrene in cultured human tissues and cells. In: Stoner G, Gelboin HV, T'so PO, eds.: *Polycyclic Hydrocarbons and Cancer,* Vol 2. New York, Academic Press, 1978, pp. 331–342.

Higginson J: The role of the pathologist in environmental medicine and public health. *Am J Pathol* 1977;86:459–484.

Hulka BS, Fowler WC, Kaufman DG, Grimson RC, et al.: Estrogen and endometrial cancer: Cases and two control groups from North Carolina. *Am J Obstet Gynecol* 1980;137:92.

Hulka BS, Wilcosky TC: Biological markers in epidemiologic research. *Arch Environ Health* 1988;43:83–89.

International Agency for Research on Cancer: Monitoring Human Exposure to Carcinogenic and Mutagenic Agents. Proceedings of a Joint Symposium Held in Espoo, Finland, 12–15 December, 1983, Berlin A, Draper M, Hemminki K, Vainio H, eds. Oxford University Press, New York, 1984.

Lipid Research Clinics Program: Lipid research clinics primary prevention trial results: I. Reduction in incidence of coronary heart disease. *JAMA* 1984;251:351–363.

Meyer U: Role of genetic factors in the rational use of drugs. In: Melmon and Morelli, eds.: *Clinical Pharmacology: Basic Principles in Therapeutics,* ed. 2. New York, Macmillan, 1978.

National Research Council, Committee on Biological Markers: Biological markers in environmental health research. *Environ Health Perspect* 1987;74:3–9.

Perera FP: Molecular cancer epidemiology: A new tool in cancer prevention. *JNCI* 1987;78:887–898.

Perera FP, Weinstein IB: Molecular epidemiology and carcinogen-DNA adduct detection: New approaches to studies of human cancer causation. *J Chronic Dis* 1982;35:581–600.

Sandler DP, Collman GW: Cytogenetic and environmental factors in the etiology of the acute leukemias in adults. *Am J Epidemiol* 1987;126:1017–1032.

Sorsa M, Norppa H, eds.: *Monitoring of Occupational Genotoxicants.* New York, Alan R. Liss, Inc., 1986.

Stolley PD, Soper KA, Galloway SM, Nichols WW, et al.: Sister-chromatid exchanges in association with occupational exposure to ethylene oxide. *Mutat Res* 1984;129:89–102.

Swift M, Reitnauer PJ, Morrell D, Chase CL: Breast and other cancers in families with ataxia-telangiectasia. *N Engl J Med* 1987;316:1289–94.

Third Task Force for Research Planning in Environmental Health Sciences: *Human Health and the Environment—Some Research Needs.* National Institutes of Health Publication No. 86-1277, 1984.

2

APPLICATIONS
OF BIOLOGICAL MARKERS

TIMOTHY C. WILCOSKY AND JACK D. GRIFFITH

Markers provide an index of events or states that may themselves be difficult or impossible to measure in their entirety. Markers may be used to indicate a susceptibility to disease, to estimate internal doses from ambient exposures, to measure biological responses in target cells, to identify early disease states, and to characterize different types of overt disease. A single marker can serve in more than one capacity, and these categories of use may overlap (Gann et al., 1985).

MARKER INTERPRETATION

The most important single determinant of a marker's usefulness is its relationship to the biological phenomenon of interest. Clearly, the biological processes that give rise to a marker must bear some direct or indirect relationship to the exposure or health outcome under investigation. Markers of gene mutation, for example, could be important for studies of cancer or reproductive outcomes, where mutations may be part of the pathogenic pathway. Markers outside the pathogenic pathway also have value. A marker of mutation could possibly be used to assess exposure in a neurotoxicity study, for example, even if gene mutation had no biological role in the neurotoxic pathway. If the neurotoxic exposure also happened to cause genetic damage, gene mutations could be used as indicators of the neurotoxin's internal dose.

The statistical, rather than biological, link between a marker and a condition of interest ultimately determines a marker's usefulness in an epidemiologic study, although an understanding of both the biological and statistical processes that underlie a marker–condition association is important to assess a marker's validity. In the absence of an adequate understanding of the biological association, the statistical association derived from empirical observations may still be used as a "black box" indicator of exposure or disease.

Validity for Different Conditions

A given marker may vary in validity for different conditions of potential interest. For example, because alcohol in the blood rapidly reaches equilibrium with air in the lungs, exhaled alcohol concentrations have found widespread use as a marker of blood alcohol levels. Because blood alcohol permeates the central nervous system, exhaled alcohol also provides a good exposure marker in the "target tissue" for neurotoxicity. From a law enforcement perspective, however, the condition of interest is typically intoxication that may result in impaired driving. Different individuals with identical internal doses of alcohol may vary widely in their degree of intoxication, however, and drugs other than alcohol can cause intoxication. As a result, the concentration of exhaled alcohol has greater validity as a marker of the internal dose or of the biologically effective dose of alcohol than as a marker of intoxication, because exhaled alcohol is more closely linked, statistically as well as biologically, to alcohol tissue concentrations than to intoxication.

Biological Relationships

The biological process that underlies the relationship between a marker and an exposure of interest can be straightforward. In some instances (e.g., the previous alcohol example), one simply measures the levels of an exogenous agent, such as a solvent that has entered the bloodstream, as an indicator of exposure. This fairly simple type of marker can have great value in estimating the internal dose of a chemical that has more than one route of entry into the body. Chemicals in blood have potential access to virtually all tissues and cells in the body, so blood levels of a chemical provide an important exposure index. Other markers, including heavy metals bound to hair or polychlorinated biphenyls in adipocytes, indicate blood levels integrated over time. Even the conceptually simple measurements of chemical levels in the blood are complicated by changes over time after the initiation and termination of the exposure. Therefore, effective use of these markers requires some knowledge of temporal relationships between ambient exposures and marker response.

For markers of early biological response, the marker may directly reflect lesions that can sometimes progress to overt disease. Potentially reversible small airways disease measured in biopsy material, for example, may precede chronic bronchitis (Cosio et al., 1977). Other times, the marker may reflect biological changes outside of some pathologic process of interest, but be closely correlated with pathogenesis. Cytogenetic markers, such as sister chromatid exchanges and chromosome aberrations, are often measured in peripheral lymphocytes, but the associated DNA lesions in mature lymphocytes do not lead to cancer. Exposures that cause a marker response in lymphocytes, however, probably also affect other tissues where malignant cell transformation can occur. Markers of exposure or response may, therefore, have varying degrees of complexity in their biological relationship with the condition of interest.

PROBLEMS THAT CAN BE ADDRESSED

Because markers vary extensively in their biological properties, the types of epidemiologic questions that markers can address are also diverse. For discussion, one can divide markers into those associated with exposure and those associated with disease.

Markers of Exposure

A true estimate of internal dose requires the integration of an agent's internal concentration over the entire time it remains in the body, so that markers in a biological material sampled at a single time point (e.g., solvent levels in a single blood sample) provide only a snapshot of part of the total dose. In this situation, the marker at least gives binary information (i.e., presence or absence) about the internal dose of the agent. Dose markers also provide qualitative or quantitative information about external exposures to an agent, as the internal dose originates from an ambient exposure. Consequently, the nonspecific term *exposure marker* describes a general class of markers that includes qualitative or quantitative markers of internal dose and biologically effective dose. Possible applications for these diverse markers are discussed in the following.

Integrate Multiple Portals of Entry

An important property of virtually all biological markers of exposure is their estimation of the internal dose resulting from all portals of entry from the environment into the body. Exposures to volatile organic compounds in drinking water (e.g., trichloroethylene or chloroform) illustrate this aspect of biological markers. Regulators have primarily focused on inhalation and ingestion as routes of exposure to these chemicals, which contaminate drinking water supplies throughout the United States (Brown et al., 1984). Skin absorption under some circumstances, however, may contribute most of the total dose (Brown et al., 1984).

Estimates derived from ambient concentrations of the amounts inhaled or ingested are prone to error, and estimates of skin absorption are also very difficult. Numerous variables, including hydration of the skin, skin temperature, skin damage, region of the body exposed, temperature and properties of the chemical, and individual variability in absorption rates due to differences in age, sex, amount of body fat, exposure history, and nutrition all influence skin absorption (Brown et al., 1984). Biological markers of internal dose intrinsically account for all these variables, as well as other routes of entry. Consequently, an epidemiologic investigation of volatile organic compounds and acute neurobehavioral effects, for example, might be conducted with much greater simplicity and precision using an internal dose marker rather than ambient exposure estimates.

Integrate Fluctuating Exposure (External and Internal)

Some markers can also improve the precision of dose estimates through temporal integration, because the ambient exposure or internal dose typically fluctuates over time. For example, accurate estimates of hyperglycemia for an individual are hampered by between-day variability and within-day variability in fasting plasma glucose levels. One or a few measurements of fasting plasma glucose may incorrectly classify a person's overall glycemic state. The measurement of nonenzymatically glycosylated hemoglobin, however, gives a glycemia index integrated over several weeks (Duncan and Heiss, 1984). Hemoglobin adducts of 4-aminobiphenyl can give a similar integrated index of cigarette smoke exposure over a 3-month period (Tannenbaum et al., 1987), whereas the fatty acid composition of triglycerides in adipose tissue reflects the dietary fatty acid intake integrated over the preceding months or years (van Staveren et al., 1986). Because short-term fluctuations in dose measured at a single time will increase intraindividual variability, using markers that integrate doses over time should reduce such variability, thereby reducing exposure misclassification in epidemiologic studies. Serial ambient or biological sampling could also reduce exposure misclassification, but some biological markers offer the convenience of dose estimates integrated over time from a sample taken at a single time point.

Relate Time of Exposure to Internal Dose

In some situations, biological markers could allow a series of dose estimates for different time points. For example, heavy metals bind to sulfhydryl groups in growing hair, so that the metal content of hair near the scalp reflects recent exposure, whereas more distal hair segments indicate earlier exposures. Markers with this property could be especially useful in studies of reproductive outcomes, where the time window of exposure can be crucial. The metal content of dentine in juvenile teeth can also indicate exposure timing, as growing children lose their teeth at different ages. This kind of marker would allow researchers to assess the health consequences of age-specific exposures. Because toenails have different lengths with corresponding age differences (Willett, 1987), toenail clippings sampled at a single time would allow approximate reconstructions of metal exposure history. Heavy metal markers in hair, teeth, and nails could help distinguish the effects of current exposures from those in past months or years on such outcomes as renal toxicity, neurotoxicity, or other conditions associated with metal exposures, although these markers have apparently not yet been used in this manner. Such markers may also offer opportunities to study temporal relationships between certain trace nutrients, such as selenium and zinc, and states of health and disease. For example, they could allow investigators to assess the putative protective effect of selenium against cancer (Ames, 1983) with regard to recent and past dietary amounts. In general, epidemiologists have yet to explore the potential use of these markers to estimate exposures at different times.

Study Acute Exposure–Outcome Associations

Because biological markers of exposure often attenuate within hours, days, or weeks after the exposure ends, their greatest epidemiologic value lies with cross-sectional studies, prospective studies of short-term outcomes, and monitoring of compliance in clinical trials. Markers of cigarette smoke exposure, for example, could be useful in studies of sidestream smoke and lung function or acute respiratory diseases in children, or to evaluate the efficacy of smoking intervention programs. Case-control studies of acute events, such as myocardial infarction, angina, or asthma attacks, could use markers to assess the role of possible precipitating exposures to carbon monoxide or other air pollutants. For example, the study by Cohen et al. (1969) of the effects of carbon monoxide on the case-fatality rate of emergency room patients with myocardial infarction might have reached more definitive conclusions if carboxyhemoglobin estimates had been available at the time the decedents and survivors were admitted. Note that, in studies of acute transient health effects, persistence in an exposure marker is a liability, as one is interested in recent, rather than past exposures.

Study Long-term Exposure–Outcome Associations

Prospective cohort studies of exposure–effect associations are possible with transient exposure markers, but the time required to complete studies of chronic disease outcomes precludes the prospective approach for many epidemiologic questions. For example, although there exists a growing interest in using DNA adducts in cancer epidemiology (Perera and Weinstein, 1982), a typical case-control study of cancer and chemical exposures could not rely on this type of biological marker. The relevant exposures occur many years before disease diagnosis, and any DNA adducts from the relevant exposure period will probably have disappeared or be indistinguishable from adducts formed more recently. The DNA adducts appear to have a greater epidemiologic value as dependent variables of a biologically effective dose in exposure studies than as independent variables to predict disease. As discussed in greater detail later, studies of DNA alterations in response to carcinogenic chemical exposures are still very valuable to the extent that DNA adducts are part of the pathogenic pathway.

Under certain conditions, transient markers, such as DNA adducts and cytogenetic markers, can be used as exposure markers in studies of diseases with long latent periods. If one knows that exposure levels for an individual remained constant over time, then markers of current exposure may provide good estimates of past exposure. The usefulness of this approach, however, may be limited, because possible metabolic changes in study participants may influence the marker, especially if due to disease among cases in a case-control study. An alternative design, the nested case-control study, can be used with great efficiency if the marker of interest is stable in stored samples. In a nested case-control design, biological samples are collected and stored for all members of a study cohort, and exposure markers are later assayed only for members who experience the outcome of interest, and for a control group of cohort members without the disease (Wald, 1985). Assays are required for only a small proportion of cohort members, minimizing assay cost. If all samples are assayed in a single batch, laboratory variation can also be minimized. Examples of this approach of using biological markers include studies of serum selenium and cancer risk (Willett et al., 1983) and maternal serum alpha-fetoprotein and birth defects (Wald, 1985). To the extent that biological sample banks are already available, such studies can be done retrospectively.

Distinguish One Pathogenic Chemical From a Complex Mixture

Theoretically, some markers can allow the identification of a single pathogenic agent present in a chemical mixture, a situation that occurs in multiexposure occupational environments and other settings. Bulky DNA adducts can sometimes be linked to specific chemical exposures using the ^{32}P-postlabeling assay (Randerath et al., 1981) or the enzyme-linked immunosorbent assay (Maugh, 1984). If epidemiologic studies show a strong association between a particular adduct and disease in the absence of other adduct–disease associations, one might plausibly argue that the parent compound of the adduct is a pathogen, because many other adduct-forming chemicals are pathogenic. This type of study may become practical as the necessary laboratory assays continue to improve.

Detect Nonspecific Exposure Hazards

Nonspecific markers, such as urine mutagenicity or sister chromatid exchanges, may also have value in a multiexposure environment to characterize different jobs with respect to their carcinogenic exposure potential. Nonspecificity may sometimes be an asset in that a marker can give an integrated estimate of total genetic damage from several different exposures. Even if the actual chemical exposures are unknown, as occurs when reaction by-products are produced through industrial processes, a single nonspecific marker could indicate possible mutagenic hazards for a certain job. Note that nonspecific markers may even be useful to assess the internal or the biologically effective dose of a specific chemical in a single-exposure environment, as confounding from other exposures will not occur.

Use Innovative Biological Specimens

The invasive nature of sampling biological material to detect some markers limits their usefulness for epidemiologic studies of free-living populations. Gann et al. (1985), however, point out that surgical specimens can sometimes be used in appropriately designed epidemiologic studies. For example, Cosio et al. (1977) studied the association between preoperative lung function and microscopic lung structure in patients undergoing biopsy. Epidemiologic studies of oncogene activation using routinely stored fixed pathology specimens may also be possible (Wald, 1985). Autopsy specimens from accident victims and other decedents have been used to examine the association between lifetime exposure to air pollution and emphysema (Ishikawa et al., 1969), as well as to study the atherosclerotic changes associated with coronary heart disease risk factors (Solberg and Strong, 1983). Reproductive epidemiologists may find new uses for ovarian follicular fluid from women undergoing in vitro fertilization (Trapp et al., 1984), amniotic fluid collected during amniocentesis, or placental material. When relatively inaccessible biological material is collected for other purposes, epidemiologists should be alert to potential opportunities.

Enhance Knowledge of Disease Mechanism

In some instances, biological markers can elucidate details in the pathologic process from exposure to disease. Some animal carcinogens, such as dioxin, apparently do not form DNA adducts (Poland, 1982), whereas others, such as diethylstilbestrol, cause cancer but not mutation (Barrett et al., 1981). Markers that indicate molecular interactions with known carcinogens, such as DNA adducts and the hypoxanthine–guanine phosphoribosyl transferase (HGPRT) marker, suggest the biochemical mechanism of carcinogenesis; the former indicates adduct formation in genetic material, and the latter indicates gene mutations. Similar responses to other chemicals not currently known to be carcinogenic could point to an unrecognized carcinogenic potential.

Markers of internal dose can also identify possible common metabolic pathways for different toxic chemicals. n-Hexane and methyl n-butyl ketone, for example, are both metabolized to the same neurotoxic compound, 2,5-hexanedione (Spencer et al., 1980). If additional chemicals were also metabolized to this same toxic compound, they would likely be neurotoxins even in the absence of observed adverse health effects.

Epidemiologic studies that use internal dose markers have the unusual opportunity of assessing real-world exposure situations using the exquisite measurements typically associated with laboratory experiments. Unlike their experimental counterparts, these epidemiologic studies avoid questions about dose and species extrapolation, while describing pathogenesis on the biochemical level of detail. As discussed later, biological markers of susceptibility and disease offer similar opportunities to improve epidemiologic studies.

Susceptibility Markers

Some markers may indicate either a susceptibility to future disease or some aspect of existing disease. Because susceptibility markers are associated with a higher risk of disease only in the presence of pathogenic exposures, they primarily serve as effect modifiers in epidemiologic studies. Low $alpha_1$-antitrypsin activity, for example, increases the risk of emphysema among cigarette smokers (Klayton et al., 1975). Low activity by itself, however, does not necessarily increase the risk of pulmonary disease in the absence of ambient exposures. Susceptibility markers in epidemiologic studies could increase both the precision and strength of putative exposure–disease associations by avoiding the dilution effect that occurs in populations with a large proportion of nonsusceptible persons.

As with markers of internal dose and early biological response, susceptibility markers may also provide clues about disease mechanisms. In a study of N-acetyltransferase phenotypes in bladder cancer patients, for example, Cartwright et al. (1982) reached tentative conclusions about exposure-specific metabolic pathways. Specifically, the preponderance of slow acetylators among bladder cancer patients exposed to dyes suggests that occupational exposure to N-substituted aryl compounds in the dyes caused the disease, as the rate of acetylation influences the detoxification of these compounds. In contrast, bladder cancer patients who smoked showed no excess of the slow acetylation phenotype, leading to the conclusion that aromatic amines in cigarette smoke apparently did not cause their cancer. Acquired susceptibilities from nutritional deficits of antioxidants or vitamins, for example, may also give insights into disease mechanisms.

Markers of Preclinical and Overt Disease

Disease markers can strengthen epidemiologic studies in a variety of ways. Markers of preclinical disease can sometimes reduce the required follow-up time in prospective cohort studies, because the preclinical disease endpoints will become apparent earlier than will the subsequent overt disease. For example, liver toxins may alter the level of various enzymes long before liver dysfunction becomes apparent. Furthermore, because some preclinical endpoints fail to progress to overt disease, the preclinical endpoints will be more numerous, increasing the study's statistical power (Gann et al., 1985). Additional applications of disease markers are presented later.

Eliminate Persons With Preclinical Disease From Cohort Studies

Cohort studies of exposure–disease associations typically attempt to exclude individuals with existing disease, because the associations may differ for prevalent and incident disease cases. In some instances, the disease may affect the exposure measurement so that the antecedent–consequent nature of the exposure–disease association is unclear. For example, associations between low cholesterol and cancer (International Collaborative Group, 1982) and between very lean body mass and different causes of death (Sorlie et al., 1980) have been attributed to undiagnosed diseases present at the time of the baseline measurements. That is, because unrecognized diseases might have caused the low cholesterol or lean body mass, they may not be actual risk factors for disease incidence. Markers of occult disease with a high positive predictive value can be used to exclude people with existing preclinical disease from follow-up studies, minimizing these types of antecedent–consequent uncertainties. For preclinical diseases with a high prevalence, such markers would be especially important to reduce disease misclassification at the inception of a cohort study.

Improve Estimates of Disease Induction Periods

As discussed by Rothman (1981), a substantial amount of time can elapse between a pathogenic exposure and preclinical disease, and additional time often precedes disease diagnosis. The individual durations of these two time periods, that is, the disease induction period after exposure and the predetection latency period, cannot be estimated from dates of exposure and disease diagnosis alone. Markers of preclinical disease, however, would enable an epidemiologist to estimate both the induction and latent period, so that the pathogenic stages become more clearly defined. Autopsy studies, for example, might reveal that a cardiovascular toxin causes rapid growth of atherosclerotic plaques, although a clinical endpoint, such as myocardial infarction, may not occur for many years.

Identify the Stage of Disease Where Exposure Has its Effect

Preclinical disease markers may help clarify the role of specific exposures at various phases in multistage disease processes. For example, markers of asymptomatic neoplasms in epidemiologic studies might allow investigators to distinguish promoters of malignant transformation in previously initiated cells from promoters of tumor progression in malignant cells. That is, markers may indicate the stage of the cells before the action of the promoters. This type of study could possibly be implemented in cancer screening programs, where risk factors could be compared between patients with small and larger asymptomatic tumors (e.g., for occult and clinically apparent prostatic cancer). Such markers as alpha-fetoprotein or fetal antigens may allow early cancer diagnosis (Perera and Weinstein, 1982). Nuclear magnetic resonance is finding use in the detection of subtle plasma lipoprotein changes associated with early cancer development (Fossel et al., 1986). In reproductive epidemiology, markers of very early fetal loss (Wilcox et al., 1988) could allow studies of environmental hazards that affect the conceptus at early stages of development.

Create More Homogeneous Categories of Disease

Markers of overt disease can strengthen epidemiologic studies by reducing disease heterogeneity. Broad disease categories, such as cancer, cardiovascular disease, and musculoskeletal disorders, include subtypes with distinct etiologies. As these diseases are subclassified into more numerous and more homogeneous categories, the ability of epidemiologic studies to identify exposure–disease associations should improve. Rheumatoid arthritis, for example, may be seropositive or seronegative for rheumatoid factor (Gilliland and Mannick, 1983), and lymphomas can be categorized by antigen markers (Hait et al., 1985). A specific nutrient or chemical exposure may increase the risk of one disease subtype but not others; in leukemia, for example, benzene exposure increases the risk of the myelogenous but not the lymphatic subtype (Infante et al., 1977).

Developments in oncogene research may lead to particularly interesting epidemiologic opportunities. Seemingly identical tumors may contain different activated oncogenes (Fujita et al., 1984), and environmental exposures eventually may be linked to the activation of specific oncogenes, although examples do not yet exist. Activated oncogenes have also been discovered in atherosclerotic plaques (Scott, 1987), so that new lines of oncogene research may become pertinent to cardiovascular disease epidemiology.

Earlier discoveries of enzyme monotypia and heterogeneity in atheromas of women heterozygous for the X-linked isoenzymes of glucose-6-phosphate dehydrogenase (Pearson et al., 1978) suggest that this biological marker can distinguish subpopulations of atherosclerotic lesions within the same arterial segment. The atheroma subpopulations could have distinct etiologies, although epidemiologists have not pursued this possibility. Epidemiologists, however, have used markers extensively to study the determinants and health implications of various dyslipoproteinemias (e.g., type IIa hypercholesterolemia with elevated levels of low density lipoprotein–cholesterol and normal triglyceride levels). Refinements in lipoprotein characterization continue, particularly for the high density lipoprotein subfraction.

In summary, biological markers not only offer potential gains in the precision of exposure and disease measurements, but some also present opportunities to study disease mechanisms. Depending on their properties, markers may either improve exposure and disease measurements in studies that use traditional epidemiologic study designs, or they may allow entirely new approaches for epidemiologic investigations of pathogenesis on the molecular or tissue level. The choice of a marker will depend upon the problem under investigation. Practical constraints, such as availability of biological material, may preclude the use of a given marker. A discussion of criteria to evaluate a marker's potential usefulness appears in Chapter 3.

ETIOLOGIC FRACTION AND DISEASE FREQUENCY

The concept of etiologic fraction is useful to determine an exposure marker's importance to public health. It reflects both the prevalence of exposure and the added risk of disease due to the exposure (Kleinbaum et al., 1982). In essence, the etiologic fraction describes the proportion of disease cases in a population that is attributable to some risk factor of interest. A large etiologic fraction for a given disease and exposure in a population might arise under different circumstances: a highly prevalent exposure with a modest relative risk; a rare exposure with a very high relative risk; or an intermediate combination of exposure prevalence and relative risk. Another measure of potential impact closely related to etiologic fraction is the prevented fraction (Kleinbaum et al., 1982), a measure used when an exposure produces a decrease in disease risk.

By definition, exposure markers with a high etiologic fraction or prevented fraction for a common disease will have great public health importance, as the marker will be associated with a substantial proportion of the population's disease burden. In urban populations with a high prevalence of lead exposure, for example, erythrocyte protoporphyrin and other markers of lead exposure may have great public health value. In rural populations where the prevalence of lead exposure is low, such markers would have little relevance to the total disease burden. Nonspecific exposure markers, such as sister chromatid exchanges or urine mutagenesis, may reflect exposures to a large variety of toxic chemicals, although the individual chemicals may each have only a modest exposure prevalence. Exposures to the chemical groups as a whole in a population may be quite common, so that nonspecific exposure markers will be associated with a large etiologic fraction for cancer or other disease. Nonspecific markers may, therefore, have considerable value for public health research in general, even though their lack of exposure specificity would be a liability in individual epidemiologic studies.

From a public health standpoint, markers associated with a large etiologic fraction for a disease have little importance unless the disease itself is both common and severe. Although rare diseases are certainly important to victims and their families, they have little impact on the population as a whole. In general, markers of common diseases or markers associated with a large etiologic fraction for a common disease have greater importance than do markers for rare diseases or infrequent exposures.

SUMMARY

Numerous markers of exposure, susceptibility, and disease have potential value for epidemiologists. By definition, all types of markers show a statistical association with some event or state of interest. Although the exact biological relationship between a marker and condition of interest may be unclear, even a crudely quantified marker–condition association may sometimes offer substantial advantages over alternative approaches to exposure and disease measurement.

Exposure markers provide especially rich opportunities for epidemiologic applications. Because some markers integrate exposures from multiple portals of entry or exposures that occur over time, a single marker measurement can give a fairly complete picture of a person's exposure status. Markers sometimes allow the innovative use of biological materials that previously had no value to epidemiologists. Some molecular markers of biologically effective dose also offer insight into biochemical mechanisms of pathogenesis.

As with exposure markers, susceptibility markers can suggest biochemical mechanisms of pathogenesis. By characterizing the metabolic state of persons with disease susceptibility, markers indicate the biochemical pathways leading from exposure to disease. Susceptibility markers can also allow the exclusion of nonsusceptible individuals from epidemiologic study populations, thereby allowing the study to evaluate putative exposure–disease associations only among those persons at greatest risk of the disease.

In cohort studies, where participants should be disease-free at the beginning of follow-up, markers of preclinical disease allow the exclusion of persons who actually have early disease. The identification of early disease states also improves estimates of disease induction periods, and helps identify the stage-specific role of exposures in multistage disease processes. Because markers of overt disease can categorize diseases into homogeneous subgroups with distinct etiologies, these markers facilitate the detection of specific exposure–disease associations.

From a public health standpoint, the most useful markers pertain to exposures and diseases that contribute substantially to the population disease burden. Nonspecific markers that respond to a variety of environmental exposures may be especially useful, although lack of specificity is often a problem in individual studies. The great diversity in properties among markers guarantees that, while most markers will have little relevance to any given study, as a group, markers offer important opportunities to advance public health research.

REFERENCES

Ames BN: Dietary carcinogens and anticarcinogens: Oxygen radicals and degenerative diseases. *Science* 1983;221:1256–1264.

Barrett JC, Wang A, McLachlan JA: Diethylstilbestrol induces neoplastic transformation without measurable gene mutation at two loci. *Science* 1981;212:1402–1404.

Brown HS, Bishop DR, Rowan CA: The role of skin absorption as a route of exposure for volatile organic compounds (VOCs) in drinking water. *Am J Public Health* 1984;74:479–484.

Cartwright RA, Rogers HJ, Barham-Hall D, Glashan RW, Ahmad RA, Higgins E, Kahn MA: Role of *N*-acetyltransferase phenotypes in bladder carcinogenesis: A pharmacogenetic epidemiological approach to bladder cancer. *Lancet* 1982:842–846.

Cohen SI, Deane M, Goldsmith JR: Carbon monoxide and survival from myocardial infarction. *Arch Environ Health* 1969;19:510–517.

Cosio M, Ghezzo H, Hogg JC, Corbin R, Loveland M, Dosman J, Macklem PT: The relations between structural changes in small airways and pulmonary-function tests. *N Engl J Med* 1977;298:1277–1281.

Duncan BB, Heiss G: Nonenzymatic glycosylation of proteins: A new tool for assessment of cumulative hyperglycemia in epidemiologic studies, past and future. *Am J Epidemiol* 1984;120:169–189.

Fossel ET, Carr JM, McDonagh J: Detection of malignant tumors: Water-suppressed proton nuclear magnetic spectroscopy of plasma. *N Engl J Med* 1986;315:1369–1376.

Fujita J, Yoshida O, Yuasa Y, Rhim JS, Hatanaka M, Aaronson SA: Ha-*ras* oncogenes are activated by somatic alterations in human urinary tract tumours. *Nature* 1984;309:464–466.

Gann PH, Davis DL, Perera F: *Biologic markers in environmental epidemiology: Constraints and opportunities*. Presented at the Fifth Workshop of the Scientific Group on Methodologies for the Safety Evaluation of Chemicals (SGOMSEC), Mexico City, August 12–16, 1985.

Gilliland BC, Mannick M: Rheumatoid arthritis. In: Petersdorf RG, Adams RD, Braunwald E, Isselbacher KJ, Martin JB, Wilson JD, eds.: *Principles of Internal Medicine*. New York, McGraw-Hill, 1983, pp. 1977–1986.

Hait WN, Farber L, Cadman E: Non–Hodgkin's lymphoma for the nononcologist. *JAMA* 1985;253:1431–1435.

Infante PF, Rinsky RA, Wagoner JK, Young RJ: Leukaemia in benzene workers. *Lancet* 1977:76–78.

International Collaborative Group: Circulating cholesterol level and risk of death from cancer in men aged 40 to 69 years. *JAMA* 1982;248:2853–2859.

Ishikawa S, Bowden DH, Fisher V, Wyatt JP: The "emphysema profile" in two midwestern cities in North America. *Arch Environ Health* 1969;18:660–666.

Klayton L, Fallat R, Cohen AB: Determinants of chronic obstructive pulmonary disease in patients with intermediate levels of alpha$_1$-antitrypsin. *Am Rev Respir Dis* 1975;112:71–81.

Kleinbaum DG, Kupper LL, Morgenstern H: *Epidemiologic Research Principles and Quantitative Methods*. Belmont, Lifetime Learning Publ, 1982.

Maugh TH: Tracking exposure to toxic substances. *Science* 1984;226:1183–1184.

Pearson TA, Dillman JM, Solez K, Heptinstall RH: Clonal markers in the study of the origin and growth of human atherosclerotic lesions. *Circ Res* 1978;43:10–18.

Perera FP, Weinstein IB: Molecular epidemiology and carcinogen-DNA adduct detection: New approaches to studies of human cancer causation. *J Chronic Dis* 1982;35:581–600.

Poland A, Knutson JC: 2,3,7,8-tetrachlorodibenzo-p-dioxin and related halogenated aromatic hydrocarbons: Examination of the mechanisms of toxicity. *Am Rev Pharmacol Toxicol* 1982;22:517–554.

Randerath K, Reddy MV, Gupta RC: ^{32}P–labeling test for DNA damage. *Proc Natl Acad Sci* 1981;78:6126–6129.

Rothman KJ: Induction and latent periods. *Am J Epidemiol* 1981;114:253–259.

Scott J: Oncogenes in atherosclerosis. *Nature* 1987;325:574–575.

Solberg LA, Strong JP: Risk factors and atherosclerotic lesions: A review of autopsy studies. *Arteriosclerosis* 1983;3:187–198.

Sorlie P, Gordon T, Kannel WB: Body build and mortality: The Framingham Study. *JAMA* 1980;243:1828–1831.

Spencer PS, Couri D, Schaumburg HH: *n*-Hexane and methyl *n*-butyl ketone. In: Spencer PS, Schaumburg HH, eds.: *Experimental and Clinical Toxicology*. Baltimore, Williams & Wilkins, 1980, pp. 456–457.

Tannenbaum SR: Direct measurements on chemicals and their effects on humans. Presented at the Symposium on Basic Research in Risk Assessment. National Institute of Environmental Health Sciences, Research Triangle Park, NC, March 9–12, 1987.

Trapp M, Baukloh V, Bohnet HG, Heeschen W: Pollutants in human follicular fluid. *Fertil Steril* 1984;42:146–148.

van Staveren WA, Deurenberg P, Katan MB, Burema J, de Groot LCPGM, Hoffmans MDAF: Validity of the fatty acid composition of subcutaneous fat tissue microbiopsies as an estimate of the long-term average fatty acid composition of the diet of separate individuals. *Am J Epidemiol* 1986;123:455–463.

Wald NJ: Use of biological sample banks in epidemiological studies. *Maturitas* 1985;7:59–67.

Wilcox AJ, Weinberg CR, O'Connor JF, Baird DD, Schlatterer JP, Canfield RE, Armstrong EG, Nisula BC: Incidence of early loss of pregnancy. *N Engl J Med* 1988;319:189–194.

Willett W: Nutritional epidemiology: Issues and challenges. *Int J Epidemiol* 1987;16(Suppl):312–317.

Willett WC, Morris SJ, Pressel S, Taylor JO, Polk BF, Stampfer MJ, Rosner B, Schneider K, Hames CG: Prediagnostic serum selenium and risk of cancer. *Lancet* 1983:130–134.

3

CRITERIA FOR SELECTING AND EVALUATING MARKERS

TIMOTHY C. WILCOSKY

PROPERTIES OF MARKERS
Biological Classification

A variety of simple and complex biological markers exists. For some markers of internal dose, for example, the marker is simply the presence of an exogenous agent in a biological material such as blood, urine, or adipose tissue. In other instances, the marker reflects a series of intricate biological steps that produce some measurable change at the molecular, cellular, or tissue level. The biological nature of a marker largely determines its properties in epidemiologic studies, and the classification scheme outlined below provides a framework to compare the similarities and differences for the diverse assortment of biological makers. Table 3-1 presents examples of markers that fall under the different categories discussed.

Unchanged Exogenous Agents

From a metabolic standpoint, the simplest markers are exogenous agents that enter the body and are measured before they undergo any biochemical changes. For example, polychlorinated biphenyls (PCBs) can appear in adipose tissue and breast milk (Rogan et al., 1980); solvents, such as benzene, are measurable in blood and expired air (Vainio, 1985); and various heavy metals bind to sulfhydryl groups in hair, teeth, and nails (Hopps, 1977; Takagi et al., 1986). Such markers are usually used to estimate internal dose.

Although these markers are conceptually simple, they can still present formidable measurement problems in complex biological materials, such as blood and urine, where myriad other chemicals are also present. Procedures for collecting, transporting, and storing the biological material may also influence the marker's measurement. Aside from technical analytic issues, researchers must also consider a chemical's pharmacokinetics when they decide which biological material to analyze and when to collect the sample. For example, Droz and Guillemin (1986) point out that field studies

Table 3-1   Examples of Markers From Different Biological Categories

Unchanged exogenous agents
Solvents	Asbestos fibers
PCBs	Ethanol
Nicotine	Heavy metals

Metabolized exogenous agents (precursors in parentheses)
Phenol (benzene)	DDE (DDT)
Cotinine (nicotine)	BPDE I (benzo(a)pyrene)
Retinol (β-carotene)	Acrolein (cyclophosphamide)

Endogenously produced molecules (exposure/disease in parentheses)
Exposure markers
   Acetylcholinesterase (organic phospate pesticides)
   γ-glutamyl transferase (liver toxins)
   Porphyrin ratios (lead and other metals)
Disease markers
   alpha-fetoprotein (liver cancer)
   SGOT (myocardial infarction)
   Creatine kinase (muscle trauma)

Molecular changes (exposure in parentheses)
Glycosylated hemoglobin (dietary glucose)
DNA adducts (chemical carcinogens)
Protein adducts (electrophilic chemicals)
Chromosome aberrations (clastogens)
Alkylated amino acids (electrophilic chemicals)
Micronuclei (clastogens)

Cellular/tissue changes (in response to various toxins)
Cell histology	Lymphocyte ratios
Sperm mobility	Sperm counts
Macrophage activity	Red blood cell counts

using breath analysis of solvent exposures show great diversity both in sampling methods and in timing of the sampling during or after exposure. Such diversity in methodology leads to difficulty in comparing exposure estimates across studies, and the issue of timing is especially relevant to solvents due to their rapid excretion (Angerer, 1985). In general, levels of internalized chemicals decrease over time, so that a given blood level of carbon monoxide, for example, may reflect a brief high-dose exposure a few hours before sampling or a prolonged low-dose exposure (Friberg, 1985). Consequently, the use of even simple markers, such as unchanged exogenous chemicals, requires careful consideration of analytic and biological issues.

Metabolized Exogenous Agents

Many chemicals that enter the body undergo metabolic changes before excretion. Most chemical carcinogens, some chemical neurotoxins, and several other types of toxins have metabolites that are more toxic than are their precursors. For chemical toxins that undergo metabolic activation, biological markers of the active metabolites, rather than the parent compounds, give a more meaningful estimate of internal dose. Although the analytic and pharmacokinetic issues relevant to unchanged exogenous chemicals also apply to metabolized exogenous chemicals, interindividual variability in metabolism makes the situation more complex for metabolized exogenous chemicals. As a result, internal dose markers for chemicals that undergo metabolic change will probably show greater interindividual variability for a given ambient exposure level than will markers for unchanged exogenous chemicals. To the extent that the metabolites are the toxins of interest in an epidemiologic study of an adverse health effect, this relatively high variability in the internal dose relative to a given ambient exposure level is an asset, rather than a liability. This allows the study to have a greater range of internal doses for assessing possible gradients in disease response to different dose levels.

Endogenously Produced Molecules

In contrast to categories of markers where unchanged chemicals or their metabolites are measured, other markers reflect molecules produced by the body itself. A large number of endogenously produced markers are enzymes. In the case of susceptibility markers, such as alpha$_1$-antitrypsin, the marker is genetically determined and constant throughout life. Other enzymes, however, indicate toxic exposures, such as γ-glutamyl transferase, which becomes elevated in response to liver damage from alcohol and other toxins. Enzyme levels can also indicate or confirm overt disease (e.g., elevated creatine kinase and serum glutamic-oxaloacetic transaminase [SGOT] after myocardial infarction). Their use in epidemiologic studies can help reduce disease misclassification. Clinicians have long used a variety of blood and urine constituents, some endogenously produced, such as platelets, and some metabolically controlled, such as calcium, to help in the detection and diagnosis of disease. Most tumor markers, such as alpha-fetoprotein or carcinoembryonic antigen, are also endogenously produced molecules.

Unlike markers based on the measurement of exogenous chemicals and their metabolites, endogenously produced exposure markers are often present at some baseline level, even in the absence of exposure. Some enzyme markers of exposure, such as δ-aminolevulinic acid dehydratase and acetylcholinesterase, show a decrease in activity after exposure to lead and organic phosphate pesticides, respectively. Others, such as γ-glutamyl transferase and the P$_{450}$ enzyme system, increase after exposure to ethanol and other chemicals. Genetically determined susceptibility markers, such as alpha$_1$-antitrypsin, typically show activity that varies by phenotype. Investigators therefore, must either use such markers as continuous variables or impose cutpoints on the distributions to enable categorization of a person's susceptibility, exposure, or disease status (Schulte, 1987).

Molecular Changes

Some markers indicate that endogenous macromolecules, such as DNA or protein, have undergone damage, repair, or other changes. A variety of interesting and elegant markers are available to detect such changes. When the changes reflect some type of exposure, these markers can often provide estimates of the biologically effective dose of the exposure agent. For example, DNA adducts from a chemical exposure indicate the potential for genetic damage from that chemical, and adduct formation in some cells may be an early step in carcinogenic cell transformation. Two people with identical blood concentrations (i.e., internal dose) of a chemical may show different degrees of DNA adduct formation because of metabolic and kinetic differences, and the person with the greater number of adducts may have a higher probability of cell transformation. Note that, in spite of this theory's attractiveness, no epidemiologic studies to date have actually demonstrated such an effect. Adducts in such cells as mature circulating lymphocytes will not themselves cause cancer, but adduct formation in these cells is presumably correlated with adducts in target tissues where tumors can arise. Protein adducts can sometimes serve a similar role as surrogate measurements of adduct formation in target tissues. In urine, degradation products from alkylated protein and DNA can also indicate the occurrence of adduct formation (Vainio et al., 1981).

In contrast to DNA adducts, which only indicate the potential for irreversible DNA damage, other markers indicate that such damage actually has occurred. Such cytogenetic markers as micronuclei and chromosome aberrations, for example, result from chromosome breakage. Some somatic cell mutations are detectable in lymphocytes using the hypoxanthine–guanine phosphoribosyl transferase (HGPRT) assay, indicating damage at a particular locus in the DNA. The interpretation of sister chromatid exchanges is less clear, because, though they result from chromosome breakage, the actual DNA sequence may be unaffected.

Markers based on molecular changes also have epidemiologic applications for diseases other than cancer. Glycosylation of serum proteins, for example, shows promise for diabetes research (Duncan and Heiss, 1984). Markers based on molecular changes are currently undergoing intensive research.

Cellular Changes

Markers based on molecular changes have conceptual counterparts on the cellular and tissue level of biological organization. Some markers pertain to morphologic changes in cells as assessed through cell cytology and histology; others reflect functional changes, such as sperm mobility and nerve conduction velocity. Changes in cell populations can also serve as markers of exposure or effect. Sperm counts, red blood cell counts, and ratios of lymphocyte subpopulations, for example, can change in response to environmental exposures.

In essence, markers can range from simple measurements of inorganic chemicals up through complex measurements on the cellular or even organismal level. A marker's properties are largely a function of its underlying biological nature. The following section describes how metabolic characteristics of exposure markers determine the appropriate physiologic sites and timing of marker measurements.

Metabolic Characteristics

In most respects the metabolic characteristics of susceptibility, exposure, and disease markers differ substantially from each other. Genetically determined susceptibilities tend to remain stable over an individual's lifetime, and acquired susceptibilities resulting from disease, injury, or diet will generally persist as long as these conditions continue. Similarly, markers of early or overt disease can stay constant unless the disease progresses or improves. Exposure markers, however, are typically dynamic.

Depending on the marker, changes in exposure markers over time reflect the kinetics of the exposure agent, the persistence of biological changes that the agent may have caused, and the persistence of the biological material itself. For example, blood solvent levels in an exposed person will rise until either the solvent concentration reaches equilibrium or the exposure stops, and the levels decrease after exposure cessation. DNA lesions from the solvent, however, will persist until the DNA is repaired or degraded. Because the kinetics of chemical exposure agents influence many properties of both kinds of markers, whether they be unchanged exogenous agents in the blood or molecular changes in DNA, pharmacokinetic issues dominate much of the discussion that follows. Furthermore, because chemical exposures provide a convenient framework to describe marker properties, the discussion emphasizes exposure markers.

Time to Appearance

Because the level of a marker can vary substantially over time, the timing of specimen collection requires careful attention. Timing is especially important for intermittent or one-time exposures where the marker will reach a maximum response at some point after exposure initiation. For example, with solvents blood levels increase during exposure until a steady state is reached, and drop quickly after exposure ends. Hence, a solvent with poor solubility in the blood, such as n-hexane, reaches steady state very quickly, whereas a highly soluble solvent, such as 2-butanone, may take several hours of exposure to reach a steady state (Angerer, 1985).

In general, markers that are unchanged exogenous chemicals reach a maximum level in biological materials more quickly than do markers that are metabolites. Nicotine in saliva, for example, reaches a maximum within about an hour of continuous exposure to sidestream cigarette smoke, whereas cotinine, a nicotine metabolite, increases over several hours as the nicotine is enzymatically oxidized in the liver (Hoffmann et al., 1984). The nicotine marker of tobacco smoke also illustrates how the timing of marker responses can vary among biological materials, in that the maximum urinary level occurs roughly 2 hours after the maximum salivary level (Hoffman et al., 1984). Pharmacokinetic data, when available, can predict the expected changes over time of chemical levels in biological materials both during and after exposure.

Such markers as DNA adducts may be measured immediately after exposure (see Chapter 5), but other markers do not appear until days, weeks, or months after exposure. As summarized in Chapter 7, for example, micronuclei in lymphocytes are measurable within a day or less after exposure, and measurements in exfoliated buccal cells require 5–7 days for the cells to migrate to the epithelial surface from the basal layer. For heavy metal exposures, even more time must elapse to allow measurements in hair or nails.

For markers that give time-integrated dose estimates, such as hemoglobin 4-aminobiphenyl adducts as a marker of cigarette smoke exposure (Tannenbaum, 1987), the concept of "time to appearance" has little relevance, as the emphasis is on exposures over time. Markers of short-term exposures, however, fluctuate over short time periods as exposure levels increase and decrease. Measuring a marker too soon after exposure may give a misleading picture of the maximum internal dose or biologically effective dose, and as discussed later, measuring too late produces a similar problem.

Persistence

A marker's persistence after exposure ends determines whether it can be used to measure past, recent, or ongoing exposures. Although some markers remain stable after exposure (e.g., polychlorinated biphenyls in adipose tissue), most eventually diminish or disappear after exposure ends. Solvent levels in blood, for example, typically increase fairly quickly when exposure begins and drop quickly after exposure ends (Angerer, 1985). The decrease in a chemical's concentration over time after exposure cessation usually follows one of three simple kinetics models (Aitio, 1984). In the zero-order model, a constant amount of chemical is cleared from the blood (or other biological material) per unit time, whereas in a first-order model, a constant *proportion* of the chemical is cleared per unit time. The third model, a two-compartment model (some models actually have more than two compartments), describes the disappearance of chemicals from two or more tissues or fluids when each has a different half-life for the chemical (Aitio, 1984). Examples of biological compartments include blood, urine, adipose tissue, and the different organs. The persistence of markers based on in vivo measurements of exogenous chemicals, therefore, depends on the kinetics model that describes the chemicals' clearance from the body.

The half-lives of chemicals in different compartments can vary dramatically. In blood and soft tissues, for example, lead has a half-life of about 3 weeks; in bone, its half-life is approximately 5 years. The half-life of elemental mercury in the body as a whole is about 2 months; in the brain, it is several years (Friberg, 1985). Depending on a chemical's kinetics and the availability of biological materials, markers measured in one compartment could estimate doses from recent exposures, whereas those in other compartments may integrate exposures over a long period of time.

In addition to differences in marker half-life in different biological materials, different markers of the same exposure measured in the same biological material may also vary in persistence. For example, two metabolites of trichloroethylene, trichloroethanol and trichloroacetic acid, have half-lives in the blood of 12 hours and 100 hours, respectively (Vainio et al., 1981). Table 3-2 illustrates the wide range of half-lives associated with different markers of cigarette smoke exposure in the blood. Serum nicotine with its short half-life would be useful for assessing the internal dose of cigarette smoke from acute exposures, whereas hemoglobin adducts of 4-aminobiphenyl integrate the dose over a period of months.

Whether an investigator prefers a marker with a long or with a short persistence depends on the study question. In studies of acute effects from exposure, using a marker with long persistence could introduce exposure misclassification due to past exposures. Epidemiologists, however, conducting retrospective studies of chronic disease often wish to estimate exposures from decades earlier. Many elegant markers, such as DNA adducts and most cytogenetic markers, have little potential use in retrospective studies, unless they are measurable in long-lived cells like some types of lymphocytes or in stored biological samples. This problem arises because DNA adducts are usually removed spontaneously or enzymatically soon after formation, and only a small proportion persists for long periods. Protein adducts are more stable, but the proteins themselves degrade with time (NIEHS, 1986, p. 222). For cytogenetic

Table 3-2 Persistence of Selected Markers of Tobacco Smoke in Blood

Marker	Duration
Nicotine	2-hr half-life (Benowitz, 1982)
Carboxyhemoglobin	3–4-hr half-life (Rode et al., 1972)
Cotinine	19-hr half-life (Benowitz, 1982)
Thiocyanate	14-day half-life (Benowitz, 1982)
4-aminobiphenyl hemo-globin adducts	3-mo integration (Tannenbaum, 1987)

markers, the lesions may persist for the lifetime of the affected cells, but the cells, like proteins, may have short life spans. Even for cell populations with long half-lives, such as some types of lymphocytes that may live for more than 20 years, one cannot distinguish recently formed lesions from those caused by long past exposures. Only in a few situations, such as with hair samples, can current biological samples indicate the timing of past exposures.

As discussed in other sections, transience in a marker does not preclude its use in chronic disease studies if it can be measured in properly stored biological specimens. Furthermore, persistent markers that reflect cumulative doses can also be used to measure internal doses from a particular time period, if other data specify the exposure period. For example, a work history may define the period of potential exposure for someone with an exposure found only in the workplace, and a persistent marker could confirm and possibly quantify the exposure. If a marker's half-life is well characterized in different biological compartments or cell subpopulations, mathematical models may allow investigators to estimate recent and past exposures separately by modeling measurements from different biological samples. Depending on the persistence of the relevant markers, however, traditional crude estimates of exposure based on records may offer the only approach to reconstructing historical exposures.

Peak or Integrated Dose

In some instances, a marker indicates the peak exposure dose during a particular time interval, whereas in others, the marker estimates the cumulative or integrated dose. This property is a function of a marker's persistence. Markers with a very long half-life in the body after a single exposure tend to give integrated dose estimates, as the marker will still reflect the effects of the first exposure when subsequent exposures occur. Unless the marker has already attained some maximum value, later effects are added to the first. For example, in an occupational setting, daily blood concentrations of chemicals with very short half-lives are independent of each other. In contrast, the concentration of a chemical with a 7-day half-life will increase each day until the rates of the chemical's elimination and absorption become equal; the level at equilibrium is proportional to the daily dose under a first-order kinetics model (Aitio, 1984). To estimate accurately the peak dose of a chemical with a short half-life, it may be necessary to collect samples frequently, but for a chemical with a long half-life, a single analysis will indicate the average exposure over a period of time (Aitio, 1984). Polychlorinated biphenyls in adipose tissue provide an extreme example of an integrated dose marker, as these chemicals accumulate over a lifetime with essentially no excretion (Rogan et al., 1980). As mentioned earlier, because half-lives can vary among different biological compartments, a marker measurement may indicate a peak dose in one biological material, whereas in another material, a measurement gives an integrated dose estimate. For a short-term dose integration, urine has advantages over blood as chemicals or their metabolites may accumulate in urine (Droz and Guillemin, 1986).

Other types of markers also show a relationship between persistence and the ability to estimate peak or integrated dose. DNA adducts, for example, tend to estimate peak exposure levels, because most of the lesions are rapidly repaired. Protein adducts, however, reflect cumulative exposures over the lifetime of the protein because there is no lesion repair. Sister chromatid exchange frequencies in lymphocytes also reflect peak rather than integrated dose levels because of DNA lesion repair. The situation is somewhat complicated for persistent DNA lesions in such cells as lymphocytes, because the lymphocytes themselves have life spans of varying lengths (Carrano, 1986).

Some markers give neither a peak nor an integrated dose estimate because they are measured as a binary rather than as a quantitative variable. DNA adducts measured with older ^{32}P-postlabeling assays, for example, were typically evaluated as present or absent, therefore, the marker indicates the occurrence of recent exposures without assessing their magnitude. Markers in other situations also fall outside of the peak dose–integrated dose dichotomy. A biological sample collected after a marker's response has dropped from its peak level, or while its level continues to rise, for example, yields neither a peak nor an integrated dose estimate, and a binary exposure assessment may be the most appropriate interpretation. The conceptual distinction between markers of peak dose and integrated dose can be helpful to an epidemiologist designing a study, depending on whether the study question concerns acute or chronic exposures. One must recognize, however, the operational limitations of this distinction.

Metabolism and Excretion

With chemical exposures, the biological fate of the agent helps determine the appropriate markers and biological materials for exposure measurement. For chemicals that become toxic after enzymatic activation, for example, the site of activation (e.g., the liver) may yield the most sensitive biological marker to assess molecular or tissue changes. In contrast, the effects of a toxin that acts directly on cells without metabolic activation may best be measured in the portal of entry (e.g., the lungs). If the toxin is transported through the blood, markers in the blood may be adequate to estimate doses or responses in target cells nourished by the blood.

Issues concerning a chemical's absorption, metabolism, and excretion relate directly to its kinetics. In the unlikely event that complete kinetics data were available for a chemical in humans, epidemiologists could make precise judgments about the most efficient use of markers to assess exposure, as they would know the interrelationships of different markers in different biological materials at different times. The constraints of reality, however, lead to less informed decisions, although very basic information may be valuable. For example, if a nonpolar chemical of interest has a polar hydrosoluble metabolite (e.g., benzene and phenol, respectively), then the metabolite would probably be the appropriate marker to measure in urine. To the extent that data exist on the metabolism and excretion of chemicals, epidemiologists can predict which markers will have the greatest potential utility before they undertake empirical testing.

Storage Sites

With some exceptions, exogenous agents or their metabolites are transient in the body, because each biological compartment has a characteristic half-life for the agents that enter it. An understanding of storage sites can help epidemiologists choose a biological material for exposure assessment. For example, nickel compounds can remain for years after exposure in the nasal mucosa, where they may cause cancer (Aitio, 1984). A search for nickel compounds in other storage sites would be less relevant to an epidemiologic study of nasal cancer as the nose is the site of toxicity, and nickel measured there estimates the biologically effective dose.

Adipose tissue serves as a storage site for many fat-soluble chemicals, including such nutrients as fatty acids and some vitamins. Because water-soluble chemicals rarely enter adipose tissue, other biological materials (e.g., urine) provide a better matrix for marker measurements. Except for their lack of accessibility, the long half-lives of lead in bones and of mercury in the brain would make these storage sites a good source of biological material. Hair provides an unusually interesting material to measure metal exposure as estimates are possible for different exposure periods.

Because virtually all of a chemical's metabolic characteristics, including its storage sites, are a function of the chemical's kinetics, data on kinetics help tremendously in choosing markers for a study. Unfortunately, detailed data are often unavailable. Epidemiologists can still use exposure markers productively in the face of incomplete kinetics data, but the exact relationship between the marker and the exposure of interest remains unclear.

Sensitivity

Laboratory scientists define the term *sensitivity* in a variety of ways. According to one definition, an assay's sensitivity is its ability to detect differences in an analyte's concentration among samples (Kateman and Pijpers, 1981); thus, assays that can detect the smallest difference in concentration are the most sensitive. Others define sensitivity as the minimum level of an analyte that a test can detect (Lohman et al., 1985). For levels above this minimum value the test is positive, and for lower levels the test is negative. Epidemiologists use the term in yet another way as depicted in the following 2 × 2 table. This table gives a cross-tabulation of frequencies from a correct classification (TRUTH) and a classification based on an imperfect measure (TEST).

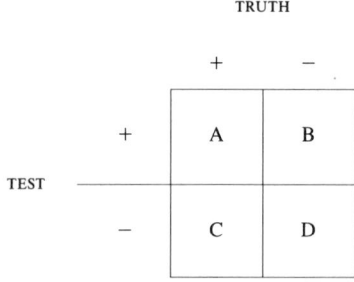

According to this scheme, cells A and D are the "true positives" and "true negatives," respectively, and cells B and C are the "false positives" and "false negatives." If the test is 100 percent correct, then cells B and C will be empty. In the epidemiologic sense, sensitivity is defined as A/(A + C), which is the proportion of people with a condition, either exposure or disease, who are correctly classified by the test as having the condition. Laboratory scientists also use this definition of sensitivity in the context of a test's diagnostic accuracy for a condition (Galen, 1977).

Because a test can achieve 100 percent sensitivity by simply classifying *everyone* as having the condition, high sensitivity is meaningless unless the test also has high specificity, defined as D/(B + D) from the preceding 2 × 2 table. That is, specificity is the proportion of people without the condition who are correctly classified. Criteria for classifying a test outcome can often be modified to increase either sensitivity or specificity at the expense of the other. A graphical approach using receiver operator characteristic (ROC) analysis can help select an optimum cutpoint to determine sensitivity and specificity levels for tests with continuous outcomes. Comparisons of ROC curves among tests often show the advantage of one test over another with regard to sensitivity and specificity (Mayewski et al., 1986).

Laboratory scientists implicitly use the concepts of sensitivity and specificity in the epidemiologic sense when they estimate a minimum detectable level for an assay. That is, an assay repeated 100 times on identical samples may sometimes be positive and sometimes negative, and analyte concentrations above the minimum detectable level should usually produce a positive test result. If the claimed minimum detectable level is actually too low, then test results will frequently be negative even when the concentration exceeds the nominal minimum. An overly high nominal minimum, on the other hand, leads to positive test results even when the concentration falls below the minimum (i.e., the positive test result implies a higher concentration than what actually exists). These two situations are similar to the complements of epidemiologic specificity (false-positive results) and sensitivity (false-negative results), and the estimated minimum detectable level is a compromise between the two types of errors.

With regard to markers, epidemiologists can encounter operational problems when they estimate a marker's sensitivity and specificity for a given exposure or disease, because marker measurements and the underlying condition of interest often follow a continuum, whereas sensitivity and specificity are defined in terms of binary outcomes. The mean number of sister chromatid exchanges (SCEs) or alkyl DNA adducts per cell, for example, always exceeds zero, and the selection of a cutpoint to distinguish the background level from an elevated level due to exposure becomes somewhat arbitrary. Furthermore, usually no binary "gold standard" exists for exposure or disease status that would allow the 2×2 classification described previously to estimate marker sensitivity and specificity. Thus, although the concepts of sensitivity and specificity are useful for marker evaluation, in many cases they must be reformulated as discussed later.

For all biological markers, there exist two components of overall sensitivity: the sensitivity of the marker to detect the underlying condition of interest (or to predict future disease in the case of susceptibility markers), and the sensitivity of the assay used to measure the marker itself. For example, protein adducts in a tissue may be more sensitive indicators of chronic exposure to chemical X than are DNA adducts, because protein adducts give cumulative dose estimates. One marker is more sensitive than the other. With regard to assays, ^{32}P-postlabeling compared with the enzyme-linked immunosorbent assay (ELISA) is more sensitive to detect DNA adducts. Operationally, one must ignore this conceptual distinction and treat different assays as if they were themselves distinct markers for a given underlying condition, as a marker only exists to the extent that it can be measured.

The distinction between markers and assays for markers may be subtle, but a marker's quantification determines how its sensitivity is assessed. For example, some chemicals that form DNA adducts also cause SCEs, and one may want to compare the sensitivity of the ^{32}P-postlabeling assay and the SCE assay to detect evidence of exposure to a chemical mutagen in a group of exposed workers. For the ^{32}P-postlabeling assay, the sensitivity (in the epidemiologic sense) is simply the proportion of exposed workers with a positive test (i.e., the test shows the presence of adducts); however, all of the workers would show at least some SCEs with current assay techniques even without exposure, so one cannot estimate the sensitivity of the assay simply by the proportion of workers with SCEs. Both markers indicate DNA lesions, but one allows a convenient binary classification of exposure status for each individual, whereas the other is measured as a continuous variable with a background level that varies among individuals.

Proportion Correctly Classified

Because some markers have continuous distributions with nonzero values among the unexposed, epidemiologists may have difficulty estimating sensitivity and specificity based on the usual 2×2 classification scheme. In some instances, however, markers with a continuous distribution can still fit into a categorical framework. With SCEs, for example, one could classify an individual as exposed or unexposed if the estimated number of SCEs per cell fell above or below some predetermined cutpoint. A high cutpoint would tend to yield false-negative results, whereas a low cutpoint would produce false-positive results. The large interlaboratory variability in baseline levels of SCEs from historical control populations, however, complicates this approach. To avoid interlaboratory variability, investigators might use the same laboratory to measure the SCE distribution in an exposed and unexposed population, and use the latter population to establish a cutpoint to define exposure.

Different procedures to define an exposure cutpoint based on an unexposed population are possible. For example, when comparing the sensitivity of the ^{32}P-postlabeling assay and the SCE assay, one could first estimate the specificity of the former assay by calculating the proportion of unexposed persons who show a negative test for adducts. Suppose, for example, that 10 percent of the occupationally unexposed population have detectable adducts from other exposures, so that the specificity of the test is 90 percent. By using as an exposure cutpoint the 90th percentile of the distribution of mean number of SCEs per cell among the unexposed individuals, one could set the specificity of the SCE assay at 90 percent. That is, 10 percent of the unexposed individuals would fall above the cutpoint and would be classified as false-positives. The 90th percentile cutpoint from the *unexposed* population could then be used as an exposure cutpoint in the *exposed* population. The proportion of exposed workers whose mean number of SCEs per cell exceeded this cutpoint would give the sensitivity of the SCE assay for detecting exposure when the specificity is 90 percent, and the sensitivity of the two assays could then be compared at the same level of specificity. If the entire distribution of the mean number of SCEs per cell among individuals in the exposed population exceeded the cutpoint, the sensitivity would be 100 percent. However, if the lower 15 percent, for example, of the distribution fell below the cutpoint, then the sensitivity would be 85 percent (i.e., 15 percent of the exposed would be incorrectly counted as unexposed).

Minimum Detectable Level

In some instances, a comparison of the minimum detectable levels for two or more markers provides the most straightforward assessment of sensitivity, as this approach avoids the imposition of an arbitrary 2×2 categorization on continuous variables. For example, one might compare the minimum blood level of a solvent that is detectable with breath versus urine analysis. To the extent that minimum detectable levels for different markers are established according to the same criteria, epidemiologists can select the marker most likely to give true-positive results without reformulating its properties in terms of categorical sensitivity and specificity.

Ability to Detect Exposure Differences

Marker sensitivity can also be assessed in terms of the ability to detect differences in exposure level. For example, Latt et al. (1981) reported the amounts of different chemicals necessary to double the background rate of SCEs. With a related approach, one could estimate the percent change in SCE levels associated with a percent change in exposure level. Then, one could compare the percent change in marker response for different markers to identify the one with the greatest sensitivity for an exposure. Consequently, all three concepts of sensitivity (viz., proportion correctly classified as positive, minimum detectable level, and ability to detect exposure differences) are useful to evaluate markers. Regardless of the procedure, however, for markers based on biological responses to external exposures, sensitivity depends on the particular exposure agent. Therefore, generalizations about the overall sensitivity of one marker as compared with another are difficult (Lohman et al., 1985).

Other approaches to compare sensitivity among markers are also possible, but for most markers the data necessary for making such comparisons will probably be unavailable. Epidemiologists are then left with qualitative statements about sensitivity, such as SCEs "respond to a wider variety of agents and require 10- to 100-fold lower doses" compared with chromosome aberrations (NTP, 1984). This kind of comparison with respect to sensitivity is probably adequate to select markers for a particular research objective. Even qualitative comparisons of markers will often be unavailable, however, and rapid advances in marker measurement technology may make earlier conclusions obsolete. Decisions about marker selection based on sensitivity may, therefore, depend on the impression of experts who are familiar with the various choices in markers.

Specificity

As mentioned in the preceding section, specificity pertains to the concepts of false-positive and true-negative results. With regard to detecting exposures, a marker has high specificity if it produces few false-positive results among the unexposed. The term is also used to denote markers that respond to only one or a few exposures. For example, only one specific chemical may produce a particular bulky DNA adduct, whereas many different chemicals can produce the same small alkyl DNA adducts. If the chemical of interest is an alkylating agent, using adducts as an exposure marker will lead to false-positive results in the presence of other alkylating agents. The operational issues concerning the quantification of specificity for marker evaluations are related to those described previously for marker sensitivity: specificity estimates in the epidemiologic sense require the use of a binary gold standard, and the marker measurement must also be dichotomous. Specificity comparisons among markers are probably assessed most conveniently in terms of the number of different exposures (and at what concentrations) to which the markers respond.

In some instances, a marker may be highly specific for a class of chemicals, such as mutagens or clastogens, but may be nonspecific for individual compounds within the class (Lohman et al., 1985). Because chromosome aberrations in lymphocytes, for example, can arise from a variety of clastogenic chemicals as well as from radiation, this marker cannot indicate exactly which exposure occurred. In other instances, the marker is specific for a single chemical, but the chemical is common to different types of exposures. Two markers of tobacco smoke exposure illustrate this point. Hemoglobin adducts of 4-aminobiphenyl give a good integrated estimate of tobacco smoke exposure, but certain occupations also allow exposures to compounds that result in 4-aminobiphenyl adducts. Similarly, both tobacco smoke and some foods lead to detectable levels of thiocyanate in saliva and blood. Using nonspecific markers in epidemiologic studies can, therefore, cause false-positive results for a particular exposure or disease, because other exposures or diseases also produce the marker response of interest.

Table 3-3 presents examples of markers with various degrees of specificity. The nonspecific markers in Table 3-3 can detect exposures that have only modest chemical similarities but produce the same biological effect. The markers with intermediate specificity detect exposures to classes of related chemicals. Most highly specific markers are based on detecting particular chemicals or their metabolites in body fluids and tissues, but some bulky adducts on macromolecules can also be linked to specific chemical exposures.

Depending on the question of interest, lack of specificity in a marker does not necessarily cause problems in epidemiologic studies. Chromosome aberrations in lymphocytes, for example, apparently reflect the effect of all clastogens that reach the blood (Lohman et al., 1985), and such a marker may be quite useful in an epidemiologic study of reproductive outcomes. In other studies where a specific exposure is of interest, a marker's lack of specificity will still not present a problem if there have been no other exposures that cause the same marker response.

For nonspecific markers, exposure misclassification occurs if members of the study population are exposed to extraneous agents that cause a marker response. The exposure misclassification can be differential or nondifferential with respect to a disease outcome. For example, suppose that an epidemiologic study of an industrial chemical exposure uses mutagenicity in urine as an exposure marker. Because cigarette smoking

Table 3-3 Examples of Marker Specificity

Low specificity (exposures in parentheses)
Chromosome aberrations in lymphocytes
(clastogens)
Mutagenicity in urine (chemical mutagens)
Hypoxanthine-guanine phosphoribosyl transferase
(HGPRT) in lymphocytes (mutagens)
Intermediate specificity (exposures in parentheses)
Total urinary amino compounds (aromatic amines)
Blood methemoglobin (aromatic amines)
Urinary nitrosoproline (nitrosamines)
High specificity
Unchanged chemicals in body tissues/fluids
Chemical-specific metabolites in body tissues/fluids
Protein adducts and DNA adducts

causes mutagenicity in urine, workers who smoke will show a positive test even without the occupational exposure. For a disease unrelated to smoking, such as leukemia, the exposure misclassification will be nondifferential (i.e., the diseased and nondiseased persons are equally likely to be smokers). In contrast, for a smoking-related disease, such as lung cancer, the study will suffer from differential exposure misclassification, as workers with lung cancer will be more likely to have a positive urine test, because of their higher prevalence of smoking, than will disease-free workers. A spurious association could, therefore, arise between the occupational exposure, as measured by the marker, and lung cancer.

Exposure misclassification, whether differential or nondifferential because of a lack of specificity in the marker, can be alleviated through a proper study design or analysis. In this example, stratification by cigarette consumption or restriction to either non-smokers or smokers would remove the effects of smoking on exposure misclassification. Smoking status could be assessed, for example, with another biological marker, such as urinary cotinine. In general, because the importance of marker specificity depends on the nature of the study question and on the prevalence of extraneous exposure (or disease) variables that affect the marker, epidemiologists must evaluate marker specificity in the context of each study setting.

Human Variability
Interindividual Variability

A major rationale for using biological markers in epidemiologic studies is that identical ambient exposures can produce different internal and biologically effective doses in different individuals; therefore, exposure estimates based on ambient monitoring can cause exposure misclassification. For example, a worker's internal dose of a solvent depends not only on its concentration in the ambient air and on the duration of exposure, but also on the worker's pulmonary ventilation and skin absorption (Angerer, 1985). Interindividual differences in the metabolic clearance of internalized agents can result in unequal biologically effective doses even when internal doses are the same (Elinder and Vesterberg, 1985). Metabolic influences have a particularly important effect on the biologically effective dose of those environmental toxins for which the metabolite, rather than its precursor, is the more hazardous compound. Additional variability exists in a person's ability to repair molecular damage from an environmental exposure. Because appropriate biological markers can take into account the effects of these sources of interindividual variability, exposure estimates from markers typically give a better picture of a person's exposure status than do ambient exposure estimates.

Some sources of interindividual variability in marker response can cause exposure misclassification. For example, suppose that an investigator uses solvent concentration in urine collected over 24 hours as an internal dose marker for the solvent in exposed workers. Two workers with identical ambient exposures could show differences in urinary solvent concentrations. If the difference in urinary concentrations reflects actual differences in blood levels between workers, then the marker is detecting a true dose gradient. The difference in urinary concentrations, however, could result from differences in the amount of solvent exhaled, or in the amount of solvent metabolized into some other chemical. In these instances, the marker would incorrectly indicate that the two workers had different internal doses of the solvent. To the extent that the differences between workers in renal function, routes of excretion, and metabolism remain stable over time, the misclassification is due to interindividual rather than intraindividual variability.

Intraindividual Variability

Variability in an individual's marker response over time adds noise to the analysis. Such variability could cause a person's biological sample at one point to indicate a low exposure state, whereas a later sample might indicate high exposure although the ambient exposure remained unchanged. Intraindividual variability can arise from a variety of sources. Random errors inherent in the laboratory assay will cause apparent changes in the marker response. Unmeasured extraneous exposures that affect a marker response will also produce intraindividual variability if the other determinants vary over time (see the preceding section on specificity for examples). Other exposures or conditions, such as dietary influences, can modify a marker response to an exposure even if these conditions themselves do not directly cause a marker response. If one hopes to obtain an overall estimate of a person's typical exposure status for a study of chronic health outcomes, intraindividual variability in the marker response will lead to exposure misclassification. In this situation, a marker with more temporal stability that gives an integrated exposure estimate would be superior to one that shows large variability. If alternative markers are not available, then repeated measurements over time of markers with high intraindividual variability will give a more precise estimate of a person's long-term exposure status.

Variability Between Groups

Epidemiologists primarily use biological markers of exposure to classify individuals' exposure status in studies of exposure–disease associations. Consequently, for such markers to be epidemiologically useful, groups of people with varying degrees of exposure must show corresponding marker variability. In other words, the marker distribution cannot be the same in exposed and unexposed groups. Ideally, the marker response will increase as a function of increasing exposure levels.

The ability of a marker to differentiate between groups is determined by its sensitivity and specificity, and these properties depend on the interindividual and intraindividual variability in marker responses and the variability between groups due to exposure or disease differences. To avoid serious exposure or disease misclassification, the intergroup variability should be relatively large compared with the other sources of variability. Because sensitivity and specificity incorporate all sources of variability, one can evaluate a marker's usefulness for classification with either sensitivity and specificity data, or with appropriate variance estimates.

In addition to the nondifferential misclassification that can arise between groups due to random error, Willett (1987) raises concerns about variability between groups that results from systematic error. For example, small differences in storing and handling of biological samples for cases and controls could bias the results of case-control studies. Laboratory drift could also cause bias if samples from cases and controls are analyzed on different days. Willett (1987) emphasizes the need to simultaneously handle specimens from sets of cases and controls (i.e., one case and one or more controls) through all steps from retrieval from storage through laboratory analysis.

Although not stated in Willett's article, the sets of specimens should ideally be collected and processed for storage at the same time, and the statistical analysis should, in some situations, maintain the matching or stratification used in the handling and assaying of the samples.

Determinants of Variability

As noted previously, variability in a marker response can occur within an individual over time. In some instances this variability reflects random errors inherent in the measurement process. Biological factors unrelated to measurement errors can also affect variability in marker responses within and between individuals, as these examples illustrate.

Synergistic Exposures

Simultaneous exposures to multiple chemicals sometimes increase the internal dose of an agent of interest. For example, exposure to tetrachloroethylene or toluene increases the blood levels of trichloroethylene after exposure, because tetrachloroethylene and toluene inhibit trichloroethylene metabolism (Angerer, 1985). Because most solvents in occupational settings are used as mixtures, situations in which one solvent affects the internal dose of another commonly arise. Ethanol-containing beverages can also increase the internal dose of other solvents (Angerer, 1985). If the extraneous exposures vary over time, the internal dose of the chemical of interest can also vary, although the ambient level of that chemical remains constant. Note that this kind of situation differs conceptually from the influence of confounding exposures on non-specific markers where extraneous exposures themselves cause a marker response. With synergistic exposures, the extraneous exposures actually increase the *dose* of the agent of interest. They have no effect on marker response in the absence of the agent of interest.

Diet

Because food intake changes the composition of blood (especially blood lipids), a person's diet can affect a marker response to a given ambient chemical exposure (Aitio, 1984). For example, because many chemicals used in the workplace are fat-soluble, high triglyceride levels in the blood after a meal increase the blood concentrations of lipid-soluble chemicals after exposure (Aitio, 1984). Plasma lipoproteins, especially the very low density lipoprotein (VLDL) particle and chylomicrons, serve as transport vehicles for fat-soluble compounds throughout the body. For highly lipophilic chemicals, such as the pesticides DDT and dieldrin, tissue concentrations are directly proportional to the concentration of lipids in the tissue (Smith et al., 1983). Similarly, people with high lipoprotein levels tend to have high blood levels of the fat-soluble vitamins transported by lipoproteins (Willett, 1987). Controlling diet before taking blood samples can remove some variability in the blood levels of lipophilic compounds (Aitio, 1984), and adjustment for plasma lipoprotein levels can improve the accuracy of estimates of dietary fat-soluble vitamins (Willett, 1987).

Some nutrients can also help induce the detoxification enzyme systems that convert some chemicals into hydrophilic metabolites before excretion (Ames, 1983). Therefore, metabolite levels after a chemical exposure can depend on diet as well as on previous chemical exposures. Ames (1983) has discussed an extensive list of nutrients that can increase or decrease the dose and effects of various chemical exposures.

Diurnal Variation

The kinetics of a chemical determine its concentration in different body compartments over time. Some chemicals also show diurnal variation in concentration superimposed on their long-term levels. Mercury, for example, has diurnal variation in its urinary concentration due to physiological changes in excretion (Aitio, 1984). The time of day at which the biological sample is collected can, therefore, influence a marker's level in some instances.

Personal Characteristics

Personal characteristics that vary from day to day in members of a study population will also influence marker response after exposure. Injured or diseased skin, for example, increases the absorption of some solvents, as do many other personal factors that change over time (Brown et al., 1984). Behaviors with potential temporal variability, such as wearing protective equipment or clothing, or the work rate, which can affect the breathing rate, also contribute to the variability in doses measured by biological markers.

In a given epidemiologic study, there will probably be more determinants of marker variability than can be controlled, measured, or even recognized. Even if a marker response fluctuates over time within an individual, it often does indicate the dose that existed in the biological sample at the time it was collected. If this is the measurement of interest, then the variability poses no problems. If one is interested in a stable estimate of longer-term exposure, however, then the variability may cause bias through misclassification or confounding, depending on the distribution of the determinants of variability with respect to true exposure and disease status. Issues of measurement error and confounding pertain to all epidemiologic studies, whether or not they employ biological markers. When using biological markers, however, epidemiologists should be alert to those sources of error most likely to exist.

Biological Materials

Marker properties typically vary among biological materials. Under ideal circumstances, one would sample the material that yielded the marker or markers with the best properties to address a particular study question. In actuality, the use of a particular biological material largely depends on its availability, and a researcher must determine if appropriate markers can be measured in the material available. Urine may be available to measure chemical exposures in an occupational cohort, for example, but urine can only be used to measure water-soluble chemicals, such as alcohol (Droz and Guillemin, 1986). If the study concerned exposure to a fat-soluble compound, such as benzene, the investigator would need to identify a water-soluble metabolite (e.g., phenol) in urine, obtain samples of a biological material, such as blood, that can carry fat-soluble compounds, or estimate exposures without using biological markers. When investigators collect biological material for an epidemiologic study, the invasiveness of the sampling procedure is the primary determinant of availability. If the material was originally collected for another purpose (e.g., surgical pathology specimens), invasiveness becomes less important than access and storage.

One motivation for using biological markers is that many health-related events occur at inaccessible sites in the body, but a marker in an accessible biological material may indicate events at these inaccessible sites of interest. The formation of DNA adducts in circulating lymphocytes, for example, may correlate with adduct formation in the liver. In general, markers in biological materials that can be collected safely with little discomfort to the donor hold greater promise for use in large-scale epidemiologic studies than do markers in less easily sampled materials.

In the context of markers, invasiveness describes the degree of intrusion into the body required to collect biological material. Urine collection is less invasive than blood collection, whereas sampling bone marrow is more invasive than venipuncture. Some materials, such as expired air, urine, and feces, are constantly excreted by the body and require no intrusion for collection. Other materials, such as saliva, sputum, and breast milk, require active collection, but no actual intrusion. In contrast, the collection of blood, amniotic fluid, or biopsy materials involves penetration of body tissues. Table 3-4 gives examples of potentially useful biological materials with varying degrees of accessibility.

In some respects, the concept of invasiveness includes aspects other than just tissue penetration. There also exist cultural and psychological components. Many individuals would be more willing to provide a blood sample than a fecal or semen sample, even though drawing blood is a more invasive procedure. In an operational sense, therefore, invasiveness includes the willingness of study participants to provide the necessary biological material as well as the physical trauma associated with specimen collection.

Sometimes biological materials collected for reasons other than epidemiologic study offer epidemiologic potential. Because clinicians routinely obtain surgical pathology specimens, autopsy specimens, blood, and other biological materials, biological samples that could not be collected on epidemiologic grounds alone may be available for epidemiologic study (see Chapter 2 for examples of such studies). Collaborative arrangements with medical staff using protocols designed for storing the samples can allow investigators to incorporate clinical specimens into epidemiologic studies.

In some instances, biological samples collected for one study can be used to address unrelated questions. For example, Willett et al. (1983) studied the association between serum selenium levels and cancer using blood samples and follow-up data collected in the Hypertension Detection and Follow-up Program. The success of studies

Table 3-4 Examples of Biological Materials Useful for Measuring Markers

Noninvasive		
Expired air	Saliva	Semen
Urine	Sputum	Hair
Feces	Breast milk	Fingernails
Invasive		
Blood	Lung tissue	Bone marrow
Amniotic fluid	Liver tissue	Bone
Follicular fluid	Adipose tissue	Blood vessels

that use biological samples collected for a different purpose depends on the stability of the marker during storage, as sample analysis may be delayed for extended periods. With creative thinking and attention to analytic details, however, epidemiologists can find opportunities to use biological markers without the overhead of specimen collection.

Target and Nontarget Tissues

A single exposure can have many different physiologic effects; some effects eventually lead to disease and others cause no apparent health problems. For example, although a chemical carcinogen may cause DNA lesions throughout the body, only lesions in some tissues give rise to cancer. DNA lesions in such cells as circulating lymphocytes do not directly cause malignancies. Markers in such nontarget cells as lymphocytes, however, may be highly correlated with lesions in disease-susceptible organs, so that the marker may predict pathogenesis in other tissues.

In general, one might expect that markers measured in target tissues (i.e., tissues that undergo pathogenic changes from the exposure) would predict disease more strongly than would markers in nontarget tissues. This expectation may be untrue for a number of reasons. For example, markers in nontarget tissues might persist longer after exposure ends than do those in target tissues, so that the target tissues show no evidence of exposure. Marker responses in nontarget compared with target tissues might also be more pronounced due to a higher tissue-specific internal dose. Blood cells, for example, may receive especially high doses of hydrophilic chemicals and low doses of lipophilic chemicals. Or the marker response in nontarget tissues may be measured with relatively low variability. Consequently, even without problems with invasive sampling, target tissues may in some instances provide an inferior source of biological material for marker measurements. In the absence of evidence to the contrary, however, target tissue is probably the material of choice to measure markers in epidemiologic studies.

One advantage of some biological markers is their ability to integrate exposures from multiple sources. Solvent levels in blood, for example, reflect skin absorption as well as inhalation. With respect to target tissues, however, this property can be a liability rather than an asset. If the risk of lung cancer is of interest, markers of the inhaled agent would have more relevance than would markers of systemic exposure from all sources (Friberg, 1985). Similarly, nickel that reaches the blood and urine has no direct relevance to nasal cancer, but some slightly soluble nickel compounds can remain in the nasal mucosa for years where they may cause cancer (Aitio, 1984).

Within a target tissue, markers that comprise part of the pathogenic pathway may be especially good predictors of disease, but, as with markers in target versus nontarget tissues, markers with tangential roles in pathogenesis may sometimes be superior in epidemiologic studies. For example, suppose that an exposure in a target tissue causes protein and DNA adducts. The DNA adducts may eventually lead to cancer, whereas the protein adducts cause no disease, but protein adducts may be a more sensitive indicator of exposure because of cumulative exposure effects. Because the markers with the greatest epidemiologic value are those with the strongest statistical, rather than biological, link to the outcome of interest, empirical studies of marker–disease associations give more compelling evidence of marker utility than do studies of a marker's role in pathogenesis.

STATE OF TESTING

The development of biological markers continues at a fast pace. New types of markers are constantly proposed and analytic techniques for existing markers improve. In the midst of this rapid progress, epidemiologists designing a study must sometimes choose between well-characterized markers with a long history of epidemiologic use and newer markers that show great promise based on preliminary evaluations. The information available for assessing a marker's potential usefulness can range from in vitro studies to large-scale epidemiologic investigations of free-living populations.

In Vitro Studies

Before a biological marker finds use in studies of human populations, it typically undergoes evaluation in nonhuman systems. Examples of in vitro systems include simple aqueous solutions, purified enzyme preparations, tissue homogenates, microsomes, cultured cells, tissue slices, and isolated perfused organs (NIEHS, 1986, p. 190). In vitro systems provide epidemiologists with the most basic source of information to evaluate marker utility, but they cannot replicate the complex metabolic pathways found in humans. Organ-specific detoxification enzyme systems in humans, for example, are often approximated in vitro using rat liver enzymes, yet the resulting metabolites of the in vitro chemical detoxification may incorrectly predict those that actually form in humans. By itself, in vitro testing provides inadequate information to evaluate markers for human epidemiologic studies, but it can yield valuable information about potential marker utility.

In the simplest applications of in vitro procedures to molecular epidemiology, techniques to measure environmental contaminants in drinking water or food, for example, are adapted to measure similar chemicals in biological samples. For example, chromatographic techniques to measure such chemicals as aflatoxins in foods have also been used to analyze tissues from humans with suspected aflatoxin exposures (NIEHS, 1986, p. 213). Methods to analyze such chemicals as N-nitroso compounds or aromatic amines in environmental samples, however, often have not been evaluated for other media, and the techniques may require extensive modifications to enable analyses of metabolites (NIEHS, 1986, p. 213). Consequently, epidemiologists who want to measure the internal dose of an environmental chemical or its metabolites must first ascertain whether the measurement technique is suitable for the biological material of interest.

On a more complex level of testing, in vitro studies using tissue homogenates or cultured cells can indicate whether a chemical is likely to form adducts with macromolecules such as DNA and proteins. In vitro evidence of adduct formation for a chemical would suggest that adducts could be used as markers of biologically effective dose for that chemical in humans. Enzymatic activation of a chemical in vitro, however, may produce metabolites and adducts that will not necessarily occur in humans.

For cytogenetic markers, such as SCEs, in vitro studies allow exploration of the marker's properties under precisely controlled conditions. The persistence of chemical-specific lesions in dividing and nondividing cells, for example, can be conveniently evaluated in cell cultures. The responses in different markers can also be compared in vitro. For example, as the dose of a chemical increases, the frequencies of SCEs and single-gene mutations also increase in cell cultures, and the relative increase in response between the two markers depends on the chemical being tested. Studies in animal models can then indicate if the cell culture studies accurately predict the marker associations and properties in vivo (NIEHS, 1986, p. 234).

On a more basic level, in vitro studies may indicate the sensitivity and specificity of a marker to detect a given chemical. Such assays as the Ames assay and SCE analysis are commonly used with cell cultures (bacterial or mammalian) to screen for genetic damage from a variety of chemicals. The in vitro literature may, therefore, indicate whether these assays can be useful for epidemiologic studies of exposure to a particular chemical.

In vitro studies provide a necessary foundation to evaluate a marker's usefulness in epidemiologic studies, but epidemiologists clearly should avoid the large-scale use of markers until they undergo scrutiny in animals and humans. Markers or assays that show undesirable properties in vitro, such as low sensitivity or high interassay variability, will probably never have epidemiologic value. The use of in vitro studies to screen for potentially useful markers may shorten the list of candidate markers for epidemiologic studies.

Animal Studies

Animal studies can validate results from in vitro studies, but more importantly, animal studies allow explorations of almost all of a marker's properties in vivo. Because markers may behave differently across species, the obvious problem with animal models concerns species extrapolation. In humans, for example, acetyl transferase shows distinct phenotypes that apparently influence the risk of bladder cancer after 4-aminobiphenyl exposure. This susceptibility marker (i.e., enzyme phenotype) has no counterpart in dogs where acetyl transferase has uniformly low activity for acetylating aromatic amines (Vainio, 1985). Similarly, studies of inhaled SO_2 using the rat model are hard to extrapolate to humans, because rats lack the mucus-producing glands in their airways that may protect against SO_2 irritation in humans (Jaeger, 1982). Calabrese (1988) summarizes the differences between humans and selected animal models with respect to several metabolic characteristics that affect responses to chemical carcinogens.

To the extent that markers in animal models accurately reflect their counterparts in humans, animal studies facilitate the development of markers for later use in human studies. For example, animal studies allow investigators to characterize marker responses to controlled levels of ambient toxic exposures and may allow them to generalize the results to humans. For example, for ethylene oxide exposures both animal and human studies show similar quantitative relationships between exposure levels and amounts of blood protein adducts. If quantitative dose–response relationships are similar between animals and humans, then the minimum ambient exposure level that produces a human marker response can be estimated from animal studies (NIEHS,

1986, p. 221). Animal studies also allow assessments of biological variability in marker responses within and among experimental animals. One might expect, however, that variability among animals will underestimate that seen in humans, as laboratory animals are often genetically homogeneous.

Animal studies allow comparisons of marker responses between relatively accessible and inaccessible tissues and cells. Because the target tissue for a particular chemical toxin may lie within the lungs or the liver, sampling the biological material would require invasive procedures. Animal studies might reveal that responses of markers, such as SCEs or DNA adducts in the liver, closely parallel the responses of these same markers in easily accessible circulating lymphocytes. To the extent that species extrapolation is appropriate, the observed marker response in human lymphocytes could then be used to predict the response in the human liver.

As with markers and assays that have been limited to in vitro testing, markers under development only in animal models are not yet suitable candidates for epidemiologic studies. For other markers, such as excised DNA adducts in urine, animal studies show promise, but the assays need refinement to detect exposure to carcinogens at the levels typical of human populations (NIEHS, 1986, p. 225). As discussed later, the markers of greatest current interest to epidemiologists are those that have undergone successful evaluations in humans.

Human Clinical Studies

Small-scale studies of markers in humans bridge epidemiologic field studies and animal studies. Such studies indicate whether the markers that show promise in animal studies actually give valid estimates of exposure or outcome in humans. The markers are themselves typically the focus of the research, rather than measurements used to answer larger questions of epidemiologic interest.

In many instances, the studies are observational in that the participants undergo exposures independent of the marker evaluation. For example, cytogenetic markers have been studied in cancer patients receiving cytotoxic drugs (Einhorn et al., 1982; Musilová et al., 1979), and in cigarette smokers (Perera et al., 1987). These same groups can be used to evaluate assays for DNA adducts. van Staveren et al. (1986) used a series of 19 24-hour dietary recalls, collected from women in another study, to assess the validity of fat tissue microbiopsies as an estimate of the long-term fatty acid composition of their diet.

For exposures that have fairly benign effects at typical ambient levels, such as sidestream cigarette smoke or other air pollutants, controlled exposure chamber studies are ethically feasible to validate biological markers of exposure. Chamber studies are useful to assess a marker's biological properties such as response gradient to different exposure doses, biological variability, and persistence after exposure cessation. Such studies can be especially valuable to estimate statistical variances for sample size estimates, and to evaluate potential confounding variables. They also allow assessment of operational problems such as biological sample collection, storage, and analysis.

Data from human clinical studies have certain advantages and disadvantages in evaluating markers for use in field studies. On the positive side, the external exposures are often carefully measured or controlled, so that biological variability in the marker response can be distinguished from variability in the ambient exposure level. Other exposures that may confound the relationship between the exposure of interest and the marker response can often be controlled or eliminated. The study populations, however, may be atypical of the groups of interest for field studies. For example, because of their disease, cancer patients receiving cytotoxic drugs may differ metabolically from healthy people. Also, their cytotoxic exposure levels will far exceed those encountered in normal occupational or environmental settings. Because ethical considerations preclude an experimental evaluation of markers for highly toxic exposures, the human studies of such markers may, in fact, be small-scale observational studies of persons with poorly characterized occupational or other unplanned exposures. In general, studies of greatest relevance to epidemiologists examine markers in the range of doses expected to be present in typical exposure environments.

A marker with clear value in small-scale human clinical studies will not necessarily be of interest to epidemiologists conducting large field studies. For example, bronchoalveolar lavage provides extensive information on how the lungs respond to inhaled vapors and particles (NIEHS, 1986, pp. 237–244). The technique, however, involves adding saline to the lungs to wash out cells and molecules of interest when the fluid is withdrawn. The procedure's invasive nature prevents its application in large free-living populations. Basic considerations, such as cost or availability of laboratory resources, may also limit the usefulness of markers with very desirable biological properties. Hemoglobin adducts, for example, give a good time-weighted estimate of 4-aminobiphenyl exposure in rats (Tannenbaum et al., 1983). In humans, small-scale studies indicate that the hemoglobin adducts may be excellent markers of active and passive cigarette smoke exposure (Tannenbaum, 1987), but the assay is expensive and not yet widely available. Thus, although human clinical studies offer an excellent opportunity to evaluate a marker's biological properties, additional properties also determine its potential value to epidemiologists.

Applied Field Studies

Applied field studies use markers to address health-related questions in observational studies of free-living human populations. This somewhat arbitrary definition distinguishes studies designed to evaluate markers from studies that use markers to examine substantive issues. Applied field studies may include: epidemiologic investigations of exposure–disease associations; disease-screening programs that identify subclinical or early-stage disease; or biological monitoring studies that measure external exposures.

Although extensive use in field studies provides evidence of a marker's potential utility, such studies typically yield little information about the markers themselves, as the evaluation of marker properties is tangential to the study's purpose. Furthermore, the field studies do not necessarily identify the most appropriate marker for a given epidemiologic problem, because they may have used markers that subsequently became obsolete, or because certain laboratory resources were unavailable to the investigator. For example, earlier cardiovascular disease studies commonly used total serum lipoprotein cholesterol as a predictor of myocardial infarction, but as technology improved, lipoprotein cholesterol subfractions became the lipoprotein markers of choice.

Field studies do, however, circumvent the major disadvantages of small-scale clinical studies. Exposures in field studies reflect those found in free-living populations. Field study populations are intentionally chosen to answer public health questions rather than purposefully selected to provide biological material. Successful field studies using a particular marker clearly demonstrate that operational difficulties associated with the marker are manageable in applied settings. In a sense, field studies serve as a feasibility screen for markers, and markers with a record of success are frequently the markers of choice.

Synthesis of Test Data

Ideally, an epidemiologist confronted with a study question that lends itself to using biological markers can review the literature to identify the most suitable markers. Unfortunately, the picture is often incomplete. The state of testing for a given marker may be exposure-specific or specific to a single biological material, so that earlier studies only predict what a researcher might encounter under specific exposure and sampling conditions. For example, because abnormal porphyrin ratios in blood and urine are a better marker of lead exposure than are blood lead measurements, porphyrins are used routinely as a screen for lead toxicity. In vitro and animal studies indicate that other metals also affect porphyrins, but human data remain sparse or nonexistent (Raloff, 1987). Consequently, although an epidemiologist can effectively evaluate the use of porphyrins as markers of lead exposure, their usefulness as markers of other metal exposures is less certain. In the absence of good competing markers for other metal exposures, however, a researcher may attempt to use porphyrins both because results from animal studies are promising and because porphyrins are a proven marker for lead.

Many issues concerning the relationships of marker responses in humans, animals, and in vitro systems fall within the realm of pharmacokinetics—the absorption, distribution, and elimination of chemicals in the body. Such information indicates when and in which biological materials a marker should be measured. Although the pharmacologic literature extensively characterizes the kinetic properties of drugs, the rigorous use of pharmacokinetics in toxicology and environmental health is fairly recent (NIEHS, 1986, p. 187). Appropriately designed pharmacokinetic studies maximize toxicologic information from an experiment, but many toxicity studies suffer from a lack of standardization. Differences in dosages, types of animals, and other experimental conditions reduce the meaningful information gained. Furthermore, large numbers of toxic chemicals will probably never undergo detailed pharmacokinetic studies in animals, whereas the toxicity of many chemicals precludes their controlled evaluation in humans (NIEHS, 1986, pp. 187–190). Due to the lack of standardized pharmacokinetic studies, epidemiologists must, therefore, expect to use incomplete information from a variety of sources when they evaluate a marker's potential value for a given study question.

Although results from in vitro studies coupled with pharmacokinetic models have been used successfully to predict the kinetics of chemicals in animals and humans (NIEHS, 1986, p. 190), few epidemiologists have the expertise to use in vitro data to evaluate markers in this way. In vitro studies, however, can provide more simple information that epidemiologists can readily use. For example, in vitro studies may indicate that a chemical of interest reacts with certain biochemicals or produces cellular or tissue changes, suggesting a marker or biological material for measuring the chemical exposure. Chemical X, for example, may form covalent adducts with serum albumin in vitro and cause SCEs in cultured lymphocytes; these markers may also detect chemical X exposures in humans.

If animal toxicology data are available for an exposure marker, the animal studies compared with in vitro studies should give more information about a marker's biological properties. Pharmacokinetic differences between the animal model and humans will preclude simple direct extrapolation about the marker's biological properties in humans. A comparison of different markers within the same animal model, however, may allow qualitative conclusions about their expected relative merits in humans. In essence, one can attempt to draw parallels among chemicals and across species to obtain a rough idea of a marker's relevance to a particular human study.

Only human studies, however, can provide the pharmacokinetic data that epidemiologists and other researchers would like. In reality, detailed pharmacokinetic data for toxic chemical exposures in humans are often limited to studies of accidental or occupational exposures where the dose and other exposure details are poorly characterized (NIEHS, 1986, p. 190). Thus, a marker's properties in humans may only be measured ad hoc, so that properties that seem to differ among various exposed populations are due merely to unquantified exposure differences. Ironically, one of the problems that biological markers of exposure can help overcome, reliance on poorly measured ambient exposure data, hampers the evaluation of the markers themselves. Even if a marker can give very precise and valid estimates of exposure, investigators may find that the lack of precise ambient exposure measurements makes this ability difficult to demonstrate in human populations alone. Therefore, the combination of in vitro, animal, and human data will give the best picture of a marker's performance.

SUMMARY

The diverse assortment of biological markers can be roughly classified into three groups: measurements of chemicals (or their metabolites) that enter the body; measurements of endogenously produced molecules; and measurements of molecular or cellular changes. Although some markers are conceptually simple, their measurement can be complex. The biological nature of markers largely determines their properties, and these properties determine the usefulness of markers in epidemiologic studies.

With regard to metabolic characteristics, exposure markers differ substantially from markers of susceptibility or disease. The kinetics of exposure agents have a major influence on the properties of exposure markers. Important marker properties related to exposure kinetics include time to appearance of the marker after exposure begins, persistence of the marker after exposure ends, and sites within the body where the marker response occurs.

Markers differ dramatically in their ability to detect low-dose exposures and to measure specific exposures in multiexposure environments. Because markers vary substantially in their quantitative and qualitative relationships with ambient exposure levels, comparisons of exposure sensitivity and specificity among markers can be difficult. Lack of consistency in the use of terms across scientific disciplines compounds the problem. Quantitative comparisons among markers, however, are possible if sufficient data exist. The quantification of variability in marker responses within individuals is especially important, because large intraindividual variability compared with the variability between exposure groups leads to a high degree of exposure misclassification.

Numerous exposures can influence the response of a marker to other exposures. Simultaneous chemical exposures, diet, and various personal characteristics can alter the degree of a marker response to a given ambient exposure. A careful study design will remove the effects of many extraneous variables.

Because a single exposure can have many different physiologic effects, marker responses to an exposure can often be measured in a variety of different tissues. In some instances, the site of measurement may also be the site where the exposure causes pathologic changes. Sometimes the marker responses in tissues distant from the site of pathogenesis are highly correlated with the pathologic changes. Because of statistical relationships between marker responses in target and nontarget tissues, markers in accessible materials like blood may be good indicators of dose or response in less accessible tissues.

Even if a marker has desirable properties, it has little or no epidemiologic value until its properties have been demonstrated and quantified in humans. Epidemiologists must sometimes choose between well-characterized markers and newer markers that show promise based on preliminary data. The synthesis of results from in vitro studies, animal studies, and human studies helps with this choice. With careful consideration of all available information, epidemiologists can select the markers that best meet their needs.

REFERENCES

Aitio A: Kinetic considerations in monitoring exposure to chemicals. In: Berlin A, Draper M, Hemminki K, Vainio H, eds.: *Monitoring Human Exposure to Carcinogenic and Mutagenic Agents.* Lyon, IARC Scientific Publ No. 59, 1984, pp. 127–133.

Ames BN: Dietary carcinogens and anticarcinogens: Oxygen radicals and degenerative diseases. *Science* 1983;221:1256–1264.

Angerer J: Biological monitoring of workers exposed to organic solvents: Past and present. *Scand J Work Environ Health* 1985;11(Suppl 1):45–52.

Brown HS, Bishop DR, Rowan CA: The role of skin absorption as a route of exposure for volatile organic compounds (VOCs) in drinking water. *Am J Public Health* 1984;74:479–484.

Calabrese EJ: Comparative biology of test species. *Environ Health Perspect* 1988;77:55–62.

Carrano AV: Chromosomal alterations as markers of exposure and effect. *J Occup Med* 1986;28:1112–1116.

Droz PO, Guillemin MP: Occupational exposure monitoring using breath analysis. *J Occup Med* 1986;28:593–602.

Duncan BB, Heiss G: Nonenzymatic glycosylation of proteins: A new tool for assessment of cumulative hyperglycemia in epidemiologic studies, past and future. *Am J Epidemiol* 1984;120:169–189.

Einhorn N, Eklund G, Franzen S, Lambert B, Lindsten J, Söderhäll S: Late side effects of chemotherapy in ovarian carcinoma: A cytogenetic, hematologic, and statistical study. *Cancer* 1982;49:2234–2241.

Elinder CG, Vesterberg O: Environmental and biological monitoring. *Scand J Work Environ Health* 1985;11(Suppl 1):91–103.

Friberg LT: The rationale of biological monitoring of chemicals with special reference to metals. *Am Ind Hyg Assoc J* 1985;46:633–642.

Galen RS: Selection of appropriate laboratory tests. In: Young DS, ed.: *Clinician and Chemist: The Relationship of the Laboratory to the Physician*. Washington, D.C., Am Assoc Clin Chem, 1977, pp. 69–105.

Hoffmann D, Haley NJ, Adams JD, Brunnemann KD: Tobacco sidestream smoke: Uptake by nonsmokers. *Prev Med* 1984;13:608–617.

Hopps HC: The biologic bases for using hair and nail for analyses of trace elements. *Sci Total Environ* 1977;7:71–89.

Jaeger MJ: Chapter 3, Toxic effects of SO_2 on the respiratory system. In: McGrath JJ, Barnes CD, eds.: *Air Pollution—Physiological Effects*. New York, Academic Press, 1982, pp. 81–105.

Kateman G, Pijpers FW: *Quality Control in Analytical Chemistry*. New York, John Wiley and Sons, 1981.

Latt SA, Allen J, Bloom SE, Carrano A, Falke E, Kram DK, Schneider E, Schreck R, Tice R, Whitfield B, Wolff S: Sister-chromatid exchanges: A report of the gen-tox program. *Mutat Res* 1981;87:17–62.

Lohman PHM, Jansen JD, Baan RA: Comparison of various methodologies with respect to sensitivity and specificity in biomonitoring occupational exposure to mutagens and carcinogens. In: Berlin K, Vainio H, Draper M, eds.: *Monitoring Human Exposure to Carcinogenic and Mutagenic Agents*. Lyon, IARC, 1985, pp. 259–277.

Mayewski RJ, Mushlin AI, Griner PF: Chapter 1, Principles of test selection and use. In: Griner PF, Panzer RJ, Greenland P, eds.: *Clinical Diagnosis and the Laboratory*. Chicago, Year Book Medical Publishers, 1986, pp. 1–16.

Musilová J, Micholová K, Urban J: Sister chromatid exchanges and chromosome breakage in patients treated with cytostatics. *Mutat Res* 1979;67:289–294.

National Institute of Environmental Health Sciences: *Human Health and the Environment - Some Research Needs*. Report of the Third Task Force for Research Planning in Environmental Health Science. U.S. Government Printing Office, 1986, Washington, D.C.

National Toxicology Program Board of Scientific Counselors: Report of the NTP Ad Hoc Panel on Chemical Carcinogenesis Testing and Evaluation. *NTP Board of Scientific Counselors* 1984; Aug 17:1–106.

Perera FP, Santella SM, Brenner D, Poirier MC, Munshi AA, Fischman HK, Ryzin JV: DNA adducts, protein adducts, and sister chromatid exchange in cigarette smokers and nonsmokers. *JNCI* 1987;79:449–456.

Raloff J: Embedded sentinels of toxicity. *Sci News* 1987;131:123–125.

Rode A, Ross R, Shepard RJ: Smoking withdrawal programme. *Arch Environ Health* 1972;24:27–36.

Rogan WJ, Bagniewska A, Damstra T: Pollutants in breast milk. *N Engl J Med* 1980;302:1450–1453.

Schulte PA: Methodologic issues in the use of biologic markers in epidemiologic research. *Am J Epidemiol* 1987;126:1006–1016.

Smith LC, Voyta JC, Kinnunen PKJ, Gotto AM, Sparrow JT: Chapter 36, Triglyceride metabolism by lipoprotein lipase. In: Perkins EG, Visek WT, eds.: *Dietary Fats and Health*. Champaign, Ill, American Oil Chemist's Society, 1983, pp. 598–611.

Takagi Y, Matsuda S, Imai S, Ohmori Y, Masuda T, Vinson JA, et al.: Trace elements in human hair: An international comparison. *Bull Environ Contam Toxicol* 1986;38:793–800.

Tannenbaum SR, Skipper PL, Green LC, Obiedzinski MW, Kadlubar F: Blood protein adducts as a monitors of exposure to 4-aminobiophenyl. *Proc Am Assoc Cancer Res* 1983;24:69.

Tannenbaum SR: Direct measurements on chemicals and their effects on humans. Presented at the Symposium on Basic Research in Risk Assessment. National Institute of Environmental Health Sciences, Research Triangle Park, NC, March 9–12, 1987.

Vainio H, Sorsa M, Rantanen J, Hemminki K, Aitio A: Biological monitoring in the identification of the cancer risk of individuals exposed to chemical carcinogens. *Scand J Work Environ Health* 1981;7:241–251.

Vainio H: Current trends in the biological monitoring of exposure to carcinogens. *Scand J Work Environ Health* 1985;11:1–6.

van Staveren WA, Deurenberg P, Katan MB, Burema J, de Grott LCPGM, Hoffmans MDAF: Validity of the fatty acid composition of subcutaneous fat tissue microbiopsies as an estimate of the long-term average fatty acid composition of the diet of separate individuals. *Am J Epidemiol* 1986;123:455–463.

Willett WC, Morris SJ, Pressel S, Taylor JO, Polk BF, Stampfer MJ, et al.: Prediagnostic serum selenium and risk of cancer. *Lancet* 1983:130–134.

Willett W: Nutritional epidemiology: issues and challenges. *Int J Epidemiol* 1987;16:312–317.

4

URINE MUTAGENICITY ASSAYS

SUSAN M. RYNARD

INTRODUCTION

Chemical mutagens can be defined as agents capable of causing heritable changes in genetic material (Sorsa et al., 1982). Various bacterial mutagenesis techniques can be used to analyze urine, feces, and breast fluid for such mutagenic chemicals. For over 15 years the presence of mutagens in human body fluids has been used as an indicator of systemic exposure to a wide range of mutagenic chemicals. Because mutagenesis testing reveals the presence of many types of mutagens in the analyzed sample, the procedure is especially useful in detecting multiple or unspecified mutagenic agents. Currently, the urine mutagenesis assay is one of the most widely used techniques to monitor populations for mutagenic exposures.

As a sample body fluid, urine has several advantages. It is a major route of elimination for xenobiotics. Urinary material consists of substances already concentrated by the kidneys (Eisenstadt, 1983). Urine is an easy body fluid to collect, and its long-term storage is somewhat simpler than that of blood, feces, or breast milk or fluid. Accordingly, the vast majority of human studies in mutagenesis have been conducted on urine specimens. The outstanding disadvantage in using urine as a specimen for mutagenic testing is the relatively short cycle of urine production and excretion. Because urine is manufactured continually and expelled every few hours, it is unsuitable as an indicator of long-term or cumulative exposures. An additional problem is the possibility that certain mutagens may be underrepresented in urine.

BIOLOGICAL BASIS OF URINE MUTAGENESIS TESTING

The principal methods of testing urine for mutagenicity are the Ames test and a derivative method, the fluctuation test. The biological basis of both tests is the ability of a test solution to induce specific mutations in selected bacteria. The mutations may be either *base-pair* or *frameshift* mutations (McCann, 1983). In base-pair mutations, one nucleotide base in a matched pair within a DNA strand is replaced by another base. If this substitution occurs at a critical location in the gene, the resulting protein product is dysfunctional (Fig. 4-1). In a frameshift mutation, a nucleotide is either added or deleted in a sequence of base pairs. As a result, the reading frame shifts for every point after the alteration (Fig. 4-2). Again, the result can be the inability to function in producing a critical product (McCann, 1983).

In the early 1970s, Ames and his colleagues developed numerous strains of *Salmonella typhimurium,* each designed to exhibit specific mutations that can be mutated back to a normal state ("reverted") by a wide variety of mutagens. Several strains, each with its own unique mutations and suitable for detecting particular mutagens, were designated as the *tester strains* of the mutagenesis assay.

The enabling mechanism of the Ames test for mutagenicity is the dependence of *Salmonella* on the amino acid histidine. Tester strains are genetically engineered mutants unable to produce this essential substance. When incubated on agar plates enriched with histidine, the bacteria will grow until the histidine in the media is exhausted. If a mutagen is mixed with the bacteria before incubation, those bacteria reverted by the mutagen will be able to produce histidine for themselves, and thus continue growing after the added histidine is gone. The presence of the mutagen can then be detected by the *Salmonella* colonies that develop (Ames et al., 1975). The assay's ability to quantitate mutagenicity varies widely, depending on the compound tested; some investigators report only qualitative results obtained with the Ames method (Tennant et al., 1987). The fluctuation test for mutagenicity is based on the same principle, but uses an additional organism, *Escherichia coli,* which has been altered to be deficient in its ability to produce tryptophan (Sorsa et al., 1981). The fluctuation test also employs test tubes or wells rather than plates as containers. Table 4-1 summarizes methods of performing both tests, which are more fully discussed later.

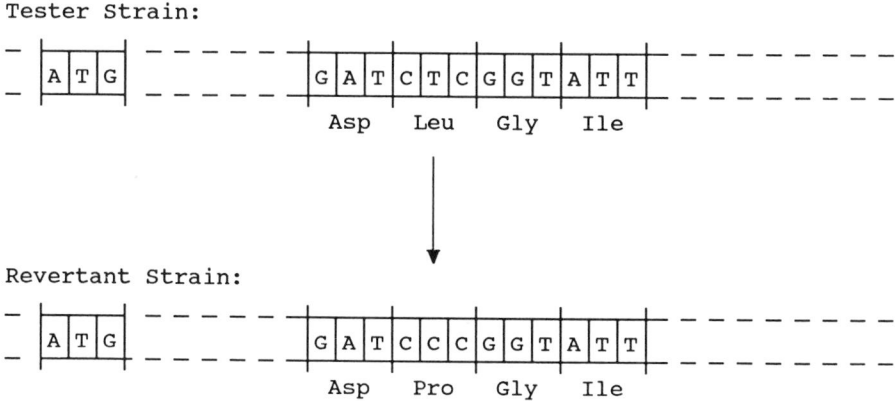

Tester Strain:

Asp Leu Gly Ile

Revertant Strain:

Asp Pro Gly Ile

Figure 4-1. Base-pair mutation. (after McCann, 1983)

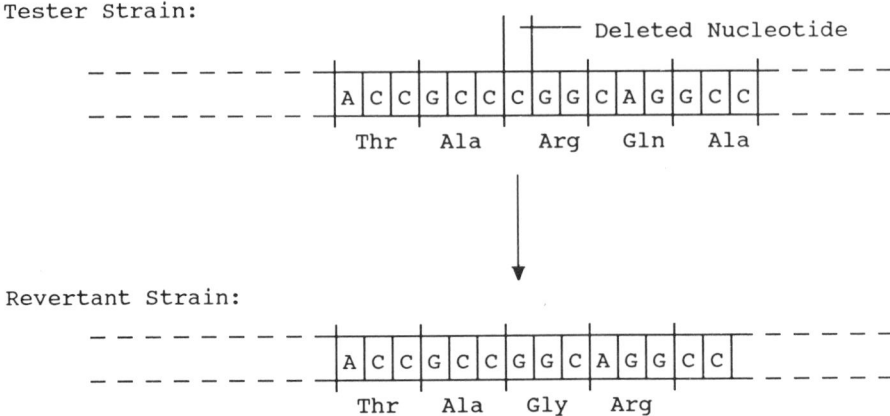

Figure 4-2. Frameshift mutation. (after McCann, 1983)

ISSUES IN SPECIMEN COLLECTION AND PREPARATION

Methods of sample collection and preparation vary slightly among investigators. Understanding of some key points in specimen preparation, however, is crucial to the valid interpretation of study results. The major issues are sample concentration, choice of elution fluid, and enzymatic sample activation.

Sample Concentration

Sample concentration is a technique employed to reduce total volume while retaining all mutagens present in the specimen. Concentration is desirable because the small

Table 4-1 Specimen Preparation and Testing Protocols

A. Collect random or timed urine specimen. Preserve chemically or by refrigeration
B. Activate specimen with S-9 liver extract and/or β-glucuronidase. Incubate overnight at 37°C
C. Concentrate specimen
   1. Pass through XAD-2 resin column
   2. Wash column
      a. with distilled water
      b. with solvent (e.g., acetone)
   3. Evaporate eluate
   4. Resuspend dried residue with solvent [e.g., dimethylsulfoxide (DMSO)]

Ames Method
A. Mix sample concentrate with *Salmonella* tester strains and histidine
B. Plate onto solid agar
C. Incubate 48 hrs at 37°C
D. Score by subtracting number of colonies on control plates from number of colonies on test plates

Fluctuation Method
A. Dispense fluid medium into about 50 test tubes/sample wells
B. Inoculate with tester organisms
C. Add sample concentrate to half of tubes
D. Incubate 72–96 hours at 37°C
E. Read turbidity by comparison with standard
F. Compare difference between controls and samples with Chi-square or *t*-test

volumes of liquid mixed with the test organisms may not contain sufficient amounts of mutagen if they are unconcentrated. Up to several hundred milliliters of urine are slowly poured through a column containing XAD-2 resin, which selectively adsorbs nonpolar molecules from the sample (Eisenstadt et al., 1983). The column is rinsed with distilled water and refilled in a wash step (eluted) with a solvent that is then evaporated. The resulting dried specimen concentrate is resuspended, usually with dimethylsulfoxide (DMSO). This elution product, containing the mutagen "collected" by the XAD-2 column, is then used to perform the mutagenesis assay. Although most studies employ this technique, some use unconcentrated urine.

Elution Techniques

An important question in sample concentration is the choice of solvent used to extract bound molecules from the concentration column. An inappropriate extraction procedure could underrepresent the amount of mutagen present in a specimen, or even result in no mutagenic material being recovered from the column. Ames recommended that the solvent used be suitable for the suspected mutagens (McCann and Ames, 1975). For general screening, like that done in most studies using human urine, he suggested an extraction procedure applicable to a wide variety of metabolites. The most common choice is a solvent, such as acetone or methylene chloride, with resuspension of the dried extract in DMSO (Eisenstadt et al., 1983; Maron et al., 1981).

Activation/Deconjugation

Activation of the urine sample with enzymes and microsomal liver preparations is a recommended specimen preparation technique (McCann, 1983). This step is based on the fact that many chemicals are not themselves mutagenic, but are transformed into mutagenic forms through hepatic activity (McCann, 1983). Activating the specimen by adding a microsomal extract of rat or human liver (known as S-9 extract) allows the transformation of promutagens into mutagenic forms in vitro. It should be noted that S-9 activation is not the exact equivalent of metabolization by the target organ, but rather is an in vitro surrogate.

Similarly, some conjugated metabolites—molecules that have been bound with other substances by the liver to aid in eliminating them from the system—are nonmutagenic when excreted in urine, but were mutagens in vivo. Adding enzymes, such as β-glucuronidase, to the urine sample deconjugates these substances and permits detection of their mutagenic nature in the body (Falck, 1982). Everson (1986) notes, however, that a potential problem in activating specimens is that mutagenicity may be wrongly attributed to biologically inactive substances that have been activated only in vitro.

Additional Considerations

Exposures of interest in studies using urine mutagenesis testing include cigarette smoking, dietary items, therapeutic drugs, and occupational exposures. There is some evidence that the time of day may be a factor in the mutagenicity of casual urine samples collected from tobacco smokers: in two studies, the mutagenicity of samples collected in the evening was greater than that of samples taken the following morning (Yamasaki and Ames, 1977; van Doorn et al., 1979). Because mutagenicity seems to be a short-lived phenomenon, and because presumed peak values may be of as much interest as average values over time, single urine samples are employed at least as often as timed 24-hour specimens. In occupational exposure monitoring, a major use of urine mutagenicity testing, 24-hour urine collection is extremely impractical (Aitio and Järvisalo, 1985) and is seldom used. Some studies attempt to correct for the low mutagenic potential of extremely dilute urines by adjusting sample volumes so that they are equivalent to a stated concentration of creatinine, an excreted substance commonly used as a measure of renal function. Using differing volumes of urine sample and reporting results per millimole of creatinine minimizes the effect of differences in the renal function of each individual.

The final factor to be considered in specimen collection and preparation is endogenous urine histidine. Certain people, such as those on high protein diets, may excrete histidine, which increases the overall bacterial growth on the test plates and possibly increases the rate of spontaneous reversion. When the sample is concentrated by column extraction, there is evidence that the distilled water wash step greatly reduces retention of urine histidine (Yamasaki and Ames, 1977; Recio et al., 1982). Alternatively, techniques are being developed to quantitate the amount of background growth, which identifies urines containing endogenous histidine (Everson, 1986).

AMES TEST PROCEDURE

The urine sample is centrifuged or filtered to remove particulates. When indicated, enzymatic deconjugation of the sample is performed by 37°C incubation overnight with β-glucuronidase. The specimen is then extracted by the XAD-2 elution column and solvent-extraction procedure described previously. This step also sterilizes the specimen, preventing growth of unwanted organisms that might be present in the urine.

Tester strains of *Salmonella typhimurium* are mixed with the specimen and with media containing enough histidine to permit a few generations of growth. Most of the literature is based on tests of five *Salmonella* strains: TA100 and TA1535 (base-pair mutations), and TA1538, TA98, and TA1537 (frameshift mutations). Currently, the recommended strains for general screening are TA97 (replacing TA1537), TA98 (replacing TA1538), TA100, and TA102 (Maron and Ames, 1983). Dr. Bruce Ames will supply these organisms on request.* It is important to understand that the different tester strains are specific for either base-pair or frameshift mutation; test organisms should be carefully selected to insure detection of the specific DNA damage that is suspected or should be employed in test panels designed to detect both mutation types.

The test plate is then incubated for 48 hours at 37°C. During incubation, those bacteria that revert to histidine production by specimen mutagens will establish colonies. Spontaneously reverted bacteria will also colonize the test plates. The test is scored by subtracting the number of spontaneously mutated colonies occurring on

---

*As of this writing, Dr. Ames' address is Department of Biochemistry, University of California, Berkeley CA 94720.

control plates from the total number of colonies on test plates (Ames et al., 1975; Maron and Ames, 1983; McCann, 1983; Everson, 1986).

Sensitivity and Specificity

In a survey of selected agents, Ames and colleagues estimated the sensitivity of the Ames test at 90 percent, specificity at 87 percent, and positive predictive value at 92 percent (McCann, 1983). These figures were based on tests with known carcinogens directly added to the tester strains. In another report of direct testing of carcinogens, Tennant et al. (1987) estimated sensitivity at 45 percent (95% C.I. 30-61), specificity at 86 percent (95% C.I. 68-96), positive predictive value at 83 percent (95% C.I. 63-95), and negative predictive value at 62 percent (95% C.I. 50-73). Estimates of sensitivity and specificity vary considerably, depending on the compounds being tested. In addition, sensitivity is probably increased and specificity decreased by the use of S-9 liver extract in the Ames test. Because compounds are unlikely to be metabolized to the same extent in human tissues, S-9 activation could result in a larger number of false-positive results when interpreted for humans.

Thus, substances identified as mutagens by the Ames method are likely to cause mutations in vivo, at least to the extent that S-9 activation reflects target tissue metabolization. Because the test is designed to detect only specific point mutations, however, a negative result may not indicate the absence of all mutagenic activity within a specimen. McCann (1983) lists several important carcinogens that have tested negative in the Ames mutagenesis assay: carbon tetrachloride, DDT, dieldrin, and other chlorinated hydrocarbons. Some of these agents have been detected as mutagens in different short-term assays, whereas others are believed to produce mutagenic metabolites with half-lives too short to be identified by any current short-term methods. It should also be recalled that nonmutagenic agents may be involved in carcinogenesis, as is the case with asbestos. This mineral fiber is thought to cause cancer through its physical properties as an irritant. Another example is diethylstilbestrol (DES), which most likely promotes carcinogenesis in already initiated cells. Failure to detect entire classes of potentially mutagenic or carcinogenic compounds is a significant disadvantage of the Ames procedure.

Interindividual and Intraindividual Variability

One factor that greatly influences variability in the Ames test is the metabolic capability of study subjects. One can expect to find both interindividual and intraindividual variability unrelated to exposures of interest, based on short-term or long-term fluctuations in hepatic and renal function. For a general discussion of variability, see "Human variability" and "Determinants of variability" in Chapter 3.

FLUCTUATION TEST PROCEDURE

The fluctuation test is based on the same biological principle as the Ames test: reversion of mutated bacteria. The most commonly used organism in this procedure is *E.*

coli, and tryptophan is the product of the gene that reverts back to its normal state. Some investigators also employ Ames' *Salmonella* strains as test organisms in this procedure.

Sample collection and preparation is a modified version of the Ames protocol. A fluid medium containing tryptophan is dispensed into about 50 test tubes or wells, which are then inoculated with the tester strains of *E. coli*. Current recommended strains are WP2 uvrA, and CM561 exrA (Green et al., 1976). The concentrated urine specimen is then added to half the tubes. After 37°C incubation for 72–96 hours, reverted bacteria will have grown to a sufficient volume to produce a qualitatively assessed level of turbidity (positive versus negative) in the tubes compared to a standard. The difference in the number of positive control tubes and test tubes is evaluated by a Chi-square or Student's *t*-test (Green et al., 1976; Collings et al., 1981; Falck, 1983).

An automated method for this assay has recently been developed (Falck et al., 1985). A major advantage, apart from labor savings, is the ability to monitor the kinetic activity of sample wells. By detecting the shape of the growth curve, one can gain more information about the mutagens present in the sample; one can also detect toxicities that prevent the tester strains from surviving.

OTHER URINE MUTAGENESIS TESTS

Two other procedures occasionally are used to analyze the mutagenicity of urine: sister chromatid exchange (SCE), presented in Chapter 6, and a forward-mutation assay that measures mutations in the hypoxanthine-guanine phosphoribosyl transferase (HGPRT) genetic locus of mammalian tester cells. In the sister chromatid exchange method, urine is used as the test substance in an attempt to induce mutations within human lymphocyte cell lines. With the HGPRT assay, mammalian cells are mixed with urine and scanned for mutations that permit cell survival under test conditions. Details of the method are beyond the scope of this chapter.

STUDIES OF URINE MUTAGENICITY IN HUMANS

The investigation of urine mutagenicity in humans has been conducted in three major categories: life-style exposures, such as tobacco smoking and dietary factors; exposures resulting from disease or medical therapy; and occupational exposures. Few of these studies were designed as epidemiologic research. Many early investigations were planned to test modifications of the method, and others reflect the genetic and toxicologic interests of their authors. In general, sample sizes are very small, often because the study involved some experimental exposure. Possible systematic biases are rarely if ever addressed, and potential confounders (apart from smoking) are only occasionally taken into account in design or data analysis. Tables 4-2 through 4-5 summarize the urine mutagenesis studies.

Tobacco Smoking and Urine Mutagens

Cigarette smoking is the most widely reported life-style exposure that produces mutagenic urine. Because of smoking's known carcinogenicity, smokers have often been chosen as subjects in tests of methodologic refinements. Table 4-2 summarizes results of the tobacco smoke studies.

In a test of specimen extraction procedures, Yamasaki and Ames (1977) assayed urine samples from 10 cigarette smokers (including three who did not inhale) whose tobacco consumption ranged from 15–44 cigarettes per day, along with urine samples from 21 nonsmokers. All participants denied taking medications and consumed "normal diets." Morning and evening specimens were collected and frozen until analysis, when the samples were concentrated using XAD-2 resin columns eluted with acetone and resuspended with DMSO. Samples were activated with S-9 liver homogenate extract and β-glucuronidase.

Smokers' urines showed significant mutagenicity to *Salmonella* strain TA1538 (up to 700 revertant colonies/25 ml urine), whereas nonsmokers produced no mutagenic specimens. A background of up to 50 revertant colonies/25 ml urine was considered negative. Some of the lowest mutagenic responses were shown by the noninhaling smokers and two low-tar brand smokers. Pooled specimens from one smoker were concentrated twice and showed a higher level of mutagenicity as more urine was added to the test plates. For nonsmokers and noninhalers, morning and evening mutagenicity were essentially the same, whereas the samples of inhaling smokers were always mutagenic in the evening and less or nonmutagenic the following morning.

In an 8-week long study, Jaffe et al. (1983) collected urine samples each week from 13 smokers and five nonsmoking controls. They did not monitor diet and medications or give specimen collection times. Specimens from the five nonsmokers showed no mutagenic activity. Specimens from smokers, however, demonstrated a 10-fold range in values, from 0.14–1.4 revertants/μmole creatinine. Although there was a positive association overall between tobacco consumption and mutagen excretion, no dose-response could be observed on the basis of either the tar content of the cigarettes or the number of cigarettes smoked.

Table 4-2 Mutagenicity Studies of Exposure to Tobacco

Reference	Sample preparation	Sample activated with	Tester strains	N	Reported results
Yamasaki & Ames	XAD-2/acetone/DMSO	S-9/β-glucuronidase	TA1538	31	+
Jaffe et al.	XAD-2/acetone/DMSO	S-9	TA98	18	+
Van Doorn et al.	XAD-2/acetone/DMSO	S-9	TA1538	20	+
Mohtashamipur et al.	XAD-2/methanol/DMSO	S-9	TA98	12	+
Recio et al.	XAD-2/acetone/DMSO	S-9	TA98	35	+
Falck et al.[a]	XAD-2		TA98/WP UVRA	39	+
Bos et al.	XAD-2/acetone/DMSO	S-9	TA1538	18	+
Aeschbacher & Chappuis	XAD-2/acetone/DMSO	S-9/β-glucuronidase	TA98/TA100	27	+

[a]Fluctuation method.

Van Doorn et al. (1979) studied mutagenicity in five nonsmokers and 15 smokers, all of whom were men taking no medications and on normal diets. Smokers were evenly divided into three groups: those who smoked 1–10, 11–20, or more than 20 cigarettes/day. Smokers of less than 10 cigarettes/day showed no significant difference from the five nonsmokers in urine mutagenicity, approximately 0.3–0.4×10^6 reverted bacteria/mmol creatinine. Urine mutagenicity in those who smoked 11–20 cigarettes was significantly different from that of nonsmokers ($p < .05$), roughly 2.5×10^6 bacteria/mmol creatinine. Samples from those who smoked over 20 cigarettes/day were significantly more mutagenic than samples from those who smoked 11–20 cigarettes ($p < .01$), about 3.5×10^6 bacteria/mmol creatinine. Similar gradients were reported for concentrations of urinary thioethers, such as mercapturic acids, which are nontoxic and nonmutagenic by-products of potentially carcinogenic alkylating substances present in cigarettes.

A threshold effect was also reported by Mohtashamipur et al. (1985). In this study, designed to test the effectiveness of three sample concentration methods, 12 subjects of both sexes were divided into "nonsmoking" and smoking groups (but nonsmoking is defined here as 1–5 cigarettes/day). Using a XAD-2/methanol/DMSO concentration protocol with S-9 activation and *Salmonella* TA98, the investigators found no mutagenicity in the urine samples of the "nonsmoking" group. Smokers produced mutagenic urine (up to 60 mean revertants/plate), but the investigators could make no correlation between the number of cigarettes smoked and amount of mutagenicity.

Recio et al. (1982) collected evening urines from 16 nonsmokers and 19 smokers who smoked an average of one pack per day. Samples were plated at three concentrations per subject: 40, 60, and 80 μL of concentrate (corresponding to 10, 15, and 20 ml of urine). Again, no significant mutagenicity was found among nonsmokers. A large variation in mutagenicity was reported for smokers, ranging from 31–162 revertants/plate (mean 80 revertants/plate). Although two low-tar brand smokers and a pipe smoker scored some of the lowest mutagenic values, Recio could find no relationship overall between number of cigarettes (self-reported by subjects) or amount of tar and urine mutagenicity. Recio also presents results of a series of assays on a single smoker who increased his cigarette consumption over 8 successive days. The result is a fairly linear dose-response between number of cigarettes and level of urine mutagenicity.

In a study of the fluctuation test, Falck (1982) examined three groups of Finnish military recruits. Group A consisted of 13 men who smoked medium-tar cigarettes; group B had 14 low-tar smokers, and group C comprised 12 nonsmokers. Because all subjects were recent service inductees and were living on-post, they were comparable in age, general health, and extraneous exposures encountered during the study period. Cigarettes were supplied daily to each subject, and consumption was comparable between the two smoking groups. Evening urine specimens were collected at the end of the first, fourth, and seventh weeks, and were then concentrated in XAD-2 resin columns. Each specimen was split into parts, half of which were S-9 activated and half which were not. The samples were then dispensed into test tubes containing suspensions of either *Salmonella* TA98 or *E. coli* WP2 uvrA. Only activated samples of smokers' urine showed mutagenic activity in the *Salmonella* mixture (creatinine-adjusted means of 17.7 ± 6.0 for group A, 17.3 ± 5.9 for group B, and 6.5 ± 4.1 for group C, $p < .001$ for both groups A and B when compared with group C). No correlation could be found between urinary mutagens and the amount of tar per cigarette.

In a study of passive smoking, Bos et al. (1983) enclosed eight nonsmokers in a poorly ventilated room for 6 hours with 10 heavy smokers. The subjects voided just before the start of the experiment and collected all urine for the succeeding 12 hours. Twelve-hour samples were also collected the day before and the day after the exposure. In addition, Bos and colleagues sampled the room air the day before, the day after, and during the test by bubbling about 500 L of air through cylinders of chilled hexane. The air samples were then evaporated to dryness, and resuspended in DMSO. Both air and urine samples were plated with *Salmonella* TA1538. The study showed statistically significant differences between values for urine from nonexposed and exposed nonsmokers (mean colony number of 2.8 and 3.7, $p < .02$). The increase in nonsmokers' urine mutagenicity was judged to be about 4 percent of the urine mutagenicity of the active smokers in the experiment. Mutation assays of room air produced values up to 10 times higher for smoky samples than for samples taken when the room was empty.

Aeschbacher and Chappuis (1981) compared the urine mutagenicity of cigarette smokers and coffee drinkers in two experiments. In the first, they divided 15 subjects into three groups: two nonsmoking groups (six persons each), one of which drank instant coffee, and a group of three who both smoked and drank coffee. The experiment lasted 4 days, during which all subjects followed a standard diet, drank coffee as assigned (12 g instant coffee per day), and smoked as usual (20–30 cigarettes per day). All urine was collected during this period, with acetic acid preservation and refrigeration of each subject's pooled specimens. Half of each pooled urine was deconjugated with β-glucuronidase, then both conjugated and deconjugated aliquots were concentrated and activated. The investigators found a dose-response relationship between the amount of smokers' urine concentrate plated and the number of revertants, ranging from 137 colonies/plate for a DMSO control to 315 colonies/plate with 100 μL of sample concentrate. There was no mutagenicity found in the urine of nonsmokers, regardless of coffee consumption.

In the second experiment, 12 nonsmokers and 6 smokers were given 1 L of water to drink, and their urines were collected and preserved. A week later the subjects ate a standard breakfast and drank 1 L of coffee, then fasted for 7 hours. Smokers consumed cigarettes as desired (ranging from 7 to 18). All urine was collected with preservative. As in the first experiment, all nonsmokers' urines were negative. There was only a slight increase in the urine mutagenicity of the smokers after they drank coffee rather than water; 68 ± 11 colonies/plate compared with 54 ± 7 colonies/plate at 200 μL of sample concentrate. In both experiments, the deconjugation step reduced the number of revertant colonies detected, perhaps because the high sample volumes resulted in concentrates with bacteriocidal potency.

Diet and Mutagenicity

Several studies, summarized in Table 4-3, have examined the urine mutagenicity of foods and food preparation methods. Baker et al. (1982) conducted two series of experiments with five subjects. In the first, the participants fasted for 24 hours and were allowed only nonalcoholic liquids, including coffee, milk, soft drinks, and juices.

Table 4-3 Mutagenicity Studies of Dietary Exposures

Reference	Exposure	Sample preparation	Sample activated with	Tester strains	N	Reported results
Baker et al.	Fried pork	XAD-2/acetone/ DMSO	S-9/β-glucuronidase	TA98/TA100/TA1535/ TA1537/TA1538	5	+
Dolara et al.	Fried pork	XAD-2/acetone/ DMSO	S-9	TA1538	8	+
Sousa et al.	Fried ground beef	XAD-2/acetone/ DMSO	S-9/β-glucuronidase	TA98/TA100	4	+
Sousa et al.	Red wine/ grape juice	XAD-2/acetone/ DMSO	S-9/β-glucuronidase	TA98/TA100	5	−

They then consumed a morning meal of either fried or microwaved pork or bacon, followed by another 24-hour liquid diet. All urine for the entire 48-hour period was collected as individual samples and frozen. In the second test, subjects ate a light lacto-ovo-vegetarian meal the preceding evening, then breakfasted on bacon. Urines were collected before breakfast and for 4 hours after.

Neither study detected any increase in urine mutagenicity in samples taken after microwave-prepared meals. The first test, a 48-hour experiment, showed that most mutagenicity was detected in the first 2–4 hours after ingestion of the fried foods, although activity continued for up to 24 hours. For both experiments, the mutagenicity of the subjects' urine was about 30 percent that of the mutagenicity detected in assays of the fried foods themselves.

Dolara et al. (1984) modified the Baker fasting protocol by adding two experimental groups: one group followed a lacto-ovo-vegetarian diet for 1 day before eating the test meal; the other group was permitted food during the urine collection period after the test meal. Dolara found a slight to moderate increase in mutagenic activity after the test meal in all of the test groups. The recovered urine mutagens accounted for only about 0.6 percent of the ingested dose, according to assays of food samples. Dolara notes that differences in the degree of char on the meat surfaces could help explain the variation between his results and Baker's.

Results similar to Baker's were reported for the ingestion of fried beef by Sousa et al. (1985,B). In addition, Sousa tested the mutagenicity of red wine and grape juice consumed by five nonsmoking subjects (Sousa et al., 1985,A). He detected no urine mutagenesis in *Salmonella* TA98 or TA100, with or without S-9 activation. Deconjugation with β-glucuronidase also produced no activity. In contrast, extracts of the beverages themselves showed mutagenicity. Concentrated urines spiked with beverage concentrates were also mutagenic.

Liver Disease and Urine Mutagens

In mammals, metabolic transformation of xenobiotics is a major protective role of the liver. Substances absorbed into the bloodstream are enzymatically converted to forms that improve biological availability or facilitate elimination. During this process, potentially mutagenic agents may be activated or frank mutagens may be altered to inactive products. Thus, liver diseases, such as cirrhosis, may have important implications for the metabolism and excretion of mutagens.

There are two possible mechanisms by which liver dysfunction could influence mutagen metabolism. First, organ damage disrupts the production of enzymes needed to degrade mutagenic agents in the system. In addition, severe liver damage may lead to portal-vein shunting, a condition in which some of the portal vein blood is put into the systemic circulation without being processed by the hepatic system. Both situations thus result in potentially prolonged systemic contact with mutagenic agents. Table 4-4 summarizes studies of mutagenicity in liver disease.

Conflicting reports of urine mutagenicity in cirrhosis have been published by Gelbart and Sontag (1980) and Everson et al. (1983). Gelbart and Sontag concentrated 12-hour urines from five nonsmoking cirrhotic patients and compared them with urine concentrates from 12 healthy smokers and 15 healthy nonsmokers. They found 60-390 revertants/25 ml urine in the urine of the cirrhotics, 70-200 revertants/25 ml urine among smokers, and essentially negative results among nonsmokers. The authors note that three of the five patients had alcoholic cirrhosis with slight elevations in some liver enzymes. None of the patients was drinking at the time of the study, but all were in poor general health and poorly nourished.

In contrast, Everson et al. (1983) reported no increase in mutagens in the urines of 12 cirrhotics (including one smoker) or 9 patients with other liver disease (including three smokers). Five smokers (four apparently healthy and one with rheumatoid arthritis) were also analyzed. Each of the liver disease patients was taking numerous medications and exhibited some abnormal laboratory values. Twelve-hour urines were collected, concentrated, and tested with and without S-9 extract activation. Only the smokers showed an increase of mutagenicity, and no dose-response could be established based on amount of concentrate plated.

Exposures From Medical Therapy

Urine mutagenicity has been investigated in a number of medical therapeutics including: cancer chemotherapeutics, coal tar, metronidazole, niridazole, and praziquantel (Table 4-4). Minnich et al. (1976) assayed random urines from patients receiving cancer chemotherapeutic agents. Mutagenic activity was observed for 19 patients receiving cyclophosphamide and four on 5-fluorouracil, whereas no increase was reported for patients receiving melphalan or one person taking mitomycin C.

To evaluate the effect of coal tar and ultraviolet (UV) light, Wheeler et al. (1981) collected urines from 2 healthy nonsmoking volunteers and 12 nonsmoking and 2 smoking psoriasis patients being treated with UV light and coal tar. Of the 14 psoriatic patients, 12 displayed urine mutagenicity, ranging from 42-496 revertants/20 ml urine among nonsmokers to 213–1,100 revertants/20 ml urine for the two smokers. The volunteers, who received UV and coal tar treatments 1 week apart, also displayed urine mutagenicity levels of 16–493 revertants/20 ml urine.

Metronidazole and niridazole were found to be mutagenic by Legator et al. (1975). Six patients receiving metronidazole provided urine samples 1 hour after taking the drug each day for 10 days. Up to a 12-fold increase in mutation frequency over control plates resulted, with the most activity starting at about day 8. Speck et al. (1976) reported that paper chromatography of mutagenic urine from patients who received metronidazole yielded the unmodified drug and at least four of its known urinary metabolites. In the Legator study just mentioned, a urine sample of the single

Table 4-4 Mutagenicity Studies of Disease States/Therapeutic Exposures

Reference	Exposure	Sample preparation	Sample activated with	Tester strains	N	Reported results
Gelbart & Sontag	Cirrhosis	XAD-2/acetone/DMSO	S-9/β-glucuronidase	TA100	32	+
Everson et al.	Cirrhosis/other liver disease	XAD-2/acetone/DMSO	S-9	TA100/TA1538	26	−
Minnich et al.	Cytotoxic drugs	None	S-9/β-glucuronidase	TA1537	24	+/−
Wheeler et al.	Coal tar/UV light	XAD-2/acetone/DMSO	S-9	TA98	16	+
Legator et al.	Metronidazole/niridazole	Freeze-drying	S-9	TA1535/TA1538	7	+
Obermeier & Frohberg	Praziquantel	XAD-2/acetone/DMSO	S-9/β-glucuronidase	TA98/TA100	3	−

niridazole patient showed a 50-fold increase in mutagenicity on day 2 after treatment. Roxe et al. (1980) attribute the mutagenic effect of niridazole to the metabolic activation of the pigments excreted by patients receiving this drug.

The antihelminth praziquantel was investigated by Obermeier and Frohberg (1977). Three patients submitted five urines each, which were activated with S-9 extract and deconjugated with β-glucuronidase and arylsulfatase. No increase in urine mutagenicity could be detected in *Salmonella* TA98 and TA100.

Occupational Exposures

Many occupations have been examined for possible mutagenic exposures. Exposure to anticancer drugs among nurses and pharmacists is the focus of the largest number of studies. Other subjects of investigations include worker exposures in chemical manufacturing, the rubber industry, foundries, and exposure to iron oxide particles (Table 4-5).

Exposures Among Health-care Workers

Falck et al. (1979) used the fluctuation assay to examine urine mutagenicity among nurses handling cytostatic drugs. Urine samples from 7 nonsmoking nurses, 10 nonsmokers receiving chemotherapy, and 32 unexposed nonsmoking controls, were tested. Mutagenicity of patients was significantly higher than that of nurses, but the nurses' urines were significantly more mutagenic than those of controls (p < .001).

In a similar study design, Bos et al. (1982) collected 24-hour urines from 32 nurses or patient care personnel exposed to cytotoxic drugs and from 29 controls not in contact with patients. The study included both smokers and nonsmokers. In tests with *Salmonella* TA100, mutagenicity among exposed nonsmokers was not increased compared with nonsmoking controls. Among smokers, exposed subjects were significantly more mutagenic than controls, who smoked a similar amount.

In three more investigations of cytostatic drug exposure, Staiano et al. (1981), Nguyen et al. (1982), and Everson et al. (1985) reported opposite, although not necessarily conflicting, results. Neither Staiano nor Everson found an increase in urine mutagenicity in hospital pharmacists working with vertical laminar flow hoods that draw aerosols up, preventing worker contact. Nguyen et al., however, reported a doubling of mutagenicity in the urines of four of six pharmacists working with a horizontal laminar flow hood, which protects materials inside from bacterial contamination but directs aerosols toward the worker.

Manufacturing and Industrial Exposures

Among Italian factory workers exposed to petroleum coke and pitch, Pasquini et al. (1982) found increased urine mutagenesis during and after work hours, but not before work or on Sunday, a day off. Ten exposed male workers and 16 unexposed controls from the same plant provided urines on Monday and Friday mornings on arising, and on Monday and Friday at the end of work. Both exposed and unexposed groups contained smokers. With tester strain *Salmonella* TA98, exposed workers showed significantly more mutagenicity than controls in urine specimens collected during or after work. Before work, and for a 12-hour specimen collected on a Sunday, the two groups showed essentially no difference.

Table 4-5 Mutagenicity Studies of Occupational Exposures

Reference	Exposure	Sample preparation	Sample activated with	Tester strains	N	Reported results
Falck et al.[a]	Cytotoxic drugs	XAD-2/acetone/DMSO	S-9	TA98/WP2 UVRA	49	+
Bos et al.	Cytotoxic drugs	XAD-2/acetone/DMSO	S-9	TA100/TA1538	61	+/−
Staiano et al.	Cytotoxic drugs	XAD-2/acetone/DMSO	−	Not given	8	−
Nguyen et al.	Cytotoxic drugs	XAD-2/acetone/DMSO	−	TA98/TA100 TA1535/TA1538/TA1975	9	+
Everson	Cytotoxic drugs	XAD-2/acetone/DMSO	S-9	TA98/TA1538	26	−
Pasquini et al.	Petroleum coke/pitch	XAD-2/acetone/DMSO	S-9/β-glucuronidase	TA98	26	+
Kreibel et al.	Chemical plant/coke oven	XAD-2/methylene chloride-acetone/DMSO	S-9	TA100/TA1538	198	+
Dolara et al.	Chemical manufacturing	XAD-2/methylene chloride/DMSO	S-9	TA100/TA1538	70	+
Laires et al.	Mineral oils/iron oxide	XAD-2/acetone/DMSO	S-9/β-glucuronidase	TA98/TA100	33	+
Falck et al.[a]	Rubber industry	XAD-2/acetone/DMSO	S-9	TA98/WP2 UVRA	36	+
Ahlborg et al.[a]	Chemical	XAD-2	S-9	TA98/WP2 UVRA	109	+
Scarlett-Kranz et al.	Sewage treatment	XAD-2/DMSO	S-9	TA100	236	+

[a]Fluctuation method.

In chemical plant and coke oven workers, Kreibel et al. (1983) found increased revertants for smokers regardless of occupational exposure, as well as an increase in mutagenicity among exposed nonsmokers in one of four test configurations. They collected urine samples from 198 persons, including 101 chemical workers, 43 coke plant workers, and 54 controls. Fifty-one percent of the chemical workers, 65 percent of coke plant workers, and 20 percent of controls smoked. The authors characterize their results as showing "modestly but significantly higher" mutagenicity levels in the urines of both chemical workers and coke oven workers. They caution, however, that smoking was the main determinant of urine mutagenicity in the study.

Dolara et al. (1981) obtained 24-hour urines from 35 workers at two small chemical plants and selected a control group of 35 nonexposed subjects from the same age group. All participants were men, and some in each group smoked. Concentrated specimens were plated with *Salmonella* TA1538 and TA100 with and without S-9 activation. In TA1538 comparisons among nonsmokers, exposed workers were significantly different from controls only when the specimen concentrate was activated. Smokers of both exposed and nonexposed groups were not significantly different in either configuration of TA1538. With TA100, smokers and nonsmokers in the control group showed significant urine mutagenicity, but both classes of workers far exceeded controls in mutagenesis ($p < .01$).

Laires et al. (1982) conducted a study of exposure to mineral oils and iron oxide particles. They collected urine samples at the end of the working day from two groups of people: 17 workers exposed to both oils and iron oxide and 16 workers exposed to mineral oils only. Both study groups contained smokers. Mutagenicity was significantly higher in the workers exposed to both mineral oils and iron oxide ($p < .002$). Among nonsmokers in both study groups, the urinary mutagenicity of those exposed to iron oxide was significantly higher than the urinary mutagenicity of those exposed to mineral oils alone ($p < .04$).

Using the fluctuation test, Falck et al. (1980) asked 20 rubber industry workers (nine of whom smoked) and 16 factory office controls (including seven smokers) to provide specimens after working 4 days of a 5-day week. Mutagenesis with the *E. coli* WP2 uvrA tester strain was marked among exposed workers regardless of smoking status. Among exposed workers, the mean values were 727.1 and 501.1 revertants/mmol creatinine for smoking and nonsmoking workers, respectively, versus 13.2 and 34.7 revertants/mmol creatinine for smoking and nonsmoking controls, respectively. Results of *Salmonella* tests, however, implicated smoking over occupational exposure: smokers had mean values of 717.1 and 298.2 revertants/mmol creatinine for exposed and nonexposed workers, respectively, versus 149.8 and 25.1 for nonsmoking workers and controls, respectively. All results were statistically significant.

Ahlborg et al. (1985) examined workers in a plant producing a large variety of chemicals and explosives. Twelve areas of specific exposure were identified, each involving different employees. One hundred and nine workers completed questionnaires on smoking and alcohol use, diet, health, and medications. Each worker provided three urines: one after 4 weeks vacation, one before work, and one at the end of a work shift. Half of each concentrated sample was activated with S-9; *E. coli* WP2 uvrA and *Salmonella* TA98 were the tester strains employed in this fluctuation assay. When all subjects were considered together, mutagenicity was significantly increased for the occupationally exposed group using TA98 without S-9 activation, but no significant differences were observed for other test configurations. The increase is almost totally explained by a large rise in urine mutagenicity in workers handling trinitrotoluene (TNT). Examining each exposure separately showed that two groups had an increase in mutagenicity measured using activated TA98 (workers handling TNT and those handling hexaminetetranitrate), but the differences failed to reach statistical significance.

In a study of toxic wastes from industrial sewage, Scarlett-Kranz et al. (1986) compared 164 sewage treatment workers from 14 New York State plants with 72 water treatment workers. Each subject completed a questionnaire on smoking and drinking habits, length of employment, and position in the plant. Random urine samples were concentrated and plated with *Salmonella* TA100, both with and without S-9 activation. The frequency of urine mutagenicity was significantly higher among sewage workers than among water treatment workers, both with and without sample activation. Models using presence/absence of mutagens as the dependent variable were constructed (one each for activated and unactivated samples) to assess such possible confounders as smoking, alcohol use, or exposure to wood stove smoke at home. The activated sample model produced an adjusted odds ratio of 12.9 (95% C.I. 4.5–37.4) for employment in a sewage treatment plant. Smoking was not significant in the model; the authors theorize that the approximately equal percentage of smokers in each occupation or the time of specimen collection (end-of-shift, when presumably few opportunities to smoke had occurred during the day) minimized the effect of smoking in these data. In the model for unactivated samples, the adjusted odds ratio is 2.2 (95% C.I. 1.2–4.3) in favor of water treatment employment.

ISSUES IN THE INTERPRETATION OF URINE MUTAGEN STUDIES

Results of mutagenicity studies using the Ames or fluctuation tests can only be regarded as approximate, even apart from a consideration of study design issues. McCann (1983) discusses reasons for this, which are fundamental to the method. First, it must be remembered that the exact amount of mutagenicity shown by the sample cannot be determined, because the rates at which mutagenic constituents are converted into active forms by S-9 extract and the rates at which these metabolites decay are both unknown. Second, calculation of results should be based on the number of bacteria at risk for reversion. This number, however, is unavailable: only the number plated is known. Thus, a urine containing large amounts of a mutagen or other substances highly toxic to the tester strain may be scored incorrectly because the toxic urine killed a high proportion of tester organisms. The automated fluctuation procedure discussed earlier can monitor the kinetic activity of the test. A warning thus provided by abrupt shifts in the growth curves of tester strains may provide at least a partial solution to this problem.

Beyond methodologic problems, the basic relationship between in vivo mutagenesis and the presence of urine mutagens is not understood. Schulte (1987) notes that xenobiotic exposures result in a wide range of measurable biological responses. A consensus has yet to be reached on which of these responses reflect actual pathologic processes and which are adaptive. Until the presence of urinary mutagens can be more directly linked to specific disease, interpretation of positive mutagenicity tests must remain conservative. Presently, most investigators view positive tests only as indicators of exposure to possible mutagens.

Even given the limitations of the procedure, the inconsistency of findings in studies of urine mutagenicity are nonetheless striking. Positive studies vary considerably in their estimates of mutagenicity for similar exposures, and several exposures have been studied repeatedly with conflicting results. Everson (1986) advances five possible reasons for variation in mutagenicity results:

1. Heterogeneity in the nature and extent of exposure of different study populations to the agent or process being studied.
2. Variable exposure of study populations to unstudied confounders.
3. Differences in assay techniques causing false-positive or false-negative results.
4. Confounding by toxic or growth-promoting substances in sample extracts, resulting in toxicity to or growth of tester strains.
5. Inadequate or inappropriate statistical analysis of data.

He points out that factors 1, 2, and 5 are traditional concerns of the epidemiologist and will become even more important in the interpretation of mutagenicity testing as methodologic improvements address factors 3 and 4. Everson also notes that positive results in assays of urine mutagenesis might be interpreted as indicative of a superior ability to eliminate systemic mutagens, thus reducing in vivo exposure. He reasons that if mutagens are abundantly present in urine, they may be evidence of faster or more complete elimination from the body. If so, the mutagen's time in contact with target tissues may well have been less than average.

Another problem is that only mutations at specific genetic loci are detectable. Although one can partly address this by using multiple organisms, one cannot capture the full spectrum of mutagenic potential with these organisms. Finally, mammalian systems may differ in important aspects from genetically altered tester organisms like *Salmonella* and *E. coli*, for instance in the action of DNA repair systems and in vivo metabolic activation of promutagens. Brusick (1982) notes that basing direct estimates of risk on this method is inappropriate, both because of these organismic differences and because of the secondary nature of urine as an indicator of exposure.

SUMMARY

1. Mutagens are substances capable of causing heritable genetic changes. Mutagenicity testing detects the presence of a wide spectrum of mutagens in body fluids such as urine, feces, and breast milk.

2. Mutagenesis testing can be performed on any body fluid. Because of the ease of collection and storage, urine is most commonly used. Collection and handling of samples is noninvasive, relatively simple, and inexpensive.

3. The physical and chemical properties of a specific mutagen govern the rate at which it is metabolized within the body and then excreted. The metabolic characteristics of mutagens may vary somewhat, depending on the body fluid being tested. In general, however, mutagenicity will begin to appear within hours after exposure to the

agent of interest. Persistence of mutagens in urine is evidently brief: many studies report diminished mutagenicity within 24 hours or less after exposure.

4. For some mutagenic agents, reports of specificity and sensitivity of the urine mutagenesis assay are high, although published estimates vary. Not all mutagens are detectable through these tests, however; chlorinated hydrocarbons, for example, are potent mutagens that are not revealed by mutagenesis testing. Nor will the test differentiate between several potentially confounding exposures; it only reveals the cumulative effects of all recent detectable exposures. The fact that not all carcinogens are mutagenic may be an additional consideration in evaluating the appropriateness of mutagenicity testing.

5. Interindividual variability is high in mutagenesis assays, at least partly as a result of differences in subjects' liver and kidney function, which directly affects the metabolization and excretion of xenobiotics.

6. Details of sample preparation and test methodology may affect the validity and comparability of results. Areas of concern include sample extraction and activation and tester strains employed.

7. Simulating mammalian function in bacteria by adding enzymes and microsomes in vitro may not accurately model these processes in vivo. Both false-positive and false-negative results may occur.

8. The relationship between the presence of urine mutagens and in vivo mutagenesis has not been established. Most investigators interpret positive test results narrowly, as evidence of exposure to a potential mutagen.

Urine mutagenesis testing provides a useful tool in the evaluation of broad categories of potentially mutagenic exposures in occupational or community settings. The test is relatively simple, it is inexpensive to perform, and it can be carried out on samples that are easy to obtain and handle. It detects mutagenic activity that results from a broad range of exposures, a distinct advantage for most applications. Although sensitivity and specificity vary with the compounds detected, urine mutagenesis testing compares favorably with other short-term mutagenesis tests (Tennant et al., 1987).

Disadvantages of the assay include: interindividual and intraindividual variability, its inability to detect some classes of mutagenic chemicals, and disparities between microsomal sample activation with S-9 compound and the actual behavior of metabolized compounds in vivo.

Until very recently, human studies of urine mutagenesis testing have been limited to methodologic or pilot studies. Of those reviewed here, only the study by Scarlett-Kranz et al. (1986) could be described as a well-designed and properly analyzed epidemiologic study. The human studies literature, then, is limited in its value for drawing overall conclusions. Currently, a more serious limitation to the use of mutagenesis testing may be the lack of valid interpretations for positive results of the assay. At present, no definite link has been forged between mutagenic urine and disease. The most pressing need for further study in urine mutagenesis is the validation of a clear relationship between mutagenicity in human urine and morbidity.

REFERENCES

Aeschbacher HU, Chappuis C: Non-mutagenicity of urine from coffee drinkers compared with that from cigarette smokers. *Mutat Res* 1981;89:161–177.

Ahlborg G Jr, Bergström B, Hogstedt C, P Einistö, Sorsa M: Urinary screening for potentially genotoxic exposures in a chemical industry. *J Ind Med* 1985;42:691–699.

Aitio A, Järvisalo J: Biological monitoring of occupational exposure to toxic chemicals: collection, processing, and storage of specimens. *Ann Clin Lab Sci* 1985;15:121–139.

Ames BN, McCann J, Yamasaki E: Methods for detecting carcinogens and mutagens with the *Salmonella*/mammalian microsome mutagenicity test. *Mut Res* 1975;31:347–364.

Baker R, Arlauskas A, Bonin A, Angus D: Detection of mutagenic activity in human urine following fried pork or bacon meals. *Cancer Lett* 1982;16:81–89.

Bos RP, Leenaars AO, Theuws JLG, Henderson PT: Mutagenicity of urine from nurses handling cytostatic drugs, influence of smoking. *Int Arch Occup Environ Health* 1982;50:359–369.

Bos RP, Theuws JLG, Henderson PT: Detection of mutagens in human urine after passive smoking. *Cancer Lett* 1983;19:85–90.

Brusick D: Value of short-term mutagenicity tests in human population monitoring. In: Bora KC, Douglas GR, Nestmann ER, eds.: *Chemical Mutagenesis, Human Population Monitoring and Genetic Risk Assessment*. New York, Elsevier Biomedical Press, 1982, pp. 125–135.

Collings BJ, Margolin BH, Oehlert GW: Analyses for binomial data, with applications to the fluctuation test for mutagenicity. *Biometrics* 1981;37:775–794.

Dolara P, Mazzoli S, Rosi D, Buiatti E, Baccetti S, Turchi A, Vannucci V: Exposure to carcinogenic chemicals and smoking increases urinary excretion of mutagens in humans. *J Toxicol Environ Health* 1981;8:95–103.

Dolara P, Caderini G, Salvadori M, Erringale L, Lodovici M: Urinary mutagens in humans after fried pork and bacon meals. *Cancer Lett* 1984;22:275–280.

Eisenstadt E: Biological assays for mutagens in human samples. *Ann Rev Public Health* 1983;4:391–395.

Eisenstadt E, Kado NV, Putzrath RM: Detection of mutagens in body fluids. In: McElheny VK, Abrahamson S, eds.: *Banbury Report No. 13*. Cold Spring Harbor Laboratory, Cold Spring Harbor, NY, 1983, pp. 33–38.

Everson RB, Flack PM, Sandler RS: Urinary excretion of mutagens in cirrhosis: limited evidence of an association. *Environ Res* 1983;32:118–126.

Everson RB: Detection of occupational and environmental exposures by bacterial mutagenesis assays of human body fluids. *J Occup Med* 1986;28:647–655.

Everson RB, Ratcliffe JM, Flack PM, Hoffman DM, Watanabe AS: Detection of low levels of urinary mutagen excretion by chemotherapy workers which was not related to occupational drug exposures. *Cancer Res* 1985;45:6487–6497.

Falck KL: Urinary mutagenicity caused by smoking. *Mutagens in our Environment* 1982:387–400.

Falck KL, Gröhn P, Sorsa M, Vainio H, Heinonen E, Holsti L: Mutagenicity in urine of nurses handling cytostatic drugs. *Lancet* 1979;i:1250–1251.

Falck KL, Sorsa M, Vainio H: Mutagenicity in urine of workers in rubber industry. *Mutat Res* 1980;79:45–52.

Falck KL, Partanen P, Sorsa M, Suovaniemi O, Vainio H: Mutascreen®, an automated bacterial mutagenicity assay. *Mutat Res* 1985;150:119–125.

Gelbart SM, Sontag S: Mutagenic urine in cirrhosis. *Lancet* 1980;i:894–895.

Green MHL, Muriel WJ, Bridges BA: Use of a simplified fluctuation test to detect low levels of mutagens. *Mutat Res* 1976;38:33–42.

Jaffe RL, Nicholson WJ, Garro AJ: Urinary mutagen levels in smokers. *Cancer Lett* 1983;20:37–42.

Kriebel D, Commoner B, Bollinger D, Bronsdon A, Gold J, Henry J: Detection of occupational exposure to genotoxic agents with a urinary mutagen assay. *Mutat Res* 1983;108:67–79.

Laires A, Borba H, Rueff J, Gomes MI, Halpern M: Urinary mutagenicity in occupational exposure to mineral oils and iron oxide particles. *Carcinogenesis* 1982;3:1077–1079.

Legator MS, Connor TH, Stoeckel M: Detection of mutagenic activity of metronidazole and niridazole in body fluids of humans and mice. *Science* 1975;188:1118–1119.

Maron D, Katzenellenbogen J, Ames BN: Compatibility of organic solvents with the *Salmonella*/microsome test. *Mutat Res* 1981;88:343–350.

Maron DM, Ames BN: Revised methods for the *Salmonella* mutagenicity test. *Mutat Res* 1983;113:173–215.

McCann J: *In vitro* testing for cancer-causing chemicals. *Hosp Pract* September 1983;73–85.

McCann J, Ames BN: The detection of mutagenic metabolites of carcinogens in urine with the *Salmonella*/microsome test. *Ann NY Acad Sci* 1975;269:21–25.

Minnich V, Smith ME, Thompson D, Kornfeld S: Detection of mutagenic activity in human urine using mutant strains of *Salmonella typhimurium*. *Cancer* 1976;38:1253–1258.

Mohtashamipur E., Norpoth K, Lieder F: Isolation of frameshift mutagens from smokers' urine: experiences with three concentration methods. *Carcinogenesis* 1985;6:783–788.

Nguyen TV, Theiss JC, Matney TS: Exposure of pharmacy personnel to mutagenic antineoplastic drugs. *Cancer Res* 1982;42:4792–4796.

Obermeier J, Frohberg H: Mutagenicity studies with praziquantel, a new antihelminthic drug: time-, host-, and urine-mediated mutagenicity assays. *Arch Toxicol* 1977;38:149–161.

Pasquini R, Monarca S, Sforzolini GS, Conti R, Fagioli F: Mutagens in the urine of carbon electrode workers. *Int Arch Occup Environ Health* 1982;50:387–395.

Recio L, Enoch H, Hannan MA: Parameters affecting the mutagenic activity of cigarette smokers' urine. *J Appl Toxicol* 1982;2:241–246.

Roxe M, Siew C, Siddiqui F, Lang I, Rao GS: Mutagenic activity of urinary pigments from patients on antischistosomal therapy with niridazole. *Mutat Res* 1980;77:367–370.

Scarlett-Kranz JM, Babish JG, Strickland D, Goodrich RM, Lisk DJ: Urinary mutagens in municipal sewage workers and water treatment workers. *Am J Epidemiol* 1986;124:884–893.

Schulte PA: Methodologic issues in the use of biologic markers in epidemiologic research. *Am J Epidemiol* 1987;126:1006–1016.

Sorsa M, Falck K, Norppa H, Vainio H: Monitoring genotoxicity in the occupational environment. *Scand J Work Environ Health* 1981;7(suppl 4):61–65.

Sorsa M, Hemminki K, Vainio H: Biologic monitoring of exposure to chemical mutagens in the occupational environment. *Teratogenesis, Carcinog Mutagen* 1982;2:137–150.

Sousa J, Nath J, Ong T: Dietary factors affecting the urinary mutagenicity assay system: I. The absence of mutagenic activity in human urine following consumption of red wine or grape juice. *Mutat Res* 1985a;156:171–176.

Sousa J, Nath J, Tucker JD, Ong T: Dietary factors affecting the urinary mutagenicity assay system: II. Detection of mutagenic activity in human urine following a fried beef meal. *Mutat Res* 1985b;149:365–374.

Speck WT, Stein AB, Rosenkranz HS: Mutagenicity of metronidazole: presence of several active metabolites in human urine. *J Natl Cancer Inst* 1976;56:283–284.

Staiano N, Gallelli JF, Adamson RH, Thorgeirsson SS: Lack of mutagenic activity in urine from hospital pharmacists admixing antitumour drugs. *Lancet* 1981;i:615–616.

Tennant RW, Margolin BH, Shelby MD, Zeiger E, Haseman JK, Spalding J, Caspary W, Resnick W, et al.: Prediction of chemical carcinogenicity in rodents from *in vitro* genetic toxicity assays. *Science* 1987;236:933–941.

van Doorn R, Bos RP, Leijdekkers CM, Wagenaas-Zegers MAP, Theuws JLG, Henderson PT: Thioether concentration and mutagenicity of urine from cigarette smokers. *Int Arch Occup Environ Health* 1979;43:159–166.

Wheeler LA, Saperstein MD, Lowe NJ: Mutagenicity of urine from psoriatic patients undergoing treatment with coal tar and ultraviolet light. *J Int Dermatol* 1981;77:181–185.

Yamasaki E, Ames BN: Concentration of mutagens from urine by adsorption with the nonpolar resin XAD-2: Cigarette smokers have mutagenic urine. *Proc Natl Acad Sci USA* 1977;74:3555–3559.

5

PROTEIN AND DNA ADDUCTS

JAY M. GOLDRING AND GEORGE W. LUCIER

INTRODUCTION

Adducts are stable complexes of reactive chemicals and cellular macromolecules that contain one or more covalent bonds between the two moieties. The chemicals may originate in the environment, as benzo(a)pyrene, a product of incomplete combustion does, or they may be intentionally introduced into the body, as drugs are; one example is *cis*-diaminedichloroplatinum, a crosslinking agent used in cancer chemotherapy. Some endogenous chemicals, such as hormones, may also form adducts. The cellular macromolecule may be DNA, RNA, or protein.

DNA adducts, which are thought to play a major role in carcinogenesis, are the primary focus of this chapter. In adduct formation, covalent bonds are formed between the chemical and one or both DNA strands. Chemicals that bind to both strands are known as *crosslinking agents* because with them the two DNA strands are bound to each other, which may alter the DNA replication process.

Adduct Formation

Absorption and Transport

The probability that a particular chemical will form an adduct depends on many biochemical and pharmacokinetic parameters (Fig. 5-1). First, the chemical must be absorbed into the body. Rates of absorption are highly variable and depend on such parameters as the physical nature of the chemical, its concentration, and its route of exposure (oral, dermal, or inhalation).

In the case of chemicals that are metabolically activated to a form capable of binding DNA, the absorbed chemical must be transported to the site of activation. Chemicals that do not require activation must similarly remain reactive until they reach a cellular macromolecule. In either case, an absorbed chemical must reach the site of

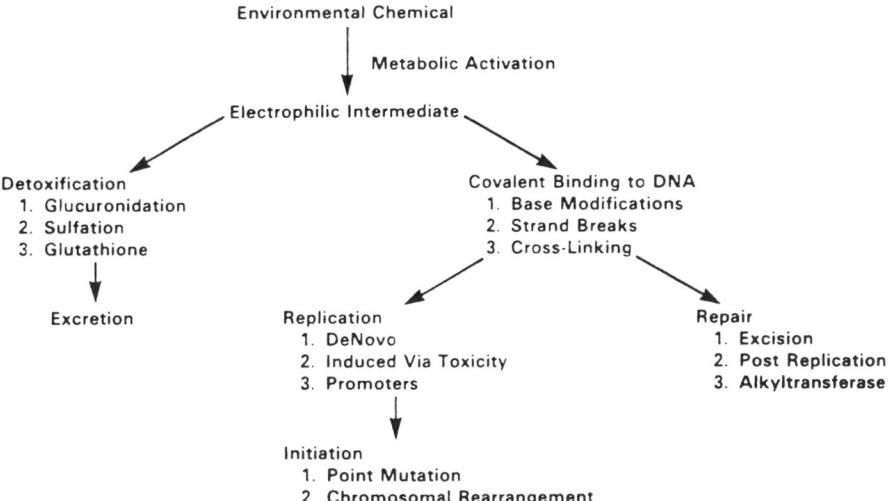

Figure 5-1. Series of events after exposure of a cell to a metabolically activated environmental chemical (such as benzo(a)pyrene). Note that cell initiation is only one of many possible endpoints. (From Belinsky et al., 1987.)

adduct formation before being inactivated by such processes as enzymatic detoxification, excretion, or sequestration in fat.

Metabolic Activation

To form adducts, a chemical must be stable enough to reach its target before breaking down, yet must be reactive enough so that the reaction can take place. Some chemicals, such as the nitrogen mustards, fulfill these conditions intrinsically (i.e., they can form adducts within the cell without enzymatic transformation). These compounds are electrophilic molecules that can react directly with nucleophilic moieties in the cell. Such agents are relatively uncommon in the environment, but have been used as chemical warfare agents and also may be important industrial contaminants.

Many other chemicals are unreactive by themselves and must first be metabolized to enable them to form electrophilic moieties. Examples include the polyaromatic hydrocarbons (PAH), some drugs and pesticides, some industrial solvents, and food contaminants, such as mycotoxins and nitrosamines. These chemicals are relatively nonpolar compounds that are widely dispersed in the environment. The process by which these compounds are converted to reactive metabolites is known as metabolic activation.

One example of metabolic activation involves conversion of these relatively nonpolar chemicals to less lipophilic products by reaction with oxygen. Enzymes of the mixed-function oxidase (MFO) system, also known as the cytochrome P_{450}-containing complex, catalyze this reaction. The oxidized chemicals may be further metabolized by conjugation with endogenous agents such as glucuronic acid, sulfate, or glutathione. Conjugation reactions are generally considered detoxification reactions because they render the chemical water soluble and excretable. In some cases, however, conjugation reactions can produce a DNA-reactive metabolite, as happens in the case of ethylene dibromide (Koga et al., 1986).

The amount of adduct formed by a given chemical in a particular tissue or cell type reflects a balance between metabolic activation and deactivation (Fig. 5-1). Many factors, including age, gender, hormonal status, disease conditions, and prior exposure which selectively induces or inhibits these enzyme systems, may affect this balance.

An example of a chemical that is metabolized in the above manner is benzo(a)pyrene (BaP), an environmentally important polyaromatic hydrocarbon (Fig. 5-2). BaP may first be metabolized to the 7,8-epoxide by the MFO system. The epoxide is then hydrated by another microsomal enzyme, epoxide hydrase. The hydrated epoxide is further oxidized by the MFO system to the 7,8-dihydroxy-9,10-epoxy-7,8,9,10 tetrahydrobenzo(a)pyrene (BPDE). This extremely reactive compound is presumed to be the ultimate carcinogen in this reaction sequence.

Because ultimate adduct-forming chemicals are reactive by nature, the time required for reaction between the chemicals and the cellular macromolecules is usually short. High concentrations of 4-nitroquinoline oxide adducts occur within 1 hour in rat lung and liver tissue after a single in vivo dose (Romagna et al., 1985). For a full review of pathways of metabolic activation, see Hodgson and Guthrie (1982).

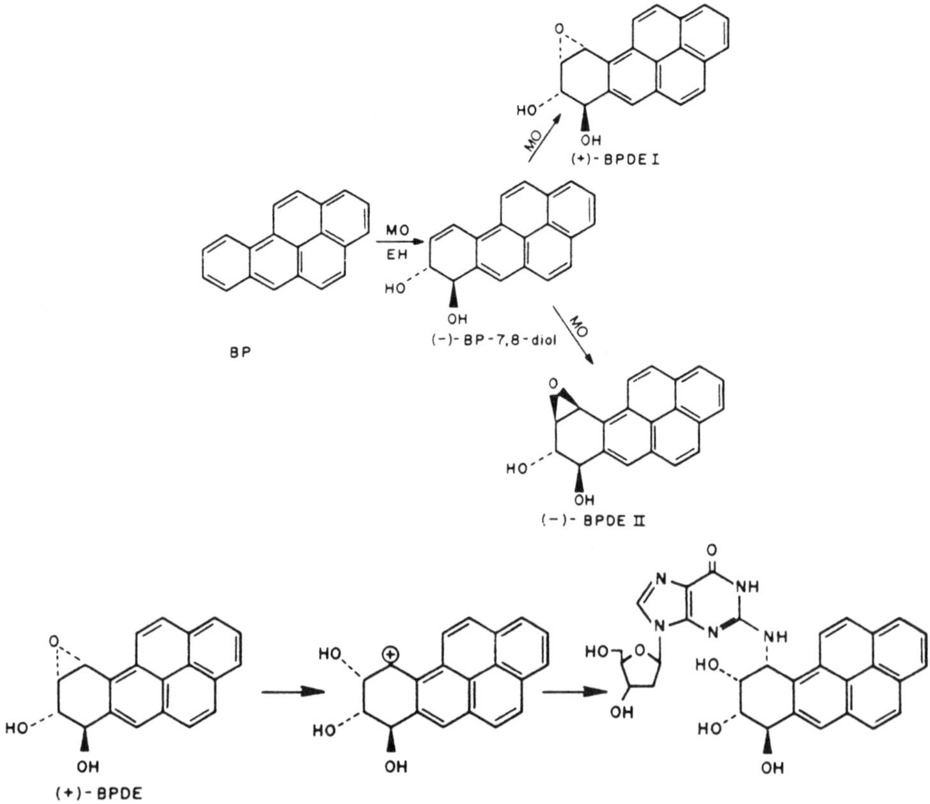

Figure 5-2. Metabolic activation of benzo(a)pyrene to 7,8-dihydroxy-9,10-epoxy-7,8,9,10-tetrahydrobenzo(a)pyrene (BPDE) and subsequent covalent binding to guanosine. MO, mixed-function oxidase; EH, epoxide hydrolase. (From Stowers and Anderson, 1985.)

Role of Adducts in Carcinogenesis

The Relationship Between Adducts and Mutations

Current theories of chemical carcinogenesis suggest that mutations may be important steps in formation of some cancers. DNA adducts may induce mutations by causing errors in the replication of genomic DNA sequences.

Exactly how a mutation can lead to cancer is currently the subject of intensive investigation. Experiments on mammary cancer induction in rats suggest that modifications in specific genes may be associated with tumor induction (Zarbl et al., 1985). At other sites in the genome, adducts may cause nondetectable changes or no change at all. A recent review article (Bishop, 1987) points out that specific mutations in particular genes may be associated with tumor induction. For a review of the role of these genes in carcinogenesis, see Chapter 9 of this book.

Many chemicals appear to cause cancer without producing mutations in short-term tests or without binding covalently to DNA (Tennant et al., 1987). Chemicals that do not form DNA adducts can still be carcinogenic. In general, however, the presence of DNA adducts or mutagenic activity, or both, predicts a carcinogenic response (Wogan and Gorelick, 1985; Tennant et al., 1987).

The effects of a particular adduct on one or more of the cell's 10^{10} base pairs are determined by the concentration and location of the adduct and the specific genes it affects.

Stages of Carcinogenesis

Chemical carcinogenesis can be divided into several stages. Several experimental models divide these into "initiation," "promotion," and "progression."

Initiation is thought to involve some kind of change in the DNA that can be passed onto daughter cells (Trosko et al., 1985). Initiation appears to be a necessary, but not sufficient, step on the path to tumor formation. Such DNA changes can be one consequence of DNA adduct formation.

Promotion is the process that involves clonal expansion of initiated cells. Often multiple doses of a promoting chemical are necessary for promotion. In general, promoters do not cause adducts (Trosko et al., 1985); instead they seem to alter the regulation of normal cellular processes, perhaps through mechanisms that involve increased cell proliferation, loss of normal intercellular communication processes, or altered communication process within the promoted cell.

Progression is the final major step of carcinogenesis and is characterized by a clinically identifiable tumor that arises from preneoplastic cells. As a phase in tumor development, it is distinct from promotion, and probably involves heritable changes and growth factor pathways, although the mechanisms of progression, like promotion, are poorly understood (Barrett and Wiseman, 1987).

To further complicate matters, some chemicals, called *complete carcinogens,* appear to act both as initiators and promoters, causing both heritable mutations and selective proliferation of damaged cells. Thus, when assessing the fate of an adduct-containing cell, investigators must consider all chemical exposures to that particular cell and its progeny.

ISSUES CONCERNING THE USE OF ADDUCTS IN EPIDEMIOLOGIC STUDIES

As the introduction to this chapter explains, the likelihood of adduct formation after chemical exposure and the fate of the adduct depend on many metabolic and pharmacokinetic factors. These factors vary among individual persons, even between cells within the body of a single person. These differences must be considered in the design and interpretation of epidemiologic studies that use adduct measurements.

Adduct Heterogeneity

Some chemicals form a variety of adducts, only some of which may lead to mutations. For example, only a small fraction of N-methyl-N-nitrosourea (NMU) adducts, those on a specific position of guanine, cause mutations, whereas the major adduct of this chemical is nonmutagenic (Singer, 1985). The location of mutation induced by adducts may determine cell initation (Glickman et al., 1987).

The sum total of all adducts in a particular cell or cell population does not necessarily indicate the risk of tumor formation. The relationship of adducts to the probability of initiation depends both on the nature and the site of the adduct, that is, on which gene in which tissue.

Differences in Cell Sensitivity to Adduct Formation and Persistence

Tissue Specificity of Adduct Formation

The distribution of adducts is highly variable and depends on the type of chemical and the route of intake. For some chemicals, adducts appear to form preferentially in tissues exposed to the highest levels of active metabolite. For example, aflatoxin B_1, which must be activated by the MFO system, preferentially forms adducts in hepatocytes, where high concentrations of MFO enzymes are found (Wogan and Gorelick, 1985). The methylating agent 4-(N-methyl-N-nitrosoamino)-1-(3-pyridyl)-1-butanone (NNK), a metabolite of nicotine, primarily attacks DNA in the Clara cells of the lung because there are large amounts of a specific form of cytochrome P_{450} in these cells (Belinsky et al., 1987).

For some carcinogens, tissue specificity cannot be ascertained by differential adduct concentrations. For example, benzo(a)pyrene-derived DNA adduct concentrations are similar in all tissues, although tumors are formed at selective sites such as lung and mammary gland (Stowers and Anderson, 1985).

The levels of adducts present in a tissue that contains many different cell types may be misleading. For example, NNK adduct levels in Clara cells may not be reflected by adduct levels in whole lung homogenate. For predictions of cancer risk, it might be necessary to measure adduct levels in specific cell types whenever feasible.

Estimates of Adduct Persistence

Persistence of a particular adduct depends on the rate of enzymatic repair of the adduct or on cell turnover, or both. Adduct frequency is reduced when a cell dies or undergoes mitosis. As a result, adducts in tissues that are replaced rapidly, such as surface epithelia, can only be detected within a short time after exposure. In longer-lived tissues, such as lymphocytes, rates of DNA repair are important in determining adduct levels.

Estimates of persistence also depend on the particular chemical and on the organ under study. In one strain of mice, the half-life of BPDE–DNA adducts, as measured by administration of a radiolabeled compound, was 18 days in lung and 9 days in liver tissue (Kulkarni and Anderson, 1984). Belinsky et al. (1986) studied formation and disappearance of NNK adducts in various rat tissues after 12 days of chronic treatment and found that maximal adduct concentrations occurred within 4 days and then declined to 50 to 80 percent of peak levels. Beland and Kadlubar (1985) reviewed persistence of arylamine adducts in animal tissues in both acute and chronic studies and found wide variations between chemicals. Some adducts disappeared within a few days, whereas others persisted for weeks and even months.

One study that addressed the question of adduct persistence in humans noted that the level of BPDE–DNA adducts remained the same or decreased a small amount for 90 percent of coke oven workers retested after 3 weeks of vacation (Haugen et al., 1986).

Thus, when assessing the importance of chemical adducts in human cell populations, one must consider (1) the tendency for adducts of a chemical to form and persist in the organ(s) under study, (2) the timing of the chemical exposure, and (3) the repair and turnover rates of the tissues under study.

Formation of Adducts from Endogenous or Dietary Compounds

Some chemicals and hormones change the levels of the chemical-metabolizing enzymes that regulate the availability of DNA reactive metabolites. The hormonal status of the individual may, therefore, affect the relative amounts of adduct formation from both endogenous and exogenous chemicals.

Liehr et al. (1986) found that Syrian hamsters exposed to a variety of estrogen derivatives without exposure to other known genotoxic chemicals displayed increased levels of DNA adducts in the kidneys. Increased adduct levels correlated with the occurrence of kidney tumors. Identical patterns of adducts were formed after exposure to structurally diverse estrogens, including steroidal and nonsteroidal estrogens such as diethylstilbestrol. The chemical structure of these adducts could not be identified, but they were not moieties derived from the estrogens. These results suggest that adducts may arise from endogenous chemicals or dietary constituents.

Lucier and Rumbaugh (1983), in a review of the literature, describe possible mechanisms by which sex steroids may affect DNA adduct formation. These mechanisms include direct stimulation or repression of cytochrome P_{450}-dependent metabolism by estrogens or androgens and alteration of pituitary regulation of the hepatic monooxygenase system.

DNA adducts of unknown composition also form in rats unexposed to known genotoxins. Garg and Gupta (1988) detected age-related adducts in untreated rats.

Because the nature of these adducts is unknown, assays that detect all adducts such as ^{32}P-postlabeling (described later) might be more useful in epidemiologic studies where adducts from dietary constituents or endogenous chemicals might be expected.

Dose–Response Relationships

In humans, a positive correlation between chemical exposure and DNA adduct formation has been consistently observed in cancer chemotherapy patients who received the DNA-crosslinking agent, *cis*-dichlorodiammine platinum (II). In addition, some recent studies (described later) have detected exposure–adduct correlations in foundry workers. In general, however, information on dose–response in cases of human exposure is relatively scarce, as human doses are more difficult to determine than experimental animal doses (Perera, 1988).

Many animal studies have noted dose–response relationships between levels of DNA adducts and chemical exposure (Perera, 1988). Most of these studies have followed single-dose administration of the compounds under study. Perera (1988), however, notes that experiments on chronic administration have been performed with some methylating and ethylating agents with results that showed linearity between dose and adduct levels at low doses.

Economic considerations force animal toxicity testing to be performed at chemical doses that are far higher than those that humans typically encounter. And although the shape of the dose–response curve at low doses is not known for most chemicals it has profound implications for risk assessment (Hoel et al., 1983). Concentrations of DNA adducts can help estimate the shape of the dose–response curve at low dose exposures of chemical carcinogens.

In one study, however, a nonlinear relationship betweeen chemical exposure and DNA adduct formation was noted. Belinsky et al. (1987) measured O^6-methylguanine concentrations in rat lung after chronic NNK exposure and found that adduct formation takes place more efficiently at lower doses. Such results suggest that exposure to low doses of this chemical may carry higher cancer risks than a simple linear model would predict.

Human Variation in Adduct Formation and Persistence

There is significant variation among individual humans in relative amounts of DNA adduct formation after incubation of human cells with chemical carcinogens. This variation greatly exceeds that seen in nonhuman cells. For example, Harris et al. (1976) found wide differences in the binding of BaP to DNA in cultured bronchial cells from different humans. Gupta et al. (1988) found wide variation in the capacity of lymphocytes from different individuals to metabolize and bind a number of chemicals. Thompson et al. (1988) also found large variation in the ability to metabolize BaP among lymphocytes from different individuals.

This variation may arise from differences in amounts of chemical-metabolizing enzymes. According to Cohen et al. (1979), who found great variation in MFO activity in lung tissue explants from cancer patients, such variation may not be connected with cancer risk. Individuals may also exhibit differences in detoxification enzymes; for instance, Siedegard et al. (1988) noted that persons showed hereditary differences in levels of activity of a specific isozyme of glutathione-S-transferase, and that low activity in individuals correlated with an absence of mRNA for the specific isozyme.

The frequency and rate of repair are also highly variable among individuals, and may depend on previous chemical exposures that induce repair enzymes, in addition to genetic and dietary factors. In a study of human lymphocytes, Oesch et al. (1987) found wide individual variation in the ability to repair adducts formed from in vitro exposure to BPDE. In a group of 40 individuals, two were able to remove over 80 percent of the adducts formed in vitro after 24 hours and four removed less than 10 percent. Other members of the group showed removal rates that were fairly evenly distributed between these two extremes.

Such individual variation in DNA repair capabilities may predispose some people to develop cancers. People who carry genetic diseases characterized by deficiencies in DNA repair, such as xeroderma pigmentosum or ataxia telangiectasia, are prone to develop cancers (Knudson, 1977). Whether the relative ability to repair specific DNA lesions, such as the BPDE–DNA adduct, reflects a predisposition to chemically induced cancers, however, remains to be seen.

Surrogate Tissues

Practical considerations limit the types of tissue available for analysis in epidemiologic studies. For example, although adducts have been studied most often in blood cells and placental tissue, these are not necessarily the target tissues for carcinogens or the most sensitive tissues for adduct formation. Due to differences in metabolic activation, deactivation, and cell proliferation, questions of whether these tissues provide reliable estimates of adduct levels in target cells still remain.

Red Blood Cells (Erythrocytes)

Because erythrocytes contain no DNA, analysis of adducts in these cells is limited to protein adducts of hemoglobin. Hemoglobin is easy to obtain, and the relatively long life span of erythrocytes (120 days) permits the determination of cumulative doses in chronic exposure studies (Osterman-Golkar et al., 1976).

Although hemoglobin adducts themselves play no direct role in tumor induction, for some chemicals there are data that correlate hemoglobin adducts with other processes more directly involved in carcinogenesis. Animal studies have shown proportionality between carcinogen binding to DNA and hemoglobin for aromatic amines (Neumann, 1983) and some alkylating agents (Ehrenberg et al., 1983; Farmer et al. 1984; Murthy et al., 1984; Lee and Santella, 1988). For two aromatic amines, trans-4-dimethylaminostilbene and 2-acetylaminofluorene, large-dose ranges tested in rodents resulted in a constant protein to DNA adduct ratio (Neumann, 1980; Periera and Chang, 1981).

In humans, according to Ehrenberg et al. (1983), small alkylating agents, such as ethylene oxide, disperse uniformly throughout the body, and the amount of hemoglobin alkylation generally approximates the dose to DNA. Calleman et al. (1978) also demonstrated a general relationship between ethylene oxide dose and hemoglobin alkylation among 10 people occupationally exposed to the chemical.

These findings indicate that, for some carcinogens, determinations of the amount of hemoglobin alkylation can give estimates of the DNA adduct burden (Farmer et al., 1987).

Lymphocytes

Because of their availability, lymphocytes are very practical cell populations for analysis. Furthermore, because the life span of lymphocytes varies from a few days to

20 years (Leavell and Thorup, 1976), they are potentially useful in determining long-term exposures, although repair processes may cause adduct removal (Sharma et al., 1988).

Because lymphocytes are in contact with many body tissues, they can provide an integrated measure of exposure (Perera et al., 1987). Reactive chemical metabolites in lymphocytes may be derived either from the inherent metabolic capacity of the lymphocytes or from reactive metabolites picked up from other tissues.

Resting (nonproliferating) lymphocytes contain very low levels of chemical-metabolizing enzymes, and consequently may be much less sensitive to adduct formation than other cells (Lucier and Thompson, 1987). Moreover, the variable life span of lymphocytes makes the number of adducts persisting after a given amount of time extremely uncertain, even within the same individual. Any immune disturbance, such as a common cold, may profoundly affect numbers and life spans of lymphocytes, and controlling for these factors may prove to be a difficult task.

Placental Tissue

A few studies have used human placentas to study maternal smoking-related adducts (Everson et al., 1986; Everson et al., 1988). Placentas are readily available, contain measurable amounts of some chemical-metabolizing enzymes, and, because they experience copious blood flow over a period of time, the tissues·may provide an integrated measure of exposure.

Other Surrogates

Other surrogates that have been monitored include DNA adduct excretion in urine (Groopman et al., 1985) and adduct binding to serum albumin (Gan et al., 1988). These surrogates are relatively easy to obtain but are otherwise unsatisfactory. Urinary DNA adducts are present only in extremely low concentrations making detection difficult. The relatively short half-life of serum albumin (20 days) makes this surrogate useful only for recent exposures (Farmer et al., 1987).

Target Tissues

Studies of target tissues are not necessarily preferable to measuring adducts in surrogate tissues. Animal experiments indicate that both tissue sensitivity to adduct formation and adduct persistence appear to be related to the site of tumor induction only for some chemicals (Wogan and Gorelick, 1985). For example, adducts resulting from exposure to some arylamines form preferentially in the bladders of exposed animals (Beland and Kadlubar, 1985), the target organ for this class of carcinogens.

Adducts of other chemicals, however, do not seem to form or persist preferentially in target organ DNA. For example, benzo(a)pyrene adducts are widely distributed in the rat, regardless of the site of tumor development (Stowers and Anderson, 1985). Similarly, Beland et al. (1982) found no correlation between persistence of N-hydroxy-2-acetyl aminofluorene adducts and tissue tumor susceptibility in rats.

METHODS OF DETECTION
Sample Preparation and Storage

In analyzing tissues or cell populations for adducts, the first important step is to protect the adducts from repair or tissue autolysis. Ideally, the DNA should be extracted from blood cells or tissues as soon as possible after collection, as removing the adducts from cellular enzymes may enhance adduct preservation. Because repair or tissue autolysis may take place in the living cell within hours of sampling, cells that cannot be extracted at once should be isolated and frozen as soon as possible. For the same reason, DNA isolation and purification should take place as soon as possible after thawing. Alternatively, the DNA can be extracted and then frozen (Maniatis et al., 1982).

As we observed above, lymphocytes, erythrocytes, placental tissues, and biopsy specimens are all sources of cells for adduct analysis. For details of techniques to isolate lymphocytes, see Böyum (1968). To isolate erythrocytes, most investigators use ultracentrifugation (Tornqvist et al., 1986).

Each of the assays described needs different amounts of DNA, ranging from 100 μg for fluorescence assays to 1–2 μg for ^{32}P-postlabeling. Roughly 1 μg DNA/10^6 cells can be isolated with standard techniques (Maniatis et al., 1982). An average of 30 $\times$ 10^6 lymphocytes can be isolated from 50 ml of blood, but this number is highly variable. A new automated DNA isolation system, the Nucleic Acid Extractor, manufactured by Applied Biosystems of Forest City, California, may improve yields.

Theoretically, storing samples at $-70°C$ for long periods should not affect adduct levels, as the chemical bonds formed should be stable through this process. The effects of freezing and thawing on the stability of a wide variety of adducts, however, has not been thoroughly tested. Thus, to assure accuracy, one must also determine the stability of the adducts of interest during isolation and storage.

Chromatography and Spectrometry
Description of Techniques

When light or electromagnetic energy is directed on chemicals, some is absorbed and some is emitted. *Spectrometry* measures the amount absorbed or emitted. Spectrometry is classified by the type of energy used; the two types of interest to us are *spectrophotometry*, which uses energy derived from light, and *mass spectrometry*, in which the chemical is bombarded with a beam of electrons. With spectrophotometry, chemicals display distinct *spectra* of light absorption or emission, and mass spectrometry measures specific patterns of fragmentation produced by electron bombardment.

Spectrometry can be used only in instances in which the compound of interest possesses unique spectrometric characteristics, or the adduct it forms has different spectrometric properties from those of unmodified DNA or amino acids. Moreover, the adduct must be pure enough to prevent interference from other compounds in the sample. Such purity is usually obtained through *chromatography*.

In chromatography, the chemical mixture is passed through a matrix that separates the different components of the sample. For example, in high pressure liquid chromatography (HPLC), a liquid sample may be passed through a column at high pressure.

The material to pack the column is chosen for its ability to retain the compound of interest for a specific time. In *gas chromatography,* the sample is converted to a gas before it is applied to the column. In both cases, technicians need to refer to appropriate standards with known retention times to ensure that the columns are performing as expected.

Mass spectrometry is based on the principle that molecules, when bombarded with a beam of high energy electrons, fragment in distinct patterns. The fragments can then be separated by mass to charge ratio. Major problems with this technique are that similar patterns are formed by many chemicals and may be difficult to distinguish and that samples must be extremely pure before analysis. The latter problem is usually solved by coupling the mass spectrometer to a gas chromatograph (GC–MS).

Hemoglobin adducts. In studies of hemoglobin adducts, gas chromatography is used in conjunction with mass spectrometry.

The standard method for determination of small hemoglobin adducts briefly involves breaking hemoglobin into its constituent amino acids, purifying the amino acids that contain adducts, and injecting them onto a GC column. A number of peaks will be obtained from the GC column and each must be analyzed by mass spectrometry. For a detailed description of the method, see Farmer et al. (1983) and Tornqvist et al. (1986) for modifications of the method. For larger adducts, such as those derived from PAH, Green et al. (1984) have developed a similar method.

Alternatively, the adducted chemical may be cleaved from the protein so that the reaction products can be analyzed. For example, Shugart (1986) cleaved benzo(a)pyrene-hemoglobin adducts to give tetrols, which are highly fluorescent. The tetrols were separated from other reaction products by high pressure liquid chromatography and analyzed by fluorescence detection. However, Wallin et al. (1987) noted poor recovery of the tetrols and suggest that this method may not be appropriate. Lee and Santella (1988) have developed modifications to this technique that may help improve recovery.

DNA adducts. Two types of spectrophotometric assays have been used to detect DNA adducts: *ultraviolet (UV) spectrophotometry and fluorescence spectrophotometry.* Ultraviolet spectrophotometry measures light absorption through a given range of wavelengths, usually 250 through 550 nm. A characteristic pattern of absorbence peaks can be obtained for many chemicals. The absorbence peaks of DNA containing some types of adducts are different from those of unmodified DNA.

The principle of fluorescence is essentially that some compounds when "excited" by light of a given wavelength, emit light of another, usually longer, wavelength. Fluorescence spectrophotometry is the most widely used spectrophotometric assay for adducts of large molecules. Polyaromatic hydrocarbons are highly fluorescent themselves and this property makes them suitable for this method of analysis.

As in UV spectrophometry, some chemicals exhibit characteristic peaks of fluorescence when excited by light of another wavelength. In synchronous fluorescence spectrophotometry (SFS), excitation and emission are scanned synchronously with a fixed wavelength difference. The advantage of SFS is that fewer peaks are seen than with conventional fluorescence spectrometry (Vahakangas et al., 1985). Details of the experimental technique may drastically affect the detectability of adducts (e.g., the degree of acid hydrolysis of BPDE-adducted DNA increases the sensitivity of the assay for this adduct 20- to 30-fold [Harris et al., 1985]). For other adducts, similar steps may be necessary for increased sensitivity.

The advantages of fluorescence spectrophotometry for DNA adduct detection are first, that the DNA does not have to be hydrolyzed to make a measurement. This means that further assays can be performed on the same sample. Second, the technique is relatively sensitive: one benzo(a)pyrene adduct in 10^8 base pairs can be detected in SFS (Table 5-1; Haugen et al., 1986). Third, extensive purification is not required (Kriek et al., 1984).

But there are a number of disadvantages: the method does not distinguish between covalent adducts and intercalated compounds, which are associated with a DNA but not covalently bound. The assay is relatively nonspecific (i.e., different adducts may show similar fluorescence spectra); the broad peaks seen in most samples prevent quantitation of adducts; and the assay calls for large amounts of DNA, about 100 μg.

Human Studies

Many groups of investigators have attempted to use spectrometric techniques to detect human exposures to genotoxic chemicals. Hemoglobin adducts have been studied using mass spectrometry, whereas DNA adducts in urine, lymphocytes, and placentas have used UV and fluorescence spectrophotometry (Table 5-2).

Hemoglobin adducts. Ethylene oxide, 4-aminobiphenyl, and N-nitroso compounds are the best studied hemoglobin alkylating agents.

Associations between exposure to ethylene oxide, which is commonly used to sterilize hospital equipment, and hemoglobin adduct levels are tenuous, perhaps because the hydroxy-ethyl hemoglobin adduct formed could result from exposure to a

Table 5-1 Comparisons of DNA Adduct Detection Assays

Assay	SFS	Immunoassays	^{32}P
DNA needed	100 μg	20–50 μg	1–2 μg
Sensitivity	1 adduct/10^8 base pairs	1 adduct/10^7–10^{10} base pairs	1 adduct/10^{10} base pairs
Specificity	Fair; similar chemicals may show similar fluorescence spectra	Fair; antibodies cross react between PAH	Good
Quantitative	Yes, with appropriate standardization	Yes, only for total antibody reactivity if cross-reactivity is a problem	Yes, with appropriate standardization
Study design considerations	Spectra of adducts must be known; detects adducts of specific chemicals, not total adduct formation	Wide variation in antibody affinity, making inter-laboratory comparisons difficult	Variations in enzymes, etc., make analysis of control samples necessary
Limitations	Only good for fluorescent compounds (i.e., PAH); does not distinguish between adducts and intercalated compounds; extensive sample purification required	Antibodies must be available for chemical of interest	Identification of spots possible only if standards exist; unidentifiable spots may arise from endogenous compounds or dietary constituents

number of endogenous and dietary chemicals that contain reactive ethyl groups (Osterman-Golkar, 1983). A comparison of levels of hydroxyethylhistidine, a modified amino acid, in 36 workers in an ethylene oxide manufacturing plant and 35 controls revealed no statistically significant difference between the two (Van Sittert et al., 1985). One recent report suggests that smoking may be a confounder in studies of nonspecific hemoglobin alkylation (Tornqvist et al., 1986). These investigators found significant differences in N-hydroxyethylvaline levels between a group of 14 non-smokers and 11 smokers.

Bartsch et al. (1983) noted that certain N-nitrosoamino acids, namely N-nitrosoproline, form on exposure to nitrosating compounds found in many foods. Their preliminary evidence, which included measurements by GC–MS of populations from different geographic areas in China, showed that significant increases in urinary excretion of N-nitrosoproline among residents of certain areas could be correlated with increased ingestion of foods containing nitroso compounds.

One compound, 4-aminobiphenyl, formerly used as an antioxidant in the rubber industry, is no longer in use in many countries, including the United States, because of its carcinogenic properties (IARC, 1972). Because it is, however, ubiquitous in cigarette smoke, 4-aminobiphenyl-hemoglobin adducts have potential use as markers for cigarette smoke exposure. Several recent studies have revealed that smokers show highly significant increases in 4-aminobiphenyl-hemoglobin adducts over nonsmokers. Nonsmokers, however, also have measurable levels of these adducts, perhaps from passive cigarette smoke exposure (Bryant et al., 1987; Perera et al., 1987).

DNA adducts. Ultraviolet spectrophotometry has been used for detection of aflatoxin–DNA adducts in human urine (Groopman et al., 1986). Because many other compounds in human urine also absorb UV light, purification has been the major problem with this technique. These investigators used monoclonal antibody affinity columns to purify samples.

Fluorescence spectrometry has been used to detect BPDE–DNA adducts in lymphocytes and placentas and aflatoxin–DNA adducts in urine. A study of 41 coke oven workers and nine nonsmoking laboratory controls found BPDE-DNA adducts in the lymphocytes of 76 percent of the workers and none in the controls (Harris et al., 1985). Another study, however, found BPDE–DNA adducts in lymphocytes of only 10 per-cent of a group of 38 coke oven workers (Haugen et al., 1986). Because techniques of DNA isolation and adduct analysis used in the two studies are identical, the differences in findings may be related to the study populations.

Another study, of Africans exposed to the highly carcinogenic grain contaminant, aflatoxin, found that 10 percent of the subjects studied had detectable amounts of aflatoxin-guanine adducts in their urine (Autrup et al., 1983, 1985).

More recently, HPLC in combination with SFS has been used to identify BPDE–DNA adducts in 10 of 28 samples of human placenta (Manchester et al., 1988). The presence of BPDE–DNA adducts was unrelated to maternal cigarette smoking. The authors postulate that exposure to benzo(a)pyrene may be through dietary exposures.

For a review of studies using fluorescence spectrometry, the reader should consult Santella (1988).

Immunoassays

Laboratory Techniques

Immunoassays are widely used to detect small amounts of particular substances in cells. In an immunoassay, an antibody is created that binds specifically to the substance of interest, in this case, a carcinogen–DNA adduct. This antibody is bound to a marker to enable the investigator to locate and quantify the amount of binding and, by inference, the amount of adduct.

Solid phase assays. In solid phase assays, the carcinogen–DNA adduct of interest is injected into an animal, for example, a rabbit. The adduct then becomes an *antigen,* a foreign compound that induces an immune response in the animal. The animal then produces *antibodies,* proteins that bind specifically to the antigen. These antibodies are the *primary antibodies.*

The solution with an unknown amount of carcinogen–DNA adduct is added to known amounts of adduct bound to the matrix (such as a plastic microtiter plate) and primary antibody. Antibodies to the primary antibodies (*secondary antibodies*), such as goat antirabbit antibodies, bound to a marker, are then added. The marker is an enzyme that catalyzes the conversion of a colorless compound (such as *para*-nitrophenylphosphate) to a colored compound. After addition of the substrate, the amount of color development (measurable in a spectrophotometer) indicates the amount of carcinogen–DNA adduct.

This assay, the enzyme-linked immunosorbent assay (ELISA) (Fig. 5-3) is *competitive* (i.e., the adduct in the sample competes with the known amount of adduct bound to the matrix). Color development is thus *inversely* proportional to the amount of adduct in the sample. The ultrasensitive enzymatic radioimmunoassay (USERIA) follows the same procedure except that the enzyme catalyzes transfer of a radioactive atom from one compound to another. The amount of product is then measured. In radioimmunoassays (RIA), the antigen–antibody complexes are precipitated. The displacement of radioactive antigen reflects the amount of binding between antibodies and adducts.

Primary antibodies created by injecting animals are called *polyclonal* because the antibodies arise from many individual cells. *Monoclonal* antibodies arise from a single cell. They are produced by fusing a cell producing the antibody of interest with a cancer cell and then allowing the fused cell to grow and divide indefinitely.

The affinity of the primary antibody for the antigen (the adduct) varies widely between batches of antibody, making quantitative comparisons of results obtained by different laboratories difficult (Santella et al., 1988). As a result of this variability, estimates of sensitivity for immunoassays vary widely (Santella, 1988).

Other problems with immunoassays include the fact that specific antibodies must be developed for each adduct of concern. Moreover, primary antibodies to some PAH appear to cross-react with DNA adducts of similar chemicals, limiting the specificity of the assay. Everson et al. (1986) and Perera et al. (1987) noted that antibodies to BPDE-modified DNA cross-react with DNA modified by benz(a)anthracene and chrysene derivatives. Thus, these assays frequently measure total antigenicity of the DNA rather than a specific adduct, making quantification difficult for some adducts. See Table 5-1 for a summary of the advantages and disadvantages of immunoassays.

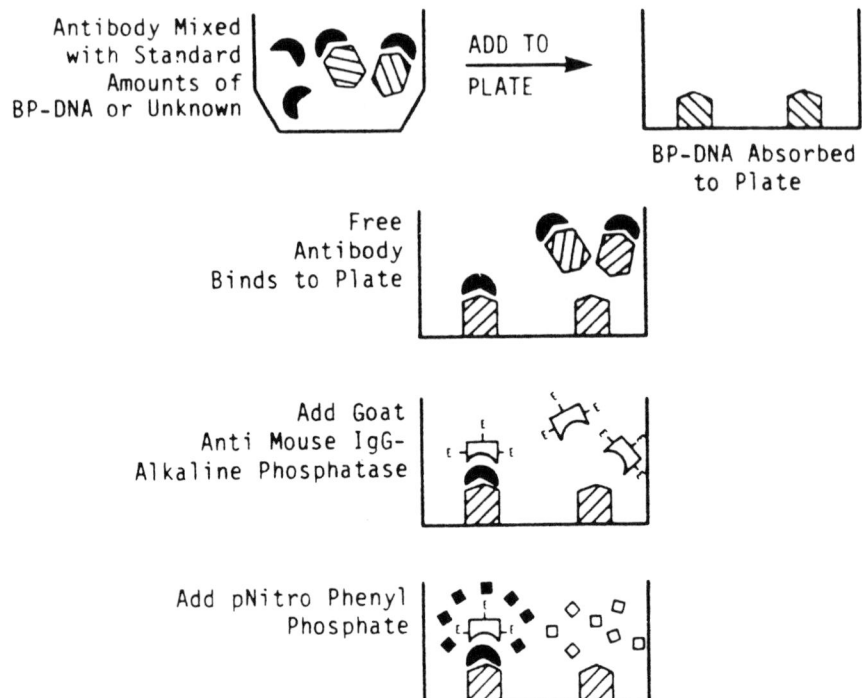

Figure 5-3. Simplified diagram of a competitive enzyme-linked immunosorbent assay (ELISA). (From Perera et al., 1986.)

Immunohistochemical assays. DNA adducts can also be measured in single cells after tissue sectioning and fixing. Sections are treated with either labeled primary antibody or primary antibody followed by labeled secondary antibody (Santella, 1988). In animal studies, the sensitivities of this technique are rather low: one adduct in 10^5–10^6 nucleotides (Santella, 1988; Table 5-1).

Human Studies

Cigarette smoking. Perera et al. (1982) first attempted to validate the ELISA method for determining tissue adduct levels. They injected mice with labeled benzo(a)pyrene and compared the levels of adducts in lung tissue as measured by scintillation counting with results obtained using ELISA. Once they obtained similar results with both methods, they measured polyaromatic hydrocarbon adduct levels, using the ELISA method, in the lung tissue of 27 hospital patients, 15 of whom had consistent exposure to cigarette smoke and 12 of whom did not. Of all patients studied, five had measurable levels of benzo(a)pyrene–DNA adducts and all were in the exposed group.

More recently, Perera et al. (1987) studied various biological markers, including DNA adducts, in the lymphocytes of 22 smokers and 24 nonsmokers. They found a small increase in mean DNA adduct levels, as measured by reactivity with antibodies to benzo(a)pyrene-diol-epoxide (BPDE-I)–DNA adducts, in smokers compared with nonsmokers. They also found a highly significant correlation between DNA and 4-aminobiphenyl (4-ABP)–hemoglobin adducts in the lymphocytes of smokers. They concluded that 4-ABP is a more direct marker of smoking than PAH–DNA adducts, as confirmed by the highly significant correlation between 4-ABP and cotinine. Everson et al. (1986) also noted a small, but statistically nonsignificant increase in adducts reacting with an antibody to BPDE–DNA adducts in the placentas of smoking women compared with controls. One recent study of autopsy specimens used immunohistochemical techniques to visualize and count cells with adducts (Shamsuddin and Gan, 1988).

Occupational groups. Associations between DNA adducts and occupational exposure to genotoxic chemicals have generally been more conclusive than those for cigarette smoke. The occupational exposures studied to date are in roofers, coke oven workers, and foundry workers.

Shamuddin et al. (1985) used the ELISA method to examine the lymphocytes of 28 roofers, 20 foundry workers, and 9 controls for benzo(a)pyrene–DNA adducts, and found 25, 25, and 7 percent positives in each group, respectively. The two positive patients in the control group were smokers.

Harris et al. (1985) found that 67 percent (18 of 27) of a sample of coke oven workers had detectable BPDE-I–DNA adducts as detected by ultrasensitive enzyme-linked radioimmunoassay (USERIA). The SFS measurements confirmed these results; 76 percent of the workers had BPDE-I–DNA adducts measurable using this assay. Adduct–antibody reactivity could not be detected in a group of nonsmoking laboratory workers. Among the coke oven workers, a slightly greater proportion of current smokers had detectable amounts of adducts (75%) than nonsmokers and former smokers combined (60%). This group also found that 27 percent of the coke oven workers had detectable levels of antibodies to BPDE–DNA adducts circulating in their blood, indicating that exposure to BPDE must have been great enough to allow the body to form its own antibodies.

Haugen et al. (1986) also compared the USERIA and SFS assays and found that USERIA assays detected BPDE-I–DNA adducts in 34 percent of a sample of 22 coke oven workers. The SFS assays, however, showed detectable adducts in only 10 percent of the same workers. The investigators noted that the most positive samples were the same in both assays and concluded that USERIA is more sensitive than SFS. Interestingly, these investigators also found BPDE-I–DNA adduct antibodies in the sera of exposed individuals.

More recently, Perera et al. (1988) used ELISA to measure PAH–DNA adduct levels by ELISA in the peripheral blood cells of 35 Finnish foundry workers and 10 controls. They classified the subjects into four exposure groups and found that adduct levels were significantly correlated with chemical exposure (p = .0001) after adjustments for cigarette smoking and time since vacation.

Dietary exposures. Umbenhauer et al. (1985), using a radioimmunoassay, reported significantly higher levels of O^6-methylguanine in the esophageal DNA of a Chinese population exposed to dietary nitrosamines than in a comparable European population with no such exposure. The researchers noted high adduct levels in 17 of 37 esophageal cancer patients from the exposed population and in none of the of 12 tissue samples from the unexposed population. They estimate the sensitivity of their technique to be about one O^6-methylguanine for every 4×10^8 unmethylated guanines, or about 100 molecules of O^6-methylguanine per human cell.

Chemotherapeutic agents. Immunoassays can also detect DNA adducts in the white blood cells of cancer patients given a chemotherapeutic agent, *cis*-diaminedichloroplatinum (II) (Poirier et al., 1985). This agent is known to bind to deoxyguanosine, forming many different types of adducts. Poirier and co-workers found positive results with the ELISA assay in 44 of 120 patients receiving the drug and none of the 18 controls. Moreover, the presence of adducts was positively correlated with response to therapy; an absence of adducts was noted in those who failed to respond.

Furthermore, a number of investigators have observed dose–response relationships between levels of drug–DNA adducts in the white blood cells of cancer patients and gradations of response to chemotherapy (Reed et al., 1987; Fichtinger-Shepman et al., 1987; Reed et al., 1988). These adducts are highly persistent; 22 months after therapy ended measurable levels were still present in kidney and spleen upon autopsy (Reed et al., 1987).

This research has wide implications. First, researchers have taken the first step toward validating the idea that DNA adducts act as a measure of a biologically effective dose. Second, the technique offers a way to screen patients before chemotherapy to find out whether or not the particular therapy is likely to be effective. If the patient forms DNA–drug adducts, the chemotherapy is more likely to be effective than if the patient does not.

^{32}P-Postlabeling

Laboratory Techniques

An additional assay currently available for detection of carcinogen–DNA adducts is the *^{32}P-postlabeling assay* (Randerath et al., 1981). In this assay (Fig. 5-4a), the cellular DNA containing the carcinogen adducts is enzymatically digested to its constituent 3'-monophosphates. Adducted monophosphates compose an extremely small fraction of the digest; the major portion is unmodified monophosphates. Two procedures can be used to enrich the mixture with adducted monophosphates: (1) incubation with P1 nuclease, which preferentially cleaves the remaining phosphate from nonadducted nucleotides (Reddy and Randerath, 1986), or (2) extraction with butanol (Gupta, 1985). The nuclease P1 procedure gives better adduct recoveries for polycyclic aromatic hydrocarbon adducts, whereas butanol extraction is preferred for certain arylamine adducts (Gupta and Earley, 1988). Both procedures should be used when dealing with unknown samples.

The mixture, enriched with adducted nucleotides, is incubated with an enzyme that attaches a radioactively labeled phosphate to 3'-monophosphates. The mixture is then dissolved in buffer solution and placed on a polyethyleneamine–cellulose thin-layer chromatography plate.

The plate is developed in buffer in two dimensions: the hydrophobicity of the modified bases allows them to remain on the plate in distinct patterns, while the unmodified bases wash through. After the plate is exposed to x-ray film, a characteris-

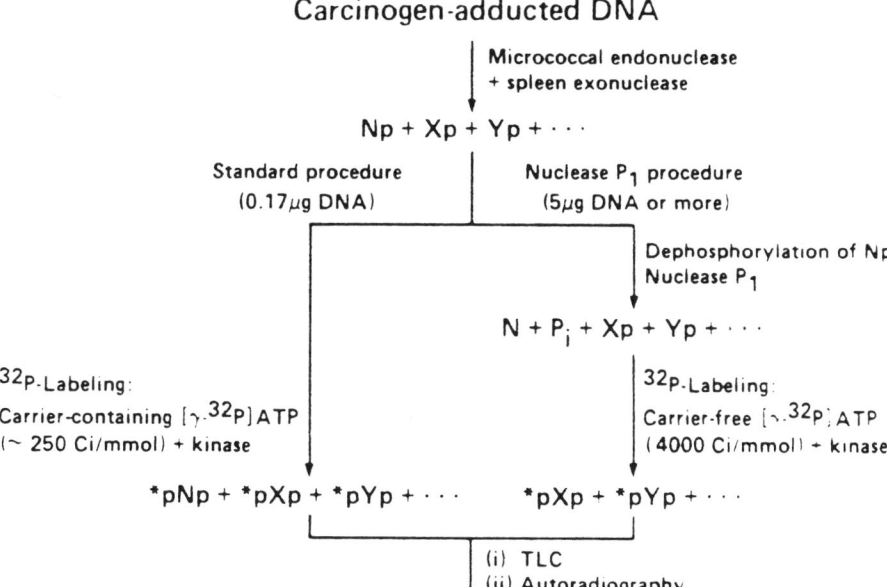

Carcinogen-adducted DNA

Figure 5-4a. Experimental strategy employed in standard and nuclease P1-enhanced procedures for ^{32}P-postlabeling analysis of carcinogen-DNA adducts. Nuclease P1 dephosphorylates 3′-monophosphates of normal nucleotides, but not adducted nucleotides, so that the latter are enriched before ^{32}P-labeling. Np indicates normal nucleotides (dGp, dAp, dCp, dm[5]Cp, and dTp). Xp, Yp denote adducted deoxyribonucleotides. (From Randerath et al., 1985.)

tic pattern of spots develops (Fig. 5-4b). The location of each spot may be attributed to a particular carcinogen–DNA adduct. To estimate adduct quantities, one excises the spots for counting in a scintillation counter. This method is extremely sensitive under optimum conditions and allows the detection of 1 adduct in 10^{10} bases.

Major drawbacks of the ^{32}P-postlabeling assay are that identities and absolute concentrations of each adduct cannot be determined without appropriate standards. For example, to identify a spot as a benzo(a)pyrene adduct and quantify it, one must first perform the assay on samples of pure benzo(a)pyrene-adducted DNA of known concentrations and determine the location of the spots. Because of the lack of standards, the composition of most spots detected in human samples remains unknown. Furthermore, the assay relies on many enzymatic steps; because enzyme activity may not be the same in different batches, adduct recovery may be highly variable. To calculate adduct amounts in the cell such information must be available.

Human Studies

Everson et al. (1986) performed the ^{32}P-postlabeling assay on placental tissue and found one unidentified adduct whose presence was strongly correlated with smoking (16 out of 17 smokers had this adduct, compared with 3 of 14 nonsmokers). The

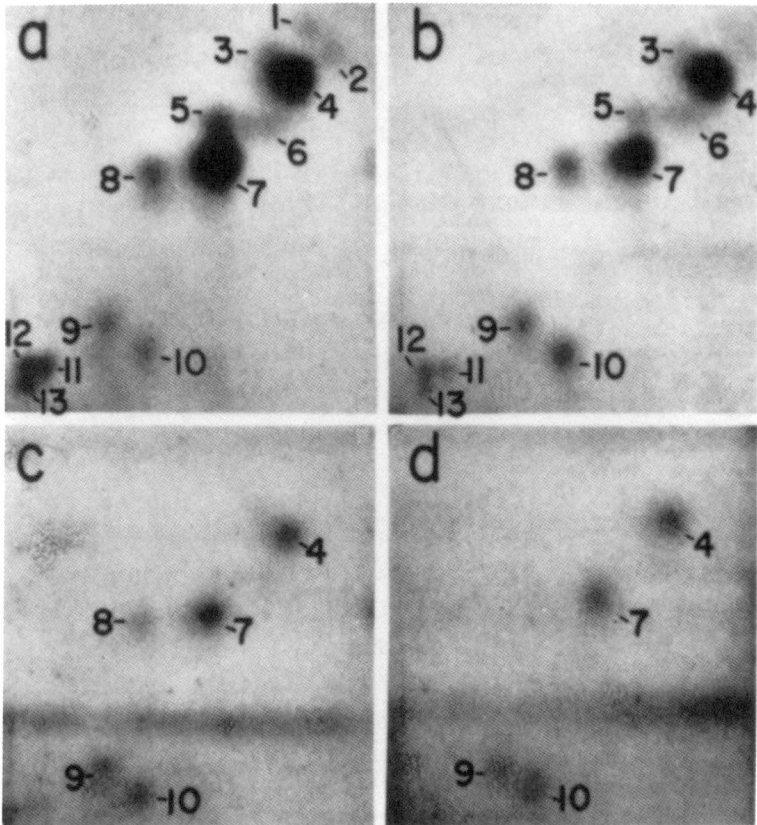

Figure 5-4b.   Actual chromatograms of DNA digests from mouse skin treated with 3-methylcholanthrene. **A.** 1 day after treatment. **B.** 6 days after treatment. **C.** 14 days after treatment. **D.** 28 days after treatment. Digest of DNA from unexposed mouse did not give any of the numbered spots. (From Randerath et al., 1985.)

amounts of the adduct, however, were only weakly related to intensity of smoking exposure, suggesting interindividual variability of adduct formation in response to tobacco smoke. In a later study of human placentas, Everson et al. (1988) found one adduct whose intensity was strongly correlated with cigarette smoke exposure. Interestingly, this adduct did not co-elute with any of the standards tested, suggesting that cigarette smoke may change the body's activation/deactivation systems to produce DNA–adduction of endogenous compounds or dietary constituents.

Phillips et al. (1986), in a study of 10 individuals, found that all had one to nine adducts per 10^8 nucleotides in bone marrow cells and similar adducts in peripheral blood lymphocytes. There was no correlation between the presence of particular adducts and cigarette smoke exposure. These adducts did not appear in four samples of fetal bone marrow. The results of this study suggest that the background DNA adduct profile among individuals is highly variable; whether this variability is the result of environmental exposures or of genetic factors remains to be studied. Jahnke et al. (1988), who performed the ^{32}P-postlabeling assay on lymphocytes from 6 smokers and

Table 5-2 Studies of DNA Adducts in Human Populations

Reference	Tissue	Population	Assay	No. positive/ total	Adduct concentrates (fmol/µg)
Perera 82	WBC[1]	Lung cancer patients	ELISA	3/5	0.10*
Autrup 85	Urine[2]	Africans (dietary)	SFS	24/335	0.3–3 pmol/25 ml urine
Harris 85	WBC[1]	Coke oven workers	USERIA	18/27	0.4–34.3
		Controls	SFS	21/27 0	NA
Vahakangas 85	WBC[1]	Aluminum workers	USERIA	1/27	6.5
Umbenhauer 85	Esophagus[2]	Chinese controls	RIA	10/37 17/37 10/37	0.0015–0.005 > 0.16 0
Poirier 85	WBC[3]	Cancer patients	ELISA	44/120	0.13–0.5
		Controls		0/18	
Shamsuddin 85	WBC[1]	Roofers	USERIA/	7/28	0.04–6
		Foundry workers	ELISA	7/20	
Groopman 86	Urine[2]	Chinese (dietary)	UV	NA	NA
Haugen 86	WBC[1]	Coke oven workers	SFS	4/38	0.5–2.2
			USERIA	13/38	0.41–0.93
Phillips 86	WBC[4]	Smokers	[32]P	4/4	0.02*
		Nonsmokers		6/6	0.02*
Dunn 86	Oral[4] Muc.	Inverted smokers	[32]P	14/15	0.3*
		Controls		10/19	
Everson 86	Placenta[1,4]	Smokers	[32]P	16/17	0.03–0.12
			ELISA	NA	1.65*
		Nonsmokers	[32]P	3/14	NA
			ELISA	NA	0.96*
Perera 87	WBC[1]	Smokers	ELISA	5/22	0.133*
		Nonsmokers		7/24	0.115*
Fichtinger-Shepman 87	WBC[3]	Cancer patients	ELISA	8/8	1–5
Shamsuddin 88	Var.[1]	Cancer patients (autopsy)	Immunohistochem	Var./5–10	NA
Everson 88	Placenta[4]	Smokers	[32]P	28/30	NA
		Nonsmokers		4/23	
Perera 88	WBC[1]	Foundry workers	ELISA	30/30	0.03–2.8
		Controls		2/10	0.03–0.3
Reed 88	WBC[3]	Cancer patients	ELISA	12/17	<0.14
				5/17	>0.14
Manchester 88	Placenta[1]	Nonsmokers	SFS	10/28	0.25*
Jahnke 88	WBC[4]	Smokers	[32]P	4/4	NA
		Nonsmokers		4/4	NA

[1]Benzo(a)pyrene or related PAH.   [2]Aflatoxin B_1.   [3]cis-Diaminedichloroplatinumm.   [4]Unknown.   *Average value.

4 nonsmokers, found no significant difference in the presence of particular adducts between the two groups. These results suggest that this variability is not related to cigarette smoking.

Phillips et al. (1988) later performed the assay on the peripheral white blood cells of Finnish foundry workers and found that cells from those exposed to higher levels of PAH were more likely to contain measurable levels of PAH–DNA adducts than those exposed to lower levels. Finally, Dunn and Stich (1986) found no difference in the levels or types of DNA adducts found in the oral mucosal cells of controls and betel nut chewers, "inverted" smokers (who place the burning end of the cigarette in their mouths) or tobacco chewers from Asia.

In any study, the research team must analyze adequate controls to insure that the spots detected are not experimental artifacts. Dunn and Stich (1986), for example, performed their DNA extraction procedure on samples that did not contain DNA to demonstrate that the spots were not experimental artifacts. An additional useful control experiment might be to perform parallel isolations of DNA that has no adducts such as calf thymus DNA. Dunn and Stich (1986) also showed that increasing enzymatic digestion did not cause the spots to disappear, suggesting that the spots do not arise from products of incomplete DNA digestion. Phillips et al. (1986, 1988) did not analyze control samples.

Comparison of Laboratory Techniques

Specifics of the laboratory techniques appear in Table 5-1. First, note that the absolute levels of adducts detected by each assay differ greatly from each other. For example, Haugen et al. (1986), in their study of coke oven workers, found 0.6–2.2 fmol BAP/μg DNA (20–70 adducts/10^8 nucleotides), using SFS. Perera et al. (1988), using anti-BPDE-I antibodies, detected a range of 0.066-1.5 fmol/μg DNA (2.2-50 adducts/10^8 nucleotides) in a sample of Finnish foundry workers. In a similar population, Phillips et al. (1988) detected 0.2–1.9 adducts/10^8 nucleotides using ^{32}P-postlabeling. Moreover, Everson et al. (1986) detected one adduct in 5×10^7 normal nucleotides in placental samples from smoking women when he used immunologic methods, but detected 1–4 adducts/10^8 nucleotides when he used the ^{32}P-postlabeling assay. Everson explains this discrepancy by suggesting that the antibody cross-reacted with other PAH–DNA adducts. Whatever the reason, the poor correlation between postlabeling, immumoassays, and SFS makes it difficult to compare results obtained by these different methods. Selection of a particular method, then depends on the resources available and the type of exposure under investigation.

ETHICAL ISSUES

Is the epidemiologist who performs studies on DNA adducts responsible for informing his or her subjects of the results? What exactly should he or she tell them?

The answers to these questions are complicated first by a lack of data on "normal" adduct levels. As mentioned in the section on ^{32}P-postlabeling, detectable levels of DNA adducts can be found in samples of fetal bone marrow from humans who have apparently no history of exposure to genotoxic chemicals. Hence, before we can draw conclusions about elevated adduct levels, we must first define the levels of background DNA adducts.

Second, what do findings of elevated DNA adduct levels in individuals actually mean? They may mean that someone has been exposed to large doses of genotoxic chemicals. Or, elevated DNA adduct levels may mean that the subject is genetically predisposed to forming adducts even with small chemical exposures. In either case, does the finding mean that the individual is at a higher risk for cancer? The answer is simply not known.

Samuels (1986) proposes a list of guidelines that he hopes will encourage the use of biological markers in a manner consistent with current knowledge of their biological role. He emphasizes using these markers to identify populations at risk and to encourage appropriate action. Data from these assays should never be used, he says, as an excuse to "reduce programs of prevention focused on controlling conditions in the workplace."

CONCLUSION

The process of chemical carcinogenesis begins with exposure to a genotoxic chemical or mixture of chemicals and ends with the appearance of a tumor. Because there are significant gaps in our knowledge of events, traditional epidemiology has focused on the beginning and end of this process in an attempt to make associations between specific exposures and cancer induction.

New techniques based on molecular biology are now available that enable the epidemiologist to measure an event that may occur somewhere in the middle: the formation of protein and DNA adducts. Encouraging results demonstrating that adduct levels may be correlated with exposure to genotoxic chemicals indicate that adduct levels may be useful as markers of chemical exposure. Because these markers may avoid errors associated with questionnaire data or estimation of individual doses from group data, they offer the opportunity to assess exposures directly and enable people to take preventive measures.

In addition, these assays may make assessment of qualitative risks at the group level possible; that is, they may allow the presence of DNA adducts to be used as an indicator of possible increased risk for cancer. Increases in particular adduct levels among a defined occupational group, for example, may indicate a possible cancer hazard. These techniques may also enable investigators to address questions concerning the process of carcinogenesis; that is, the relationship between exposure, measured by traditional methods (such as air monitoring), and the damage seen at the cellular level. Before such goals can be reached, however, much work remains to be done.

First, investigators in this field need to develop animal models to validate the relationships among exposures, the presence of particular markers, and cancer risks. Such models involve administering measured doses of the chemical and following these animal for their entire life spans. There is a need to perform parallel human and animal studies on chemicals of occupational or environmental significance to assess where humans lie in the spectrum of interspecies variability.

The magnitude of interindividual variability is another issue that must be addressed. Results from the ^{32}P-postlabeling assay demonstrate a great variability in adduct formation among humans exposed to genotoxins. Hence, there is a need to conduct research to characterize the factors that affect adduct formation and repair in given tissues. To obtain background levels, there is a need to determine average adduct levels and distributions of adduct frequency for particular chemicals in various tissues for the general population.

Technological advances have now achieved enough sensitivity to detect low levels of adducts for some types of genotoxic chemicals. A major task of modern epidemiology is to determine what the new data mean.

REFERENCES

Autrup H, Bradley KA, Shamsuddin AKM, Wakhisi J, Wasunna A: Detection of putative adduct with fluorescence characteristics identical to 2,3-dihydro-2-(7'-guanyl)-3-hydroxyaflatoxin B$_1$ in human urine collected in Murang'a district, Kenya. *Carcinogenesis* 1983;4:1193–1195.

Autrup H, Wakhisi J, Vahakangas, Wasunna A, Harris CC: Detection of 8, 9-dihydro (7'-guanyl)-9-hydroxyaflatoxin B_1 in human urine. *Environ Health Perspect* 1985;62:105–108.

Barrett JC, Wiseman RW: Cellular and molecular mechanisms of multistepcarcinogenesis: Relevance to carcinogen risk assessment. *Environ Health Perspect* 1987;76:65–70.

Bartsch H, Ohshima H, Munoz N, Pignatelli B, Friesen M, O'Neill I, Crespi, Lu SH: Assessment of endogenous nitrosation in humans in relation to the risk of cancer of the digestive tract. In: Hayes AW, Schnell RC, Miya TS, eds.: *Developments in the Science and Practice of Toxicology.* Amsterdam, Elsevier, 1983 pp. 299–309.

Beland FA, Dooley KL, Jackson CD: Persistence of DNA adducts in rat liver after multiple doses of the carcinogen *N*-hydroxy-2-acetylaminofluorene. *Cancer Res* 1982;42:1348–1354.

Beland FA, Kadlubar FF: Formation and persistence of arylamine DNA adducts *in vivo*. *Environ Health Perspect* 1985;62:19–30.

Belinsky SA, White CM, Boucheron JA, Richardson FC, Swenberg JA, Anderson MA: Accumulation and persistence of DNA adducts in respiratory tissue of rats following multiple administrations of the tobacco specific carcinogen 4-(*N*-methyl-*N*-nitrosoamino)-1-(3-pyridyl)-1-butanone. *Cancer Res* 1986;46:1280–1284.

Belinsky SA, White CM, Devereux TR, Anderson MW: DNA adducts as a dosimeter for risk estimation. *Environ Health Perspect* 1987;76:3–8.

Bishop JM: The molecular genetics of cancer. *Science* 1987;236:305–308.

Böyum A: Separation of leukocytes from blood and bone marrow. *Scand J Clin Lab Invest* 1968;21(suppl):97.

Bryant MS, Skipper PL, Tannenbaum SR, Maclure M: Hemoglobin adducts of 4-aminobiphenyl in smokers and nonsmokers. *Cancer Res* 1987;47:602–608.

Calleman CJ, Ehrenberg L, Jansson B, Osterman-Golkar S, Segerback D, Svensson K, Wachtmeister CA: Monitoring and risk assessment by means of alkyl groups in hemoglobin in persons occupationally exposed to ethylene oxide. *J Environ Pathol Toxicol Oncol* 1978;2:427–442.

Cohen GM, Mehta R, Meredith-Brown M: Large interindividual variations in metabolism of benzo(alpha)pyrene by peripheral lung tissue from lung cancer patients. *Int J Cancer* 1979;24:129–133.

Dunn BF, Stich HF: ^{32}P–Postlabeling of aromatic DNA adducts in human oral mucosal cells. *Carcinogenesis* 1986;7:1115–1120.

Ehrenberg L, Osterman-Golkar S: Alkylation of macromolecules for detecting mutagenic agents. *Teratogenesis Carcinog Mutagen* 1980;1:105–127.

Ehrenberg L, Moustacchi E, Osterman-Golkar S, Ekman G: Dosimetry of genotoxic agents and dose/response relationship of their effects. *Mutat Res* 1983;123:121–182.

Everson RB, Randerath E, Santella RM, Cefalo RC, Avitts TA, Randerath K: Detection of smoking-related covalent DNA adducts in human placenta. *Science* 1986;231:54–57.

Everson RB, Randerath E, Santella RM, Avitts TA, Weinstein IB, Randerath K: Quantitative association between DNA damage in human placenta and maternal smoking and birth weight. *JNCI* 1988;80:567–575.

Farmer PB, Bailey E, Shuker DEG: The determination of *in vivo* alkylation of haemoglobin and DNA using gas chromatography-mass spectrometry. In: Hayes AW, Schnell RC, Miya TS, eds.: *Developments in the Science and Practice of Toxicology.* Amsterdam, Elsevier, 1983, pp. 273–280.

Farmer PB, Bailey E, Campbell JB: Use of alkylated proteins in the monitoring of exposure to alkylating agents. In: Berlin A, Draper M, Hemminki K, Vainio H, eds.: *Monitoring Human Exposure to Carcinogenic and Mutagenic Agents.* Lyon, IARC Scientific Publication 59, 1984, pp. 189–198.

Farmer PB, Neumann HG, Henschler D: Estimation of exposure of man to substances reacting covalently with macromolecules. *Arch Toxicol* 1987;60:251–260.

Fichtinger-Shepman AMJ, van Oosterom HT, Lohman PH, Berends F: Interindividual human variation in cisplatimum sensitivity, predictable in an *in vitro* assay? *Mutat Res* 1987;190:59–62.

Gan LS, Skipper PL, Peng X, Groopman JD, Chen JS, Wogan GN, Tannenbaum SR: Serum albumin adducts in the molecular epidemiology of aflatoxin carcinogenesis: Correlation with aflatoxin B$_1$ intake and urinary excretion of aflatoxin M$_1$. *Carcinogenesis* 1988;9:1323–1325.

Garg A, Gupta RC: Tissue-specific DNA modifications in untreated, aged rats as detected by ^{32}P-adduct assay. *Proc Am Assoc Cancer Res* 1988;29:104.

Glickman BW, Horsfall MJ, Gordon JE, Burns PA: Nearest neighbor affects G:C to A:T transitions induced by alkylating agents. *Environ Health Perspect* 1987;76:29–32.

Green LC, Skipper PL, Turesky RJ, Bryant MS, Tannenbaum SR: *In vivo* dosimetry of 4-aminobiphenyl in rats via a cysteine adduct in hemoglobin. *Cancer Res* 1984;44:4254–4259.

Groopman JD, Donahue PR, Zhu J, Chen J, Wogan GN: Aflatoxin metabolism in humans: Detection of metabolites and nucleic acid adducts in urine by affinity chromatography. *Proc Natl Acad Sci USA* 1985;82:6492–6496.

Gupta RC: Enhanced sensitivity of ^{32}P-postlabeling analysis of aromatic carcinogen: DNA adducts. *Cancer Res* 1985;45:5656–5662.

Gupta RC, Earley K: ^{32}P-adduct assay: Comparative recoveries of structurally diverse DNA adducts in the various enhancement procedures. *Carcinogenesis* 1988;9:1687–1693.

Gupta RC, Earley K, Sharma S: Use of human peripheral blood lymphocytes to measure DNA binding capacity of chemical carcinogens. *Proc Natl Acad Sci USA* 1988;85:3513–3517.

Hanawalt PC: Preferential DNA repair in expressed genes. *Environ Health Perspect* 1987;76:9–14.

Harris CC, Autrup H, Connor R, Barrett LA, McDowell EM, Trump BF: Interindividual variation in binding of benzo(a)pyrene to DNA in cultured human bronchi. *Science* 1976;194:1067–1069.

Harris CC, Vahakangas K, Newman MJ, Trivers GE, Shamsuddin A, Sinopoli N, Mann DL, Wright WE: Detection of benzo(a)pyrene diol epoxide-DNA adducts in peripheral blood lymphocytes and antibodies to the adducts in serum from coke oven workers. *Proc Natl Acad Sci USA* 1985;82:6672–6676.

Haugen A, Becher G, Benestad C, Vahakangas K, Trivers GE, Newman MH, Harris CC: Determination of polycyclic aromatic hydrocarbons in the urine, benzo(a)pyrene diol epoxide-DNA adducts in sera from coke oven workers exposed to measured amounts of polycyclic aromatic hydrocarbons in the work atmosphere. *Cancer Res* 1986;46:4178–4183.

Hodgson E, Guthrie FE: *Introduction to Biochemical Toxicology.* New York, Elsevier, 1980.

Hoel DG, Kaplan NL, Anderson MW: Implications of nonlinear kinetics on risk estimation. *Science* 1983;219:1032–1037.

International Agency for Research on Cancer. *IARC Monographs on the Evaluation of Carcinogenic Risk of Chemicals to Man.* Volume 1, p. 74, Lyon, 1972.

Jahnke GD, Thompson CL, Walker MP, Gallagher JE, Lucier GW, DiAugustine RP: Detection of DNA adducts in human peripheral leukocytes by ^{32}P-postlabeling analysis. *Proc Am Assoc Cancer Res* 1988;29:99.

Knudson AG: Mutation and cancer in man. *Cancer* 1977;39(suppl 4):1882–1886.

Koga N, Inskeep PB, Cmarik JL, Guengerich FP: S[2–(N^7-guanyl)ethyl]-glutathione the major DNA adduct formed from 1,2-dibromoethane. *Biochemistry* 1986;25:2192–2198.

Kriek E, den Engelse L, Scherer E, Westra JG: Formation of DNA modifications by chemical carcinogens, identification, localization and quantification. *Biochim Biophys Acta* 1984;738:181–201.

Kulkarni MS, Anderson MW: Persistence of benzo(a)pyrene metabolite: DNA adducts in lung and liver of mice. *Cancer Res* 1984;44:97–101.

Leavell BS, Thorup OA: *Fundamentals of Clinical Hematology,* 4 ed. Philadelphia, W. B. Saunders Co., 1976.

Lee BM, Santella RM: Quantitation of protein adducts as a marker of genotoxic exposure: Immunologic detection of benzo(a)pyrene-globin adducts in mice. *Carcinogenesis* 1988;9:1773–1777.

Liehr JG, Avitts TA, Randerath E, Randerath K: Estrogen-induced endogenous DNA adduction: Possible mechanism of hormonal cancer. *Proc Natl Acad Sci USA* 1986;83:5301–5305.

Lucier GW, Rumbaugh K: Influence of sex steroids on experimental carcinogenesis. In: Turosov V, Montesano R, eds.: *Modulators of Experimental Carcinogenesis.* Lyon, IARC Scientific Publication No. 51, 1983, pp. 49–64.

Lucier GW, Thompson CL: Issues in biochemical applications to risk assessment: When can lymphocytes be used as surrogate markers? *Environ Health Perspect* 1987;76:187–191.

Manchester DK, Weston A, Choi JS, Trivers GE, Fennessey PV, Quintana E, Farmer PB, Mann DL, Harris CC: Detection of benzo(a)pyrene diol epoxide-DNA adducts in human placenta. *Proc Natl Acad Sci USA* 1988;85:9243–9247.

Maniatis T, Frisch EF, Sambrook J: *Molecular Cloning: A Laboratory Manual.* Cold Spring Harbor, New York, Cold Spring Harbor Laboratory, 1982.

Murthy MSS, Calleman CJ, Osterman-Golkar S, Segerback D, Svensson K: Relationships between ethylation of hemoglobin, ethylation of DNA and administered amount of ethyl methanesulfonate in the mouse. *Mutat Res* 1984;127:1–8.

Nakayama J, Yuspa SH, Poirier MC: Benzo(a)pyrene-DNA adduct formation and removal in mouse epidermis *in vivo* and *in vitro:* Relationship of DNA binding to initiation of skin carcinogenesis. *Cancer Res* 1984;44:4087–4095.

Neumann HG: Dose relationships in the primary lesion of strong electrophilic carcinogens. *Arch Toxicol* 1980; Suppl 3:69–77.

Neumann HG: The dose-dependence of DNA interactions of aminostilbene derivatives and other chemical carcinogens. In: Hayes AW, Schnell RC, Miya TS, eds.: *Developments in the Science and Practice of Toxicology.* Amsterdam, Elsevier, 1983, pp. 135–144.

Oesch F, Aulmann W, Platt KL, Doerjer G: Individual differences in DNA repair capacities in man. *Arch Toxicol* 1987; Suppl 10:172–179.

Osterman-Golkar S, Ehrenberg L, Segerbäck D, Hällström I: Evaluation of genetic risks of alkylating agents. II. Haemoglobin as a dose monitor. *Mutat Res* 1976;34:1–10.

Osterman-Golkar S: Tissue doses in man, implications in risk assessment. In: Hayes AW, Schnell RC, Miya TS, eds.: *Developments in the Science and Practice of Toxicology.* Amsterdam, Elsevier, 1983, pp. 289–298.

Perera FP: The significance of DNA and protein adducts in human biomonitoring studies. *Mutat Res* 1988;205:271–282.

Perera FP, Poirier MC, Yuspa SH, Nakayama J, Jaretzski A, Curmen MM, Knowles DM, Weinstein IB: A pilot study in molecular cancer epidemiology: Determination of benzo(a)pyrene-DNA adducts in animal and human tissues by immunoassays. *Carcinogenesis* 1982;3:1405–1410.

Perera FP, Santella R, Poirier M: Biomonitoring of workers exposed to carcinogens: Immunoassays to benzo(a)pyrene-DNA adducts as a prototype. *J Occup Med* 1986;28:1117–1123.

Perera FP, Santella RM, Brenner D, Poirier MC, Munshi AA, Fischman HK, Van Ryzin J: DNA adducts, protein adducts and sister chromatid exchange in cigarette smokers and non-smokers. *JNCI* 1987;79:449–456.

Perera FP, Hemminki K, Young TL, Brenner D, Kelly G, Santella RM: Detection of polycyclic aromtic hydrocarbon-DNA adducts in white blood cells of foundry workers. *Cancer Res* 1988;48:2288–2291.

Periera MA, Chang LW: Binding of chemical carcinogens and mutagens to rat hemoglobin. *Chem Biol Interact* 1981;33:301–305.

Phillips DH, Hewer A, Grover PL: Aromatic DNA adducts in human bone marrow and peripheral blood leukocytes. *Carcinogenesis* 1986;7:2071–2075.

Phillips DH, Hemminki K, Alhonen A, Hewer A, Grover PL: Monitoring occupational exposure to carcinogens: Detection by ^{32}P-postlabeling of aromatic DNA adduct in white blood cells from foundry workers. *Mutat Res* 1988;204:531–542.

Poirier MC, Reed E, Zwelling LA, Ozols RF, Litterst CL, Yuspa SH: Polyclonal antibodies to quantitate *cis*-diamminedichloroplatinum (II)-DNA adducts in cancer patients and animal models. *Environ Health Perspect* 1985;62:89–94.

Randerath K, Reddy MJ, Gupta RC: ^{32}P-labelling test for DNA damage. *Proc Natl Acad Sci USA* 1981;78:6126–6129.

Randerath K, Randerath E, Agrawal HP, Gupta RC, Schurdak ME, Reddy MV: Postlabeling methods for carcinogen-DNA adduct analysis. *Environ Health Perspect* 1985;62:57–66.

Reddy MV, Randerath K: Nuclease P1-mediated enhancement of sensitivity of ^{32}P-postlabeling test for structurally diverse DNA adducts. *Carcinogenesis* 1986;7:1543–1551.

Reddy MV, Randerath K: 32P–postlabeling assay for carcinogen-DNA adducts: Nuclease P_1-mediated enhancement of its sensitivity and applications. *Environ Health Perspect* 1987;76:41–47.

Reed E, Ozols RF, Tarone R, Yuspa SH, Poirier MC: Platinum-DNA adducts in leukocyte DNA correlate with disease response in ovarian cancer patients receiving platinum-based chemotherapy. *Proc Natl Acad Sci USA* 1987;84:5024–5028.

Reed E, Ozols RF, Tarone R, Yuspa SH, Poirier MC: The measurement of cisplatin-DNA adduct levels in testicular cancer patients. *Carcinogenesis* 1988;9:1909–1911.

Reynolds SH, Stowers SJ, Patterson RM, Maronpot RB, Aaronson SA, Anderson MW: Activated oncogenes in B6C3F1 mouse liver tumors: Implications for risk assessment. *Science* 1987;237:1309–1216.

Romagna F, Kulkarni MS, Anderson MW: Detection of repair of chemical-induced DNA damage *in vivo* by the nucleoid sedimentation assay. *Biochem Biophys Res Commun* 1985;127:56–62.

Samuels SW: Medical surveillance: Biological, social and ethical parameters. *J Occup Med* 1986;28:572–577.

Santella RM: Application of new techniques for the detection of carcinogen adducts to human population monitoring. *Mutat Res* 1988;205:271–282.

Santella RM, Weston A, Perera FP, Trivers GT, Harris CC, Young TL, Nguyen D, Lee BM, Poirier MC: Interlaboratory comparison of antisera and immunoassays for benzo(a)pyrene-diol-epoxide-I-modified DNA. *Carcinogenesis* 1988;9:1265–1269.

Shamsuddin AKM, Sinopoli NT, Hemminki K, Boesch RR, Harris CC: Detection of benzo(a)pyrene-DNA adducts in human white blood cells. *Cancer Res* 1985;45:66–68.

Shamsuddin AKM, Gan R: Immunocytochemical localization of benzo(a)pyrene-DNA adducts in human tissue. *Hum Pathol* 1988;19:309–315.

Sharma S, Nesnow S, Maizel A, Gupta RC: Regulation of DNA repair in human B and T lymphocytes. *Proc Am Assoc Cancer Res* 1988;29:85.

Shugart L: Quantifying adductive modification of hemoglobin from mice exposed to benzo(a)pyrene. *Anal Biochem* 1986;152:365–369.

Shuker DEG, Bailey E, Parry H, Lamb J, Farmer PB: The determination of 3-methyladenine in humans as a potential monitor of exposure to methylating agents. *Carcinogenesis* 1987;8:959–962.

Siedegard J, Vorachek WR, Pero RW, Pearson WR: Hereditary differences in the expression of the human glutathione transferase active on *trans*-stilbene oxide are due to a gene deletion. *Proc Natl Acad Sci USA* 1988;85:7293–7297.

Singer B: *In vivo* formation and persistence of modified nucleosides resulting from alkylating agents. *Environ Health Perspect* 1985;62:41–48.

Stowers SJ, Anderson MW: Formation and persistence of benzo(a)pyrene metabolite-DNA adducts. *Environ Health Perspect* 1985;62:31–40.

Tennant RW, Margolin BH, Shelby MD, Zeiger E, Haseman JK, Spalding J, Caspary W, Resnick M, Stasiewica S, Anderson B, Minor R: Prediction of chemical carcinogenicity in rodents from *in vitro* genetic toxicity assays. *Science* 1987;236:933–941.

Thompson CL, Jahnke G, Goldring J, Liu Y, DiAugustine R, Lucier GW: Analysis of metabolism and DNA adduct formation in human lymphocytes following *in vitro* exposure to benzo(a)pyrene. *Proc Am Assoc Cancer Res* 1988;29:99.

Tornqvist M, Osterman-Golkar S, Kautianen A, Jense S, Farmer PB, Ehrenberg L: Tissue doses of ethylene oxide in cigarette smokers determined from adduct levels in hemoglobin. *Carcinogenesis* 1986;7:1519–1521.

Tornqvist M, Osterman-Golkar S, Kautianen A, Naslund M, Calleman CJ, Ehrenberg L: Methylations in human hemoglobin. *Mutat Res* 1988;204:521–529.

Trosko JE, Riccardi VM, Chang CC, Warren S, Wade M: Genetic predispositions to initiation or promotion phases in human carcinogenesis. In: Anton-Guirguis H, Lynch HT, eds.: *Biomarkers, Genetics and Cancer.* New York, Van Nostrand Reinhold, 1985, pp. 13–38.

Umbenhauer D, Wild CP, Montesano R, Saffhill R, Boyle JM, Huh N, Kirstein U, Thomale J, Rajewsky MF, Lu SH: O⁶-methyldeoxyguanosine in oesophageal DNA among individuals at high risk of oesophageal cancer. *Int J Cancer* 1985;36:661–665.

Vahakangas K, Haugen A, Harris CC: An applied synchronous fluorescence spectrophotometric assay to study benzo(a)pyrene-diol-epoxide-DNA adducts. *Carcinogenesis* 1985;8:1109–1116.

Vahakangas K, Trivers G, Rowe M, Harris CC: Benzo(a)pyrene diol-epoxide-DNA adducts detected by synchronous fluorescence spectrophotometry. *Environ Health Perspect* 1985;62:101–104.

van Sittert NJ, de Jong G, Clare MG, Davis R, Dean BJ, Wren LJ, Wright AS: Cytogenetic, immunological and haematological effects in workers in an ethylene oxide plant. *Br J Ind Med* 1985;42:19–26.

Wallin H, Jeffrey AM, Santella RM: Investigation of benzo(a)pyrene-globin adducts. *Cancer Lett* 1987;35:139–146.

Wogan GN, Gorelick NJ: An overview of chemical and biochemical dosimetry of exposure to genotoxic chemicals. *Environ Health Perspect* 1985;62:5–18.

Zarbl H, Sukumar S, Arthur AV, Martin-Zanca D, Barbacid M: Direct mutagenesis of Ha-*ras*-1 oncogenes by *N*-nitroso-*N*-methylurea during initiation of mammary carcinogenesis in rats. *Nature* 1985;315:382–386.

6

SISTER CHROMATID EXCHANGES

TIMOTHY C. WILCOSKY AND SUSAN M. RYNARD

INTRODUCTION

Sister chromatid exchanges (SCEs) occur during cell replication when a chromosome duplicates its genetic material, forming a pair of chromosomes (sister chromatids) attached at the centromere. Through mechanisms that involve DNA breakage and rejoining, sister chromatids can exchange seemingly identical segments of DNA without known alteration of cell viability or function (Allen et al., 1983).

SCE analysis has been used widely as an in vitro method for assessing the mutagenic potential of chemicals (Allen et al., 1983), but interest is growing in SCEs as markers of DNA lesions in humans exposed to certain types of chemical carcinogens (NTP, 1984). Although SCEs themselves do not necessarily lead to adverse health outcomes, elevated levels of SCEs apparently indicate that cells have been exposed to a mutagen. This chapter explains the principles of the assay, considers some of the issues governing its use in epidemiologic research, and briefly discusses its application in human studies to date.

CHARACTERISTICS OF SISTER CHROMATID EXCHANGES

Important characteristics of SCEs include the mechanisms that lead to their occurrence, the agents that produce them, the time necessary for their appearance, and their persistence in the body.

Mechanism of Occurrence

Two major theoretical models of SCE formation have been proposed. The recombination model is based on chromatid exchange as part of a postreplication repair process (Bender et al., 1974; Kato, 1977), whereas the replication model involves recombination during DNA replication (Painter, 1980; Ishii and Bender, 1980). The articles cited present the details of these complex models. Although the mechanisms responsible for the appearance of SCEs are still under investigation, SCEs apparently reflect processes distinct from those that produce chromosome aberrations (Wolff et al., 1977).

Sister Chromatid Exchange-Producing Agents In Vitro

Although a variety of physical and biological agents, including viruses, ionizing radiation, clastogens, and mutagens, can produce SCEs (Gebhart, 1981), this chapter focuses on the chemical induction of SCEs. A wide range of chemicals can induce SCEs in mammalian cell lines (Latt et al., 1981). Those most likely to produce SCEs in vitro include alkylating agents and other DNA-binding agents, certain DNA-base analogs, and chemicals that interfere with DNA repair or cause single-strand breaks in DNA. In contrast, exposures that cause double-strand DNA breaks, such as bleomycin and ionizing radiation, are efficient producers of chromosome breakage but not of SCEs (NTP, 1984; Carrano, 1986).

For most of the SCE-inducing chemicals tested, induction increases linearly with dose (NTP, 1984). Studies in vitro also indicate that some chemicals, but not others, show a linear association between SCE induction and single-gene mutations. A possibility also exists that some DNA lesions can produce either a mutation or an SCE (Carrano, 1986). In general, SCEs compared with chromosome breakage are a more sensitive indicator of DNA damage; the assay responds to a wider variety of agents and responds at doses that are 10- to 100-fold lower (NTP, 1984). The marker is nonspecific in that many different chemical exposures lead to the same response.

Temporal Aspects of Exposure, Sister Chromatid Exchange Appearance, and Sampling

SCEs occur when certain DNA lesions are present during cell division. When SCEs are used as markers of DNA lesions in humans, the lesions occur in vivo, but the resulting SCEs are measured in sampled cells that have been stimulated to divide in culture. The DNA lesions should occur as soon as the exposure agent reaches the cell. If DNA repair takes place before replication, however, SCEs may not occur.

Persistence of Sister Chromatid Exchange

The persistence of detectable SCEs depends both on the rate of DNA repair and on the normal half-life of the affected cells. For different lymphocyte subpopulations, for example, the life spans range from a few months to 20 years (Carrano, 1986). When stimulated to divide in culture, a sample of long-lived cells with unrepaired DNA lesions could give a good estimate of dose integrated over time. Cells with rapid turnover or cells with transient lesions could provide estimates of more recent exposures, if such cells can be separated from the total lymphocyte population. An exposure itself may increase the rate of cell turnover and alter the proportion of long- and short-lived lymphocytes. The persistence of SCE-inducing chemicals within the body after the ambient exposure ends also affects the persistence of detectable SCEs.

The persistence of elevated SCE levels may increase with increasing dose (NTP,

1984), but few data exist to support or reject the possibility. A study of only one ciga-rette smoker suggests that a transient elevation in SCEs returns to normal after 18 hours of nonsmoking (Lambert et al., 1982). Other studies found that, for unknown reasons, SCE levels increased for several months after long-term smokers quit (Wulf et al., 1985; Tucker et al., 1988). As summarized by Lambert et al. (1982), cancer chemotherapy may increase SCE frequencies for weeks or months. Workers with acute high exposure to ethylene oxide showed a 40 percent elevation in SCEs 5 days after exposure, but their SCE levels were normal 2 years later (Laurent, 1988). Chronic ethylene oxide exposure, on the other hand, apparently increases SCE levels for at least 1 to 2 years after exposure is reduced or ends (Stolley et al., 1984; Sarto et al., 1984).

Accessibility of Tissues with Sister Chromatid Exchanges

Although SCEs can apparently occur in any type of dividing cell, most studies of SCEs in humans focus on circulating lymphocytes because they are so easily available. For cancer etiology, cells in bone marrow or other tissues are of greater interest, as cancer can arise from such cells but apparently not from mature circulating lymphocytes. Mutagenic exposures that increase SCE levels in lymphocytes, however, presumably also affect other cells that can form tumors; therefore, lymphocyte SCEs should be a good biological response marker. Because the sampling procedure for lymphocytes is less invasive than that for most other cells of interest, population studies of SCEs have typically used lymphocytes (Bloom, 1981). For this reason, the rest of this discussion focuses on SCEs in lymphocytes.

THE SISTER CHROMATID EXCHANGE ASSAY

The SCE assay is a process in which one member of each chromatid pair in replicating cells is stained differently from its sister chromatid. This differential staining enables investigators to detect genetic material exchanged between sister chromatids. The assay is based on the incorporation of 5-bromodeoxyuridine (BrdUrd), a thymidine analog, into replicating chromosomes, so that BrdUrd-sensitive staining procedures allow visualization of newly formed SCEs.

Specimen Collection and Cell Culturing

In the human lymphocyte SCE procedure, summarized in Table 6-1, 10 ml of whole blood are centrifuged to yield leukocytes (white blood cells). Roughly 20–30 percent of the white cells are lymphocytes, the cell type used in the assay (Langley, 1971). The white cells are placed in a culture medium containing nutrients, BrdUrd, and phy-tohemagglutinin (PHA); PHA is a mitogen that stimulates lymphocytes (especially T-cells) to divide. Because cells are scored during their second division metaphases in culture, the culture duration should be selected to yield a high percentage of cells in their second division (Bloom, 1981). A culture length of about 72 hours is recom-mended (Lambert et al., 1982). When comparing exposed and nonexposed groups, some investigators report the proportion of cells that have undergone one, two, and

Table 6-1 SCE Assay Procedure

A. Collect 10 ml venous blood; add PHA and separate white cells and plasma by centrifugation.
B. Establish cell culture in medium containing antibiotics, autologous human serum, and BrdUrd.
C. Incubate for at least 72 hours at 37°C; protect from light.
D. When ready to harvest cells, add colchicine to inhibit further cell division.
E. Harvest cells by centrifugation.
F. Fix cells in 3 : 1 methanol : acetic acid; drop cells on slides and air dry.
G. Stain prepared slides in fluorescent 33258 Hoechst.
H. Irradiate stained slides under UV light.
I. For permanent preparation, counterstain with Giemsa.
J. Number-code slides to assure blind analysis.
K. Analyze for SCEs.

three divisions during a specific culture length. These proportions can be interpreted as indicators of cytotoxicity or mitotic delay.

BrdUrd Uptake in DNA Synthesis

As summarized in Chapter 8, dividing cells pass through different phases. Cells preparing to replicate enter a period of DNA synthesis called the S phase. During this phase, the DNA of chromosomes is duplicated.

In the S phase under assay conditions, BrdUrd partially replaces thymidine, a DNA base that is one of the chromosome's normal components. During the first metaphase in culture, each sister chromatid has one newly formed BrdUrd-substituted DNA strand and one parent strand of normal DNA without BrdUrd substitution, as Figure 6-1 shows. After mitosis, the double-stranded DNA of chromosomes in the two daughter cells also contains one BrdUrd-substituted strand and one parent strand. During DNA synthesis in the second cell division in culture, BrdUrd again partially replaces thymidine in the newly synthesized strands of DNA in each chromatid. Then, when the daughter cells enter metaphase, one of the sister chromatids includes a parent strand of DNA and a BrdUrd-substituted strand of DNA, and the other contains two strands of BrdUrd-substituted DNA. The asymmetrical distribution of BrdUrd-substituted DNA in the second metaphase allows visualization of SCEs: the chromatid containing the parent DNA strand stains with a different intensity compared with the chromatid with BrdUrd in both strands. If an SCE has occurred, it appears as a discontinuity in the stain intensity along the chromatid (Figs. 6-1 and 6-2). Note that the SCE assay cannot detect a DNA lesion formed in vivo unless it persists until the first DNA synthesis in vitro when BrdUrd is present.

Sister Chromatid Exchange Scoring

Investigators use various approaches to score SCEs. Some researchers perform replicate cell cultures from each individual in the study and prepare multiple slides from each culture (Anderson et al., 1986). They then select cells for scoring from the multiple slides prepared for each person. Because random fluctuations in SCE numbers among slides and cultures would tend to cancel each other, this procedure helps minimize the effect of variation among slides and cultures when estimating the mean number of SCEs per cell for an individual.

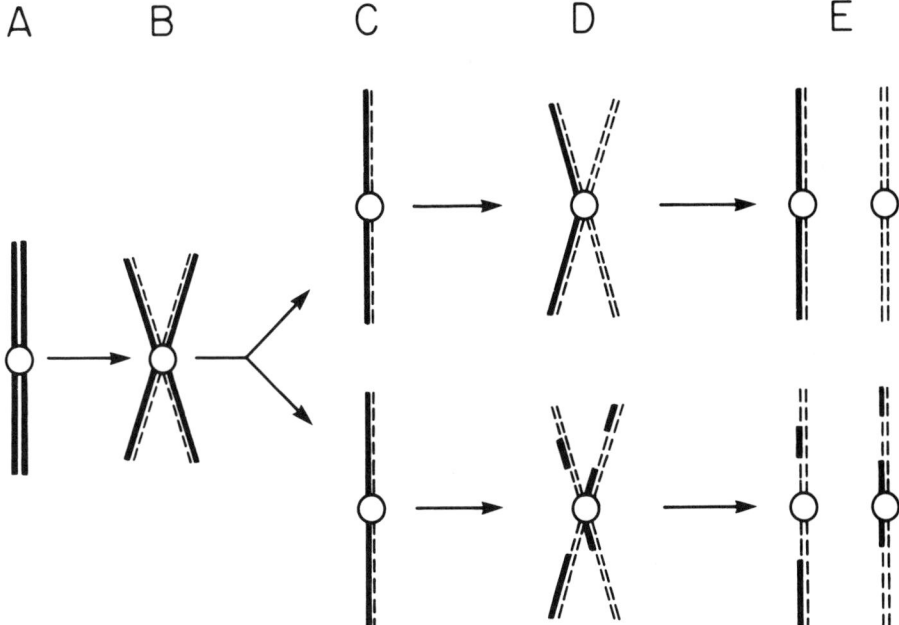

Figure 6-1. BrdUrd uptake and the visualization of SCEs. A schematic representation of a chromosome is shown for two cell cycles. **A.** During G_0, the chromosome has two arms, each having two DNA strands. **B.** When the cell enters its first metaphase in culture, each chromosome replicates in the presence of BrdUrd forming a pair of sister chromatids. Newly formed DNA strands, indicated by *dashed lines,* incorporate BrdUrd; the parent DNA strands are shown as *heavy dark lines.* Note that each sister chromatid in metaphase of the first cell cycle contains one BrdUrd-substituted DNA strand and one parent strand. **C.** After mitosis, each of two daughter cells, therefore, has one parent strand and one BrdUrd-substituted strand of DNA. **D.** When the daughter cells enter metaphase in the second cell division, one of the sister chromatids includes a parent strand of DNA and a BrdUrd-substituted strand of DNA; the other sister chromatid contains two strands of BrdUrd-substituted DNA. The asymmetrical distribution of BrdUrd-substitution in the second metaphase allows visualization of SCEs: the chromatid containing the parent DNA strand stains with a different intensity compared with the chromatid with BrdUrd in both strands. SCEs appear under a microscope as a discontinuity in stain intensity along the chromatids, as depicted in the lower chromosome, which shows three SCEs. **E.** After the second mitosis, the daughter cells have BrdUrd substitution as shown.

Although normal human cells contain 46 chromosomes, cells stained for SCE scoring may have fewer than 46 detectable chromosomes. Some researchers require that all scored cells have 46 clearly visible chromosomes (Lambert et al., 1982), whereas others score cells with 45 (Anderson et al., 1986) or even 40 chromosomes (Soper et al., 1984). Although the inclusion of cells with fewer than 46 chromosomes leads to a smaller average number of SCEs per cell for an individual, Soper et al. (1984) found this bias to be negligible in their analysis. Most investigators, however, who score fewer than 46 chromosomes normalize the SCE count to the frequency expected for 46 chromosomes.

The number of cells scored per individual varies among studies. Bloom (1981)

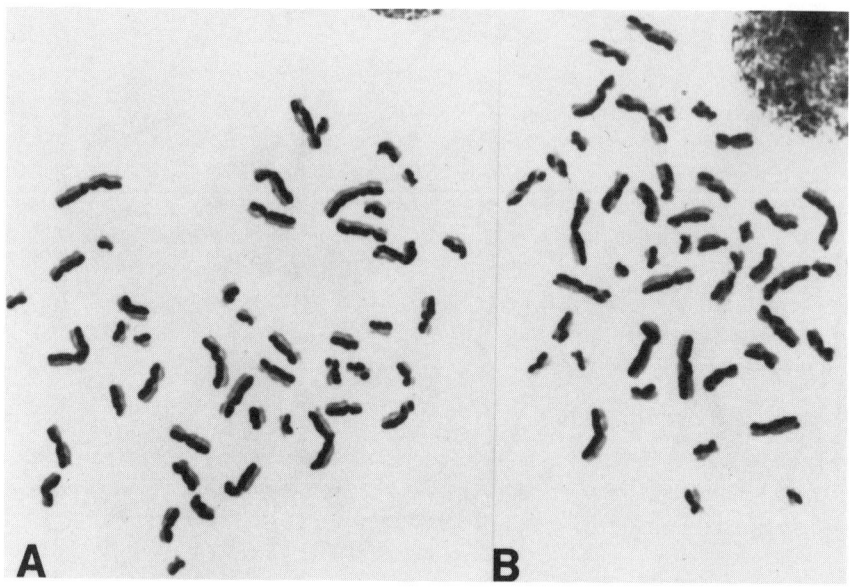

Figure 6-2. SCEs in human lymphocytes. Each panel shows differentially stained chromosomes from a human lymphocyte in metaphase. **A.** Cell from a control (unexposed) culture shows eight SCEs. **B.** Cell from a culture exposed to 0.1 mg/ml of vinyl carbamate shows approximately 40 SCEs. (Photograph from Allen et al. [1984] reprinted with permission from publisher and author.)

mentioned study hypotheses, heterogeneity of the study population, and the desired precision of results as factors that influence the number of cells scored. Many investigators score 50 cells (25 from each of two replicate cultures), as Anderson et al. (1986) and others suggest.

Hirsch et al. (1984) performed a computer simulation study that indicated that scoring 50 cells per person is appropriate. Scoring additional cells gives only modest increases in statistical power to detect differences between groups, unless variation in SCEs among cells within individuals is unusually high. Hirsch et al. point out that increasing the number of individuals in the study, scoring additional cells per person, or both can improve the ability to detect differences in SCE levels between groups. They provide tables that can be used to help estimate the number of persons and cells per person required to detect SCE percentage differences of varying magnitudes between groups.

Effects of Protocol Variations in the Assay

A number of protocol variations can influence the outcome of the assay. Important factors include the duration of sample storage before culture, the BrdUrd concentration, the time at which the mitogen is added, whether the investigator uses the macroculture or microculture technique, and other variables. The upcoming sections review these factors.

Sample Storage Before Culture

If possible, researchers should begin lymphocyte culture immediately after collecting the blood. Although heparinized blood can be stored for several days at 4–37°C, storage can lead to lymphocyte death, reduction of mitogenic response, and selective loss of cells with lesions that can result in SCE formation (Bloom, 1981). In a limited study of blood storage conditions and SCE formation, Lambert et al. (1982) found that storing blood for 8 to 24 hours caused a modest reduction in the mean number of SCEs per cell and in the number of cells with high SCE frequencies. Carrano et al. (1980) found small reductions in SCE frequencies after a week of storage in a study of four persons. More extensive studies with longer storage durations under various conditions would be helpful to design protocols for field studies of SCEs.

BrdUrd Concentration

Because BrdUrd itself causes SCEs in a dose-dependent manner, the BrdUrd concentration in the culture medium is a factor of great importance in determining the measured background level of SCEs (Lambert et al., 1976; Crossen, 1982; Lambert et al., 1982). BrdUrd induction of SCEs apparently depends on the ratio of BrdUrd concentration to the number of dividing cells per culture; within any given study, an investigator will need to standardize this ratio across cultures as much as possible (Stetka and Carrano, 1977; Bloom, 1981; Crossen, 1982). Otherwise, different numbers of cells across cultures will be competing for a given amount of BrdUrd. Because BrdUrd causes SCEs, current techniques cannot give a direct measure of the true background rate of SCEs. The artifactual background level of SCEs does not necessarily cause validity problems in comparisons of different groups, because an identical assay should produce the same baseline levels in all groups. One should remember, however, that the assays in no way measure the frequency of SCEs that actually occur among humans in vivo, because the assays are conducted on cultured cells, and the measurement procedure itself causes SCEs. Nevertheless, the marker allows investigators to make inferences about relative frequencies of in vivo alterations among individuals.

Timing of PHA Addition

To stimulate mitosis, an investigator adds a mitogen, usually PHA, to the culture. The timing of this addition, that is, whether PHA is added to whole blood before separation of cells or added directly to the culture, can affect the SCE frequency in the culture (Lambert et al., 1982). According to these researchers, differential selection of lymphocyte subpopulations may account for this observation.

Lymphocyte cultures contain T and B lymphocytes and other lymphocyte subpopulations, all of which vary in their proliferative response to specific mitogens. Because lymphocyte subpopulations vary in their half-lives, the detectable prevalence of exposure-related DNA lesions in a cell culture may depend on the types of lymphocytes that are stimulated to divide. Most human studies are based on T lymphocytes because PHA primarily stimulates this subpopulation. Although possible differential selection of lymphocytes is a nuisance in some respects, comparison of subpopulations could theoretically allow investigators to use markers in cells with different half-lives to estimate the timing of past exposures (Perera, 1987).

Macroculture Versus Microculture Technique

An alternative to the so-called macroculture technique described previously uses 0.5 ml rather than 10 ml of whole blood. In a study of 19 persons, Lambert et al. (1982) found that the microculture technique yielded a 40 percent lower mean SCE frequency compared with the macroculture. They attributed the difference to the fact that the microculture technique uses fetal calf serum as a nutrient instead of the autologous human serum typically used in macrocultures. Lambert et al. found higher SCE frequencies in cultures that used autologous serum compared with cultures that used fetal calf serum. They speculated that variation in SCE frequencies among individuals could result from different factors in their sera that influence SCEs. In contrast, Crossen (1982) found no differences in SCE frequencies between cultures that used autologous human serum and cultures that used fetal calf serum, and other researchers found lower frequencies when they used autologous serum (Gosh and Nand, 1979). Crossen (1982) suggested that different batches of fetal calf serum vary in their content of SCE-inducing factors and recommended pretesting to eliminate batches that increase SCEs. If human serum does vary with regard to SCE-inducing factors, the use of fetal calf serum in the culture medium may reduce the variance in measured SCE frequencies among humans.

Additional Variables in the Assay

In addition to BrdUrd concentration, PHA timing, and culture technique, other variations in SCE assays can also affect the measured frequency. For example, exposing the culture to light (other than red or yellow) dramatically increases SCE frequencies, and different culture media also influence frequencies (Crossen, 1982). In view of the numerous laboratory parameters that are determinants of observed SCE frequencies, the large variation in SCE scores observed across studies (Crossen, 1982) is not surprising.

In Vivo Sister Chromatid Exchange Assays

In addition to in vitro assays, extensive in vivo testing has been performed in both mammalian and nonmammalian systems. The protocols involve exposing test animals both to agents of interest and to BrdUrd (Latt et al., 1981; NTP, 1984). The major advantage of in vivo SCE assays is the incorporation of host mediation, that is, metabolism of the agent of interest. Furthermore, in vivo testing of animals also allows investigators to examine tissues that are not readily available from humans, such as germ cells or internal organ cells. In vivo assays thus permit comparisons of the sensitivity of various tissues to the mutagenic effects of agents of interest. Similarly, comparisons of in vivo animal assays with human in vitro assay data may provide insight into differences between the exposure-specific responses of humans and of animal models. Although this chapter focuses on in vitro laboratory methods and studies of human populations, in vivo testing in animal systems should be considered a valuable adjunct for evaluating SCEs.

EPIDEMIOLOGIC CONSIDERATIONS IN SISTER CHROMATID EXCHANGE TESTING

Epidemiologists must consider more than just sources of assay variability in determining the usefulness of SCEs for their research. Such issues as the sensitivity and specificity of the assay, the distribution of SCEs in individuals and groups, potential confounders, and research opportunities are concerns that need to be addressed in an evaluation of the SCE assay. These topics are discussed in the following sections.

Exposure Sensitivity and Specificity

Epidemiologists define exposure sensitivity as the proportion of exposed individuals identified by the measurement technique. This is analogous to the epidemiologic use of the term *sensitivity* in disease screening, where it denotes the correctly classified proportion of diseased persons (Mausner and Bahn, 1974). As Chapter 3 points out, other scientific disciplines use definitions of sensitivity and specificity that differ from the epidemiologic definition. For the SCE assay, estimates of exposure sensitivity in the epidemiologic sense are essentially nonexistent.

If exposure sensitivity is the measure of interest, some standard for ascertaining true exposure status must be identified. With regard to SCEs and a given chemical, *true exposure* could be defined variously as contact with any ambient level of the chemical, any level of internal dose, or at least one DNA lesion resulting from the chemical exposure. Consequently, the sensitivity of SCEs as a marker of a particular exposure depends on the definition of the exposure, as all ambient exposures will not necessarily produce internal doses high enough to cause DNA lesions. Given their biological properties, SCEs are theoretically most useful as markers of DNA lesions, rather than as more general markers of internal dose. Exposure sensitivity in the epidemiologic sense, then, ideally should be calculated to be the proportion of persons with DNA lesions who show elevated levels of SCEs.

The above definition of exposure sensitivity raises many operational problems. One must decide how many DNA lesions constitute an exposed state, what level of SCEs is higher than background, how the SCE level in one biological sample compares with the levels in other tissues and cell populations, and what the "gold standard" for estimating the true underlying prevalence of DNA lesions will be. Because of these operational issues, an epidemiologic definition of exposure sensitivity with respect to SCEs may have limited utility.

An alternative formulation of exposure sensitivity might use an approach like that of Latt et al. (1981), who reported the exposure concentrations that doubled the background level of SCEs for different chemicals in a variety of animal species and tissues. For those exposures that did double the level, the required doses of active chemical were usually about 10^{-4} to 10^{-5} mole/kg body weight, although many exceptions occurred outside of this range. In human studies, one might estimate the dose required to produce a 50 percent or other detectable percent increase in SCEs over the background level in a nonexposed group. Precise exposure information will usually be unavailable, however, so most statements about exposure sensitivity and SCEs in human populations must be qualitative rather than quantitative.

Exposure specificity in the epidemiologic sense is the proportion of nonexposed persons who are correctly classified as nonexposed by the measurement technique. Again, this definition is analogous to the epidemiologic definition of specificity used in disease screening, where it indicates the correctly classified proportion of nondiseased individuals (Mausner and Bahn, 1974). In general, the operational difficulties that apply to SCEs and sensitivity also apply to specificity. Nonmutagenic exposures in vitro usually do not cause an increase in SCEs (NTP, 1984), but, as discussed in greater detail later, confounders can cause false-positive results in human populations, because many exposures in addition to the exposure of interest can elevate the number of SCEs.

Sister Chromatid Exchange Distribution

With some exceptions, SCEs occur randomly among the chromosomes, and the number of SCEs per chromosome correlates positively with chromosome length (Block, 1982). Almost all lymphocytes from an individual contain at least one SCE as measured with current assays. A single cell may have 20 or more SCEs, however, and the distribution among cells is positively skewed (Crossen, 1982; Soper et al., 1984). That is, many cells in a sample have a small number of SCEs, but relatively few cells contain a large number; therefore, the frequency distribution of SCEs among cells within individuals has an asymmetrical shape.

Hirsch et al. (1984) and Anderson et al. (1986) examined a number of different theoretical frequency distributions to identify those that best describe the distribution of SCEs in human lymphocytes. Identification of appropriate distributions helps in selecting statistical tests for SCE differences between populations of individuals. For most people in their samples, these researchers found that the negative binomial and normal distributions adequately fit the distribution of SCEs among cells. The Poisson distribution, on the other hand, fit the data poorly, presumably because the scored lymphocytes include a heterogeneous mixture of subpopulations with differences in longevity, sensitivity to mutagens, or other biological differences (Carrano and Moore, 1982; Margolin and Shelby, 1985). The SCEs within each lymphocyte subpopulation may follow a Poisson distribution, and the negative binomial distribution can fit a mixture of Poisson distributions.

The individual means and the individual variances are significantly correlated; that is, persons with a large mean number of SCEs per cell also show a large variance in the number of SCEs per cell. As a result, Anderson et al. (1986) and Soper et al. (1984) recommended using a log transformation of each person's mean SCEs per cell as a dependent variable in analysis of variance (ANOVA) models. Hirsch et al. (1984) applied log or square root transformations to the SCE frequency for each cell.

Although the distribution of SCEs per cell is positively skewed within a given individual, the mean SCE frequency per cell among individuals follows a symmetrical normal distribution (Crossen, 1982). Researchers typically use the mean SCE frequency per cell to characterize an individual's SCE levels and base comparisons of groups on the overall mean of individuals' means. In addition, Carrano and Moore (1982) hypothesized the existence of cells with abnormally high SCE frequencies, which they termed high frequency cells. According to these investigators, the presence of high frequency cells may be at least as important as mean frequencies in analyzing SCEs, because they may reflect persistent, cumulative effects or the existence of particularly sensitive lymphocyte subpopulations, or both. They also conclude that analyses of high frequency cells have greater power to detect individuals with elevated SCE frequencies, whereas comparisons of mean SCE levels have more power to detect differences in SCE levels between groups. Margolin and Shelby (1985) have proposed the H value, an index of heterogeneity, as an appropriate measure of high frequency cells. The H value is the variance to mean ratio estimated from the SCE distribution in each person's sample of cells.

Ideally, the variability in SCE frequencies between individuals should be greater than that within individuals, and different scorers should show close agreement. Anderson et al. (1986) found substantially more variation between individuals than between replicate cultures from the same people, although they did find significant variation between replicate cultures. When they resampled 32 individuals over about 7 weeks, they found similar SCE frequencies on both occasions. Crossen (1982) found nonsignificant variations in mean SCEs per cell in 17 of 20 people sampled repeatedly at 3-month or greater intervals; he attributed the significant differences in the other three people to possible exposure to SCE-inducing factors. Tucker et al. (1987) found larger variations in mean SCE levels between individuals than within individuals resampled at daily or twice-weekly intervals, but the temporal variation was statistically significant. Because the proportion of high frequency cells varied less over time than did mean SCE levels, Tucker et al. suggest that analyses of high frequency cells may be superior to comparisons of mean SCE levels. Soper et al. (1984) also found more variation between persons than for the same persons resampled at 6-month or yearly intervals. In general, most studies indicate that SCE frequencies remain fairly constant over time if exposures and assay conditions are also constant (Crossen, 1982), although differences in SCE frequencies between samples increase with increasing time between samples (Tucker et al., 1988).

Differences in scoring may influence the variability found in SCE distributions. Soper et al. (1984) found significant interreader variability that weakened observed associations between SCEs and various independent variables. Anderson et al. (1986), on the other hand, found no significant variation in SCE scores among different readers in a laboratory with very careful quality control. Although Tucker et al. (1987) found statistically significant differences between readers, they felt that the differences were small enough to ignore in most studies.

Statistical techniques for SCE analysis are still under development. Temporal elements, choice of controls, underlying response model, and departures from the response model may be relevant areas of statistical concern (Archer, 1984). Margolin and Shelby (1985) have urged that investigators publish individual SCE data, rather than simple group means, to serve as a catalyst for the development of SCE data analysis techniques.

Potential Confounders in Studies of Sister Chromatid Exchanges

Because many different chemical exposures can increase SCE frequencies, observed differences in SCEs between groups in an epidemiologic study could result from exposures other than the one of primary interest. Cigarette smoking provides an excellent example. Smokers have about 20 percent more SCEs than do nonsmokers (Lambert et al., 1982; Anderson et al., 1986), and confounding can occur if smokers are differentially distributed among groups being compared with respect to some other exposure. Most studies have found no association between SCEs and age (e.g., Anderson et al., 1986), although some (e.g., Soper et al., 1984) found a weak positive association.

Recent studies indicate that women have roughly 10 percent more SCEs than do men (Anderson et al., 1986; Bender et al., 1988). Margolin and Shelby (1985) reviewed data from 12 major SCE studies and found a small but significant increase of 0.5 SCEs per cell for women as compared to men. Preliminary findings from Tucker et al. (1987) suggest that SCE frequencies show three different peaks during the menstrual cycle. These authors also summarize the conflicting studies of SCEs with regard to pregnancy and oral contraceptive use.

The Margolin and Shelby (1985) analysis of data from Butler's (1981) study showed differences in SCE levels by race using comparisons based on H values, but systematic scoring differences across races may have contributed to the race effect. Bender et al. (1988) found no SCE differences between whites and blacks in a larger study with careful scoring. They compared SCE means rather than H values, however, and SCE means were not sensitive to race differences in Butler's (1981) data.

Other potential confounders include vaccinations and drug therapy. Crossen (1982) summarized limited data that indicate that smallpox and measles vaccinations increase SCEs for days or weeks. Although naladixic acid therapy and treatment with melphalan resulted in elevated SCE levels, therapy with known mutagenic drugs such as metronidazole, actinomycin D, and PUVA (8-methoxypsoralen combined with ultraviolet A light) caused no significant increase in SCEs (Lambert et al., 1982). Lambert speculates that the negative findings may result from differences in metabolism between in vivo and in vitro test systems, or that clinical dosages were too low to produce detectable SCEs above background.

Opportunities for Retrospective Studies

Although some mutagenic exposures may produce only transiently elevated SCE levels, retrospective case-control studies of chronic diseases using SCEs as exposure markers are possible if cells are frozen at liquid nitrogen temperatures and properly thawed to maintain viability. Case-control studies might be nested within cohorts selected on some criterion other than exposure status, such as blood donation or clinic attendance. In such situations, although each cohort member initially provides blood samples, SCE assays are conducted only on a subset of controls and cases with a disease outcome of interest. This kind of study could answer the question of whether SCE levels in lymphocytes are themselves associated with subsequent cancer or other diseases, and the design would be more efficient than would a prospective cohort design requiring assays of all baseline blood samples. Alternatively, the nested case-control approach could make use of stored blood from a cohort with a particular exposure; the samples could be used to study the relationship between different exposure levels and the subsequent development of disease.

HUMAN SISTER CHROMATID EXCHANGE STUDIES

SCEs have been investigated in numerous human studies, including investigations of life-style factors, occupational exposures, disease states, and therapeutic exposures. Table 6-2 summarizes studies of diet, tobacco use, and medical therapy. Table 6-3 summarizes occupational SCE studies.

The investigations described here were chosen to represent a variety of exposures and populations. Compared with the literature on other markers (e.g., urine mutagenesis), these studies show such superior design elements as relatively large sample sizes, greater attention to choice of control groups, and increased control of confounders.

Diet, Trace Minerals, and Tobacco Use

Wulf et al. (1986) studied SCE frequency and diet among three geographically separate groups of Greenlandic Eskimos with a total sample of 147 persons. The different groups had different levels of seal consumption, which is a key element of traditional Eskimo diet and one with a high heavy metal content. The investigators scored 30 cells per person (some consider this a small number), and expressed the results as mean SCEs per cell. Multiple regression analyses considered sex, age, tobacco use, diet, area of residence, and blood levels of lead, mercury, selenium, and cadmium. For the regression model that included lead and mercury (but not selenium and cadmium), diet, residence, age, tobacco use, and mercury were all significantly related to the number of SCEs per cell with a linear dose–response. In both this model and one that also included selenium and cadmium, the traditional seal meat diet was the most important predictor of increased SCEs. A possible bias in Wulf's work lies in the relatively long time lag between blood sample collection and SCE testing; in many instances, 4–7 days elapsed before testing. If samples from the communities with the highest seal consumption (presumably the most remote) experienced the longest delays, and if the delays reduced SCEs, Wulf's results may understate the true association.

Adhvaryu et al. (1986) examined small groups of East Indian patients suffering from oral submucous fibrosis (SMF), a chronic fibrotic change of the oral tissues

Table 6-2 Studies of SCEs and Life-Style or Therapeutic Exposures

Reference	Exposure	Sample size	Cells scored per person	Reported results
Wulf et al. (1986)	Diet	147	30	+
Adhvaryu et al. (1986)	Tobacco/betel nut chewing	35	25	+
Kelsey et al. (1986)	Asbestos and cigarette smoking	32	50	+
Hou et al. (1985)	Acute leukemia	60	20–50	+
Kärki et al. (1986)	Multiple sclerosis	28	25	+
Aronson et al. (1982)	Drug and radiation therapy	54	50	+

Table 6-3 Studies of SCEs and Occupational Exposures

Reference	Exposure	Sample size	Cells scored per person	Reported results
Pohlová et al. (1986)	Cytotoxic drug manufacturing	57	30	+
Stiller et al. (1983)	Cytotoxic drug handling	19	25	−
Jordan et al. (1986)	Cytotoxic drug handling	36	30	−
Stolley et al. (1984)	Ethylene oxide	234	80	+
Yager et al. (1983)	Ethylene oxide	27	50	+
Mäki-Paakkanen et al. (1984)	Rubber industry	90	30	+
Nagaya (1986)	Chromium plating industry	48	25	−

thought to be a cancer precursor. Blood was drawn from 20 long-time tobacco/betel nut chewers, 10 of whom had SMF, and from 15 controls who had never used any form of tobacco or betel nut, and who had been screened for recent viral infections and current medication use. Mean SCE scores for each individual and group were calculated from 25 scored cells per person. Group means were significantly higher for chewers (both SMF patients and so-called normal chewers) than for controls, whereas SMF patients and normal chewers had essentially the same mean number of SCEs.

In a study of workers occupationally exposed to asbestos, Kelsey et al. (1986) examined 22 male asbestos-exposed workers (11 smokers and 11 nonsmokers) and 10 unexposed workers (four smokers and six nonsmokers) of the same age. Mean SCE scores were calculated from 50-cell scores, and the data were analyzed by t-tests and one-way ANOVA. Cigarette smoking significantly increased the baseline number of SCEs. Asbestos exposure was associated with a small nonsignificant increase in SCEs, and a positive interaction between asbestos and smoking approached nominal statistical significance.

Sister Chromatid Exchanges in Disease States

The SCEs have been investigated both as markers of disease states and as indicators of therapy. Several studies have shown extremely high SCE levels in patients with Bloom's syndrome. Other genetic DNA repair defects, however, apparently do not cause dramatically elevated SCE levels (Zakharov, 1982).

Hou et al. (1985) studied SCEs in 49 cases of acute leukemia and found increases among patients before therapy. Mean levels of SCEs were significantly higher for 36 acute nonlymphocytic leukemias and for 13 cases of acute lymphocytic leukemia compared with 11 healthy controls. In nine treated cases where complete remission occurred within 6 months of treatment, SCE levels were significantly lower than pretreatment levels, but significantly higher than among healthy controls.

Kärki et al. (1986) studied SCEs in patients with multiple sclerosis. Fourteen clinically established multiple sclerosis patients were matched by age and sex with healthy controls drawn from a population of laboratory workers and blood donors. Mean SCE levels were significantly higher among patients compared with controls after a standard 72-hour incubation, but prolonged incubation (9 days) reduced the relatively high level of SCEs among multiple sclerosis patients.

A study of acute and long-term effects of drug and radiation therapies in childhood cancer (Aronson et al., 1982) included SCEs and chromosome aberrations. Pretreatment cancer patients, patients undergoing therapy, posttherapy patients, and adult noncancer controls provided a total of 53 individuals. Fifty cells were scored per person. Among pretreatment patients and posttherapy patients, SCE levels were comparable with those of controls. The SCEs increased, however, among patients undergoing chemotherapy compared both with healthy controls and to pretreatment patients. The authors speculated that the considerable variability among individuals may be due to the broad representation of tumor types included in the study. The use of adults, 30 percent of whom smoked cigarettes, as noncancer controls was probably inappropriate. Data on chromosome breakage followed the same general pattern as the SCE findings.

Occupational Exposures and Sister Chromatid Exchanges

Two areas of occupational exposure have been extensively investigated for an association with SCEs: health-care workers handling cytotoxic drugs and workers exposed to ethylene oxide. Pohlová et al. (1986) investigated SCEs, chromosomal aberrations, and urine mutagenicity among 38 chemists and plant workers who were exposed to alkylating agents and other drugs during research and pilot production of newly developed cytotoxic drugs. Nineteen controls were chosen from presumably unexposed plant librarians and clerks, and matched on age and sex. All participants completed questionnaires on health history, smoking, and x-ray exposures. For the SCE assays, 30 cells were scored per participant, and differences between group means were evaluated with a t-test. Exposed workers had significantly elevated levels of SCEs (8.94 per cell compared with 5.81). Frequency of chromosome aberrations (defined as breaks) and urine mutagenicity was also significantly higher among exposed workers.

Two other studies, however, found no significant elevation in SCEs among hospital workers handling cytotoxic drugs. Stiller et al. (1983) assayed SCEs and chromosomal aberrations in 9 exposed workers and 10 unexposed controls and found no differences between exposed and unexposed participants. Six controls, however, smoked cigarettes and only two exposed workers smoked, so smoking differences could have masked SCE elevations from the drug exposures. Jordan et al. (1986) found no difference in the mean number of SCEs between two groups of 18 nurses each. One group handled cytotoxic agents an average of 3 days per work week, whereas the other never came in contact with oncology patients. All members of both groups were women, and comparable in age, smoking history, medication history, and alcohol intake. Regression analyses showed no association between mean number of SCEs and number of drug-handling days. Although the data suggested a relatively high prevalence of high frequency cells (i.e., individual cells with a large number of SCEs) among the exposed group, the difference was not statistically significant. The investigators scored only 30 cells per person. Although the reasons are unclear for the differences in results between the studies of plant workers and hospital workers, possible differences in study design and analysis, exposure levels, and drug toxicity may contribute to the disparate findings.

In a study of workers exposed to ethylene oxide, Stolley et al. (1984) identified three industrial sites with low (site I), intermediate (site II), and high (site III) exposures to the agent. At each site, workers were further characterized by potential exposure levels based on job classification. At sites I and II, the researchers chose worksite controls; at site III, they used both worksite and community controls. Blood samples were collected from a total of 234 persons at the start of the study and at 6-, 12-, and 24-month intervals. In over 91 percent of the assays, the researchers scored at least 80 cells. Age, sex, smoking history, and variability among scorers were controlled using ANOVA. At site III (high exposure), they found large differences in SCEs among high- and low-potential exposure groups that persisted throughout the 24-month study period. At site II, the investigators found a higher frequency of SCEs in the high-potential exposed group than in other groups, but found no consistent differences at site I.

Yager et al. (1983) studied ethylene oxide exposures among 14 hospital workers and 13 unexposed controls. They characterized exposure as high or low based on 6-month cumulative estimates from self-reports that were supported by hospital records that documented the use of ethylene oxide sterilizers. Age, sex, medical histories, and caffeine, alcohol,and other drug use were similarly distributed between exposed workers and controls. Although an equal number of exposed workers and controls smoked, smokers among the exposed workers smoked an average of nine cigarettes per day compared to 21 for controls. Fifty cells were scored in each assay, and data were analyzed with the Mann-Whitney U test. The mean frequency of SCEs was significantly higher among exposed workers compared with controls. Furthermore, a significant increase appeared when high-exposure workers were compared with those with low exposure.

A small number of studies have focused on SCEs and chromosome aberrations among rubber workers and metal plating workers. Mäki-Paakkanen et al. (1984) studied chromosome aberrations and SCEs among rubber workers in two manufacturing plants. They compared 55 workers exposed to complex mixtures of rubber manufacturing compounds with 35 controls from office jobs in the same factory or from a research institute. Thirty cells per assay were scored for SCEs, and a single scorer rated all the assays. Among nonsmokers, there was a significant increase in SCEs among exposed compared with unexposed persons in both factories. For both smoking workers and smoking controls, mean SCE frequencies were higher than for nonsmokers.

Nagaya (1986) compared SCEs among 24 workers in the chromium plating industry with 24 unexposed office workers matched for sex and age. An attempt was made to match on smoking history, but smokers averaged from 5–40 cigarettes per day, and "nonsmokers" included anyone who had not smoked for the previous 2 years, regardless of lifetime tobacco consumption. Twenty-five cells per assay were scored for SCEs, and urine chromium was analyzed by atomic absorption. The SCE levels and urinary chromium were not correlated, and mean SCE frequencies did not differ significantly between the chromium platers and the unexposed controls. The SCEs among smokers of both exposed and control groups, however, were significantly higher than SCEs among nonsmokers.

Numerous other studies have compared SCE levels across groups defined by lifestyle, demographic, exposure, or other characteristics, and virtually all epidemiologic studies of SCEs use them as dependent variables rather than as exposure markers in studies of exposure–disease associations. The link between SCEs and disease risk remains unclear. The fact that many mutagenic exposures cause SCEs, however, suggests that they may be associated with increased disease risk. Descriptive studies of SCEs are necessary, because the determinants of SCE levels in healthy individuals are still a subject of controversy. Only recently, for example, have most investigators agreed that SCEs vary by sex and smoking status, and studies of age and race effects are still inconclusive. The current limited state of knowledge about SCEs and their measurement suggests that their greatest contributions to epidemiology lie in the future.

SUMMARY

1. SCEs are a form of chromosomal alteration. Although a background level of SCEs exists in the absence of identifiable mutagenic exposure, an increased SCE level is generally interpreted as an exposure or response marker. Theoretically, SCEs are detectable through in vivo and in vitro assays using any cell type; most human studies, however, use circulating lymphocytes.

2. The DNA lesions thought to produce SCEs undergo repair processes that may prevent SCE formation. Therefore, the number of observed SCEs can depend, in part, on the time between exposure and the sampling of biological material.

3. The SCE assay is most useful in detecting exposures from alkylating chemicals, agents that induce single-strand DNA breakage, DNA-binding agents, and some DNA-base analogs.

4. Several laboratory issues can substantially affect the interpretation of assay data. Lag time between sample collection and culturing, standardization of culturing protocol, and scoring procedure are points that require attention. Because cell half-lives vary from days to several years, the specific cell type under study also affects assay interpretation.

5. Estimates of the sensitivity and specificity (in the epidemiologic sense) of the SCE assay for exposure assessment are not available, largely because of operational problems with the epidemiologic definition of sensitivity and specificity in the context of SCEs. One alternative definition of sensitivity is the exposure level that produces a specified percentage increase in SCEs compared with the background level.

6. Human studies of SCEs have found associations with such life-style factors as diet and smoking, occupational exposures, and therapeutic exposures. Different studies, however, often show conflicting results.

7. Given the importance of variations in laboratory methods, comparisons across studies should most likely be limited to qualitative assessments unless assay protocols are very similar or identical.

8. A clear connection between the presence of SCEs and morbidity has not yet been established. Furthermore, the assay is nonspecific in the sense that it cannot discriminate the effects of several different exposures. Thus, SCE data should be evaluated conservatively as indicators of damage to genetic material.

SCE analysis has been used primarily as an in vivo (in animals) and in vitro method of screening chemicals for genotoxic activity. It is now gaining importance as a useful marker of exposures to genotoxic agents in epidemiologic studies. Its utility is limited, however, to questions that can be addressed by a transient, nonspecific marker. Because the application of SCE analysis to epidemiologic studies began only recently, many methodologic issues require further resolution, and standardization of laboratory techniques across studies has yet to be accomplished. As their sophistication with SCE analysis increases, epidemiologists may apply this marker to investigations of a variety of research questions.

REFERENCES

Adhvaryu SG, Bhatt R, Dayal PK, Trivedi AH, Dave BH, Vyas RC, Jani KH: SCE frequencies in lymphocytes of tobacco/betal nut chewers and patients with oral submucous fibrosis. *Br J Cancer* 1986;53:141–143.

Allen JW, Sharief Y, Langenbach R, Waters MD: Tissue-specific sister chromatid exchange analyses in mutagen-carcinogen exposed animals. In: Langenbach R, Nesnow S, Rice JM, eds: *Organ and Species Specificity in Chemical Carcinogenesis.* New York, Plenum Publishing Corporation, 1983, pp. 451–472.

Allen JW, Brock K, Campbell J, Sharief Y: Sister chromatid exchange analysis in lymphocytes. In: Ansari AA, de Serres FJ, eds.: *Single-Cell Mutation Monitoring Systems.* New York, Plenum Publishing Corporation, 1984, pp. 145–163.

Anderson D, Dewdney RS, Jenkenson PC, Lovell DP, Butterworth KR, Conning DM: Sister chromatid exchange (SCE) analysis in 106 control individuals: Monitoring of occupational genotoxicants. In: Sorsa M, ed.: *Progress in Clinical and Biological Research.* New York, Alan R. Liss, Inc., 1986, pp. 39–58.

Archer PG: Some statistical and methodologic issues in cytogenetic testing. In: *Banbury Report 16: Genetic Variability in Response to Chemical Exposures.* Cold Spring Harbor, New York, Cold Spring Harbor Laboratory, 1984, pp. 369–376.

Aronson MM, Miller RC, Hill RB, Nichols WW, Meadows AT: Acute and long-term cytogenetic effects of treatment in childhood cancer: Sister chromatid exchanges and chromosome aberrations. *Mutat Res* 1982;92:291–307.

Bender MA, Griggs HG, Bedford JS: Recombinational DNA repair and sister chromatid exchanges. *Mutat Res* 1974;24:117–123.

Bender MA, Preston RJ, Leonard RC, Pyatt BE, Gooch PC, Shelby MD: Chromosomal aberration and sister-chromatid exchange frequencies in peripheral blood lymphocytes of a large human population sample. *Mutat Res* 1988;204:421–433.

Block AMW: Chapter 2, Sister chromatid exchange methodology. In: Sandberg AA, ed.: *Sister Chromatid Exchange.* New York, Alan R. Liss Inc., 1982, pp. 13–32.

Bloom AD, ed.: *Guidelines for Studies of Human Populations Exposed to Mutagenic and Reproductive Hazards.* March of Dimes Birth Defects Foundation, 1981.

Butler MG: Sister chromatid exchange in 4 human races. *Mutat Res* 1981;91:377–379.

Carrano AV: Chromosomal alterations as markers of exposure and effect. *J Occup Med* 1986;28:1112–1116.

Carrano AV, Minkler JL, Stetka DG, Moore DH II: Variation in the baseline sister chromatid exchange frequency in human lymphocytes. *Environ Mutagen* 1980;2:325–337.

Carrano AV, Moore DH: The rationale and methodology for quantifying sister chromatid exchange. In: Heddle JA, ed.: *Mutagenicity: New horizons in Genetic Toxicology.* New York, Academic Press, 1982, pp. 267–304.

Crossen PE: Chapter 11, SCE in lymphocytes. In: Sandberg AA, ed.: *Sister Chromatid Exchange.* New York, Alan R. Liss Inc., 1982, pp. 175–193.

Gebhart E: Sister chromatid exchange (SCE) and structural chromosome aberration in mutagenicity testing. *Hum Genet* 1981;58:235–254.

Gosh PK, Nand R: Reduced frequency of sister chromatid exchanges in human lymphocytes cultured with autologous serum. *Hum Genet* 1979;51:167–170.

Hirsch B, McGue M, Cervenka J: Characterization of the distribution of sister chromatid exchange frequencies: Implications for research design. *Hum Genet* 1984;65:280–286.

Hou YH, Li XR, Li DG, Zhang A: Sister chromatid exchange and cell cycle in peripheral lymphocytes in patients with acute leukemia. *Chin Med J* 1985;98:598–602.

Ishii Y, Bender MA: Effects of inhibitors of DNA synthesis on spontaneous and ultraviolet light-induced sister chromatid exchanges in Chinese hamster cells. *Mutat Res* 1980;79:19–32.

Jordan DK, Patil SR, Jochimsen PR, Lachenbruch PA, Corder MP: Sister chromatid exchange analysis in nurses handling antineoplastic drugs. *Cancer Invest* 1986;4(2):101–107.

Kärki NT, Ilonen J, Reunanen M: Increased sister-chromatid exchange rate and its regression during prolonged incubation in lymphocyte cultures from patients with multiple sclerosis. *Mutat Res* 1986;160:215–219.

Kato H: Mechanisms for sister chromatid exchanges and their relation to the production of chromosomal aberrations. *Chromosoma* 1977;59:179–191.

Kelsey KT, Christiani DC, Little JB: Enhancement of benzo(a)pyrene-induced sister chromatid exchanges in lymphocytes from cigarette smokers occupationally exposed to asbestos. *JNCI* 1986;77:321–327.

Lambert B, Hansson K, Lindsten J, Sten M, Werelius B: Bromodeoxyuridine-induced sister chromatid exchanges in human lymphocytes. *Hereditas* 1976;83:163–174.

Lambert B, Lindblad A, Holmberg K, Francesconi D: Chapter 6, The use of sister chromatid exchange to monitor human populations for exposure to toxicologically harmful agents. In: Wolff S, ed.: *Sister Chromatid Exchange*. New York, John Wiley & Sons, 1982, pp. 149–182.

Langley LL: *Physiology of Man*. New York, Van Nostrand Reinhold, 1971, p. 270.

Latt SA, Allen J, Bloom SE, Carrano A, Falke E, Kram D, Schneider E, Schreck R, Tice R, Whitfield B, Wolff S: Sister chromatid exchanges: A report of the gene-tox program. *Mutat Res* 1981;87:17–62.

Laurent C: SCE increases after an accidental acute inhalation exposure to EtO and recovery to normal after 2 years. *Mutat Res* 1988;204:711–717.

Mäki-Paakkanen J, Sorsa M, Vainio H: Sister chromatid exchanges and chromosome aberrations in rubber workers. *Teratogenesis Carcinog Mutagen* 1984;4:189–200.

Margolin BH, Shelby MD: Sister chromatid exchanges: A reexamination of the evidence for sex and race differences in humans. *Environ Mutagen* 1985;7(Suppl 4):63–72.

Mausner JS, Bahn AK: *Epidemiology: An introductory text*. Philadelphia, WB Saunders, 1974, p. 242.

Nagaya T: No increase in sister-chromatid exchange frequency in lymphocytes of chromium platers. *Mutat Res* 1986;170:129–132.

National Toxicology Program, Board of Scientific Counselors: Report of the Ad Hoc Panel on Chemical Carcinogenesis Testing and Evaluation. August 17, 1984.

Painter RB: A replication model for sister chromatid exchange. *Mutat Res.* 1980;70:337–341.

Perera FP: Molecular cancer epidemiology: A new tool in cancer prevention. *JNCI* 1987;78:887–898.

Pohlová H, Černá M, Rössner P: Chromosomal aberrations, SCE and urine mutagenicity in workers occupationally exposed to cytostatic drugs. *Mutat Res* 1986;174:213–217.

Sarto F, Cominata I, Pinton AM, Brovedani PG, Faccioli CM, Bianchi V, Levis AG: Cytogenetic damage in workers exposed to ethylene oxide. *Mutat Res* 1984;138:185–195.

Soper KA, Stolley PD, Galloway SM, Smith JG, Nichols WW, Wolman SR: Sister-chromatid exchange (SCE) report on control subjects in a study of occupationally exposed workers. *Mutat Res* 1984;129:77–88.

Stetka DG, Carrano AV: The interaction of Hoechst 33258 and BrdU substituted DNA in the formation of sister chromatid exchange. *Chromosoma* 1977;36:21–31.

Stiller A, Obe G, Boll I, Pribilla W: No elevation of the frequencies of chromosomal alterations as a consequence of handling cytostatic drugs: analyses with peripheral blood and urine of hospital personnel. *Mutat Res* 1983;121:253–259.

Stolley PD, Soper KA, Galloway SM, Nichols WW, Norman SA, Wolman S: Sister-chromatid exchanges in association with occupational exposure to ethylene oxide. *Mutat Res* 1984;129:89–102.

Tucker JD, Christensen ML, Strout CL, McGee KA, Carrano AV: Variation in the human lymphocyte sister chromatid exchange frequency as a function of time: Results of daily and twice-weekly sampling. *Environ Mol Mutagen* 1987;10:69–78.

Tucker JD, Ashworth LK, Johnston GR, Allen NA, Carrano AV: Variation in the human lymphocyte sister-chromatid exchange frequency: Results of a long-term longitudinal study. *Mutat Res* 1988;204:435–444.

Wolff S, Rodin B, Cleaver JE: Sister chromatid exchanges induced by mutagenic carcinogens in normal and xeroderma pigmentosum cells. *Nature* 1977;265:347–349.

Wulf HC, Husum B, Niebuhr E: Cessation of smoking enhances sister chromatid exchanges in lymphocytes. *Hereditas* 1985;102:195–198.

Wulf H, Kromann CN, Kousgaard N, Hansen JC, Niebuhr E, Albøge K: Sister chromatid exchange (SCE) in Greenlandic eskimos: Dose-response relationship between SCE and seal diet, smoking, and blood cadium and mercury concentrations. *Sci Total Environ* 1986;48:81–94.

Yager JW, Hines CJ, Spear RC: Exposure to ethylene oxide at work increases sister chromatid exchanges in human peripheral lymphocytes. *Science* 1983;219:1221–1223.

Zakharov AF: Chapter 1, Historical Aspects of Sister Chromatid Exchange. In: Sandberg AA, ed.: *Sister Chromatid Exchange*. New York, Alan R. Liss Inc., 1982, pp. 1–12.

7

MICRONUCLEI

MARILYN F. VINE

INTRODUCTION
What Are Micronuclei?

Micronuclei consist of small amounts of DNA that arise in the cytoplasm when chromatid/chromosomal fragments or whole chromosomes are not incorporated into daughter nuclei during mitosis, often because these fragments do not possess a centromere. Acentric fragments remain behind at anaphase, whereas chromosomal elements with centromeres are drawn toward the spindle poles (Schmid, 1975). The fragments of DNA left behind are incorporated into secondary nuclei. These, much smaller than the main nucleus of the cell, are known as micronuclei. Hence, the formation of micronuclei requires a dividing cell population. Micronuclei are about 1/20 to 1/5 the size of the main nucleus. Usually there is only one micronucleus formed per cell (Jenssen, 1982). The frequency of micronuclei is usually reported as the number of cells containing micronuclei per total cells counted.

Micronuclei may be formed as the result of agents that cause chromosome breaks (clastogens) or as the result of agents that cause damage to the spindle apparatus (Jenssen, 1982). Damage to DNA, which ultimately leads to the formation of micronuclei, may occur during various parts of the cell cycle and may result from exposure to a variety of environmental agents (see Chapter 8 for a review of the cell cycle). Methyl methanesulfonate (MMS) induces micronuclei during DNA synthesis, alkylating agents during the G_1 and DNA synthesis phases, and agents that operate on the spindle apparatus induce micronuclei during mitosis (Jenssen, 1982). Clastogenic agents, such as x-rays, often cause micronuclei to form by creating chromatid or chromosomal fragments, whereas agents that cause spindle dysfunction can lead to the formation of micronuclei from loss of whole chromosomes. Micronuclei that result from loss of whole chromosomes tend to be larger than those that result from chromosome breaks (Högstedt and Karlsson, 1985).

What Is Their Significance?

It is generally believed that any agent capable of causing structural damage to DNA is also potentially carcinogenic, as most carcinogens have been found to be mutagens (McCann and Ames, 1976). DNA damage can lead to oncogene amplification and transposition, mechanisms thought to be involved in the neoplastic transformation of cells (Stich, 1986).

The presence of micronuclei in a population of cells indicates chromosome damage that has occurred as the result of exposure to a variety of genotoxic agents that either cause chromosome breaks or spindle dysfunction. The frequency of micronuclei alone, however, cannot distinguish between these two types of damage. Thus, the frequency of micronuclei in the cells of a tissue serves as a marker of exposure and of biological response to genotoxic agents. An important characteristic of micronuclei is that they reflect damage that has occurred in the presence of the host's metabolic activation and detoxifying mechanisms.

The formation of micronuclei and the incidence of chromosome breakage or loss are believed to correlate in dividing cell populations (Heddle et al., 1983). In animal studies, micronuclei are associated with standard cytogenetic indices of chromosomal breakage (Goetz et al., 1975). Micronuclei are much easier and faster to score (Heddle, 1973), however, and are more sensitive indicators of chromosome damage than chromosome aberrations (Jensen and Hüttel, 1976; Jensen and Nyfors, 1979; Högstedt et al., 1981b). An increase in the incidence of micronuclei is associated with an increase in chromosome or chromatid aberrations (Jenssen, 1982). As noted previously, chromosomal aberrations are believed to be early steps in carcinogenesis, although there is no documented association between the frequency of chromosomal aberrations and the development of cancer.

History of the Micronucleus Assay

Micronuclei were originally discovered in red blood cells by Howell in 1891 and later characterized by Jolly in 1905. As a result, micronuclei in red blood cells are often referred to as Howell–Jolly bodies (Jenssen, 1982). Investigators have known for at least 50 years that micronuclei form in association with exposure to radiation. The first major attempt at using micronuclei as indicators of cytogenetic damage, however, was not done until fairly recently when Evans and co-workers (1959) exposed plant root tips to radiation (Heddle et al., 1983). In 1966, Schroeder (1966) showed that micronuclei occurred in bone marrow cells after cytogenetic damage by chemical mutagens. Schmid and co-workers (Boller and Schmid, 1970) and Heddle (1973) tried to determine which characteristics of bone marrow cells would best indicate cytogenetic damage in vivo. They concluded that the presence of micronuclei in polychromatic erythrocytes (PCEs) served as a particularly useful indicator of cytogenetic damage in mice (Heddle et al., 1983). Schmid and co-workers (Boller and Schmid, 1970) and Heddle (1973) independently devised a micronucleus test with mouse PCEs to detect chromosomal damage caused by genotoxic chemicals as a relatively quick and inexpensive method of screening for potential carcinogens.

Currently, there is no one micronucleus assay. Such tests can be performed on a variety of species and with different types of cells; the techniques differ depending on the cell type assayed. The assays have been performed most often with PCEs from mouse bone marrow. Bone marrow sampling, however, is highly invasive. Although the bone marrow assay has been used in occupational settings (Högstedt et al., 1981a), it is unlikely to be widely used in human populations. The bone marrow assay in humans may, therefore, be limited to hospitalized patients who have bone marrow samples taken for diagnostic or therapeutic purposes. For example, Högstedt et al. (1981b) explored the use of micronuclei in bone marrow cells as a prognostic indicator of survival among patients with acute nonlymphocytic leukemia. In general, however, such populations are unlikely to be representative of the groups to which one would like to make inferences. Because of its limited application for human studies, the bone marrow assay is not discussed further.

Micronucleus assays in humans have also been carried out using peripheral red blood cells (Schlegel et al., 1986), peripheral blood lymphocytes (Countryman and Heddle, 1976; Högstedt et al., 1983b; Pincu et al., 1984; Norman et al., 1978; 1985; Fenech and Morley, 1985, 1986; Högstedt and Karlsson, 1985; Kormos and Köteles, 1988), and exfoliated cells such as buccal mucosa cells and urinary tract cells (Stich et al., 1982, 1984, 1985; Stich and Rosin, 1983a,b; Stich and Rosin, 1984; Rosin and German, 1985; Fontham et al., 1986). The following section will review methods of performing these assays with various cell types and explore issues relating to their usefulness in epidemiologic research.

THE MICRONUCLEUS ASSAY AND PERIPHERAL BLOOD ERYTHROCYTES

Schlegel et al. (1986) studied the utility of the micronucleus assay in detecting genotoxic effects of chemical agents in peripheral blood erythrocytes (PBEs). PBEs are derived from erythroblasts, which are erthrocyte stem cells located in the bone marrow. Micronuclei are formed during the last mitosis leading to the development of PBEs. They remain in the PBEs even after the nucleus is expelled. Although perhaps not target cells of interest, PBEs may serve as indicators of exposure to genotoxic agents.

Assay Techniques (Schlegel et al., 1986)

1. Draw a sample of peripheral blood.
2. Apply to microscope slide.
3. Air dry smear.
4. Fix for 5 minutes in absolute methanol.
5. Stain with Wright's stain (for total erythrocytes) or acridine orange (for reticulocytes). (For acridine orange, immerse slides for 5 minutes in pH 7.4 sodium phosphate buffer (1% by weight) containing 0.02 mg acridine orange per milliliter. Rinse for 10 minutes in pH 7.4 phosphate buffer.)
6. Wet mount slides.
7. Examine by fluorescent microscopy using Zeiss fluorescein isocyanate filter.
8. Score micronuclei by hand at X 1000 magnification under oil in 2000 total erythrocytes per person.

Methodologic Issues

The chief obstacle in the use of peripheral blood erythrocytes is the fact that in healthy individuals the spleen removes micronucleated red blood cells from circulation. People with normally functioning spleens have very low frequencies of micronuclei (0/100,000 cells), even after treatment with a known clastogenic chemotherapy agent (Schlegel et al., 1986).

Schlegel et al. (1986) studied the effects of genotoxic agents on the frequency of micronuclei among splenectomized and nonsplenectomized individuals. Among 12 people with intact spleens who had not been exposed to radiation or chemotherapy, the frequency of micronuclei in PBEs was 0/56,000 cells analyzed. The frequency of micronuclei in PBEs of 16 people with intact spleens who had received at least 1 month of chemotherapy during the 4-month period before sampling was 0/100,000 cells. The authors note that one can detect an increased frequency of micronuclei in nonsplenectomized individuals receiving chemotherapy, if sampling is done shortly after administration of the drug. Because there is rapid removal by the spleen of micronucleated erythrocytes, the efficiency of the spleen will affect micronucleus frequencies.

Among splenectomized individuals who had not received chemotherapy, micronuclei began to appear in PBEs shortly after splenectomy. The frequency of micronuclei reached a steady state of 4/2,000 PBEs after 4 months. After chemotherapy, these people experienced an increase in frequency of micronuclei, with a higher frequency corresponding to increased duration of treatment. Those undergoing chemotherapy ultimately had micronucleus frequencies five times higher than splenectomized control levels. It was noted that micronuclei persisted in the PBEs of splenectomized individuals for about 120 days (the life span of an erythrocyte). About 4 months after the end of chemotherapy, the frequency of micronuclei returned to baseline levels.

If the exposure is not continuous, scoring total erythrocytes may not provide the information sought. Because many erythrocytes will have been derived from erythroblasts not exposed to the genotoxic agent, the assay would underestimate the effect of the exposure. The sensitivity of the assay could be improved by only evaluating newly formed reticulocytes that were derived from exposed erythroblasts in the bone marrow. Erythroblasts mature and give rise to circulating reticulocytes after about 3 to 4 days. Because reticulocytes are believed to appear in the blood within 3 to 4 days and disappear within 4 to 10 days, sampling would have to take place within 4 to 10 days after exposure to the agent. If total erythrocytes are scored, the sensitivity decreases but there is less of a chance of missing the point of highest elevation in micronucleus frequency. The other alternative is to examine micronucleus frequencies in both total erythrocytes and in reticulocytes (Schlegel et al., 1986).

Another methodologic consideration is that people who are folate deficient (even mildly so) have elevated levels of micronuclei in their peripheral blood erythrocytes (Everson et al., 1988). Therefore, investigators should control for folate levels in epidemiologic studies using the micronucleus assay with PBEs.

Summary of Advantages and Disadvantages of The Micronucleus Assay Using Peripheral Blood Erythrocytes

Advantages

1. The sampling technique for this assay, the drawing of peripheral blood, is relatively noninvasive.

2. The assay is fairly inexpensive and easy to perform.

3. A dose–response relationship has been noted between exposure (duration of

chemotherapy treatment) and frequency of micronuclei among splenectomized individuals (Schlegel et al., 1986).

4. The cessation of treatment leads to a decrease in micronucleus frequencies among splenectomized individuals (Schlegel et al., 1986).

Disadvantages

The major disadvantage of using the micronucleus assay with peripheral blood erythrocytes is that the spleen removes micronucleated erythrocytes from circulating blood. Thus, people with normally functioning spleens often do not have detectable levels of micronuclei. The efficiency of the spleen will also affect micronucleus frequencies. The use of this assay is, therefore, most likely limited to splenectomized subjects.

THE MICRONUCLEUS ASSAY AND PERIPHERAL BLOOD LYMPHOCYTES

Several investigators have explored the use of the micronucleus assay with peripheral blood lymphocytes (PBLs) (Countryman and Heddle, 1976; Norman et al., 1978, 1985; Högstedt et al., 1983b; Pincu et al., 1984; Fenech and Morley, 1985, 1986; Kormos and Köteles, 1988). Like PCEs and PBEs, lymphocytes may not necessarily be the target cell population of interest with respect to future development of disease, but the frequency of micronuclei in PBLs may serve as an in vivo index of exposure to genotoxic agents. As with PBEs, the sampling method involves drawing peripheral blood, a fairly noninvasive technique.

Methodologic Issues

Performing micronucleus assays with circulating blood lymphocytes presents a unique set of problems. In essence, the dilemma is that, although circulating lymphocytes are not a naturally dividing cell population, cell division is necessary to induce micronuclei. Inducing lymphocytes to divide in cell culture overcomes this limitation, allowing investigators to use an in vitro assay to detect genotoxic damage that occurs in vivo. But, because one cannot be certain that cell culture techniques do not themselves induce micronuclei, it is important to perform the micronucleus assay with control cells to quantify background frequencies induced by the technique.

Methods for using peripheral blood lymphocytes in micronucleus assays are currently under development. At least four different methods of preparing lymphocytes for the assay have been tested. Several investigators have scored micronuclei in lymphocytes after hypotonic treatment with potassium chloride. This method has been used to show elevated frequencies of micronuclei among patients after angiocardiography (Norman et al., 1978) and among smokers (Högstedt et al., 1983a), but it has drawbacks. The hypotonic treatment destroys the lymphocyte cytoplasm making detection of micronuclei difficult; micronuclei may also be indistinguishable from cellular debris or may become separated from the cell of origin (Högstedt, 1984).

Högstedt (1984) proposed a method of preparing lymphocytes that preserves the cytoplasm. This method offers a more precise determination of micronucleus frequencies. It has been used to detect elevated levels of micronuclei among 38 workers exposed to low levels of styrene compared with 20 controls (p=.005), controlling for age and smoking status (Högstedt et al., 1983b).

One of the major issues in developing the micronucleus assay has been determining which lymphocytes should serve as the denominator of the micronucleus frequency. Only cells that have divided at least once after exposure are competent to have formed micronuclei, and should be included in the denominator. Pincu et al. (1984) have developed a staining procedure that identifies which lymphocytes have undergone cell division. Therefore, with this technique one can determine which lymphocytes could not have developed micronuclei, improving scoring speed, and reducing the assay's variability due to differences in cell proliferation. Both x-rays (Countryman and Heddle, 1976) and certain chemicals, including bromodeoxyuridine (BrdUrd) (Boyes and Koval, 1985), used in lymphocyte cell cultures, slow cell division, delaying the time of the first mitosis and leading to an underestimate of micronucleus frequency if cells that have not divided are included in the denominator.

Still, knowing that the lymphocytes have divided does not answer the question of how many cell divisions they have undergone. Ideally, one would like to identify cells that have undergone only one cell division. The more cell divisions after the time of exposure, the more dilute the micronucleus frequencies become. This is more of an issue with acute, as opposed to chronic, exposures.

Fenech and Morley (1985, 1986) have developed the most promising method of identifying cells that have divided only once. To do this, they used a mitogen, phytohemagglutinin (PHA), to stimulate lymphocytes in culture to divide, then allowed the cells to complete nuclear division, and used cytochalasin B to block the completion of cell division. It is then possible to score micronuclei in the binucleate cytokinesis-blocked cells. Cytochalasin B was not found to cause chromosome abnormalities or induce micronuclei when cells were cultured for 48 to 72 hours at a concentration of 3.0 µg/ml. Fenech and Morley made no mention of the ability of PHA to induce micronuclei. The frequency of micronuclei found with this assay depends on the proportion of cells that are induced by the mitogen to divide (Fenech and Morley, 1985). Lymphocytes from different individuals vary in their response to PHA.

Assay Techniques for the Fenech and Morley (1985) Lymphocyte Assay

1. Draw a sample of peripheral blood from the subject.
2. Separate peripheral blood lymphocytes from whole blood on Ficoll–Hypaque gradients, wash twice in Hanks' balanced salt solution, and resuspend in McCoy's modified medium 5A containing 15 percent heat inactivated fetal calf serum.
3. Culture lymphocytes in 0.2-ml microwells at a concentration of 0.5×10^6 cells/ml.
4. Add PHA (5 µg/ml, Burroughs Wellcome reagent grade).
5. Culture cells at 37°C in a humidified atmosphere containing 10 percent CO_2.
6. Prepare cytochalasin B as a stock solution in dimethyl sulfoxide (DMSO) at a concentration of 2 mg/ml divided into small portions and stored at -70°C.
7. Thaw solution and dilute in saline.
8. Add cytochalasin B at a concentration of 3.0 µg/ml to culture 44 hours after the start of the culture.
9. Stop culture at 72 hours.

10. Centrifuge cells and prepare slides.
11. Score a minimum of 800 binucleate cells per individual (or score until 45 micronuclei are observed (Fenech and Morley, 1986)).
12. Score slides with X1000 magnification.

Specimen Sampling Schedule

Because lymphocytes circulate throughout the body, they can reflect exposures that occur at various sites. Only damage that has occurred during the life of the lymphocyte can be detected. Damage should be detectable almost immediately, perhaps within a day of an individual's exposure to the genotoxic agent (time to appearance of the marker).

The life span of lymphocytes varies from about 3 days to 20 years (Leavell and Thorup, 1976), depending on the type of lymphocyte (persistence of the marker). Ninety percent of lymphocytes have a half-life of about 3 years. The half-life of the remaining 10 percent is 1 to 10 days. Approximately 50 percent of all lymphocytes and most peripheral lymphocytes circulate between the blood, spleen, lymph nodes, and other tissues. Most of these lymphocytes are of the long-lived T-cell type. The turnover rate of all lymphocytes in the body is about 2 to 5 percent per day. Because lymphocytes have a fairly long life span and relatively low repair rates, damage can accumulate over the years (Natarajan and Obe, 1982). With acute exposures, sampling should occur as close as possible to the time of exposure, as lymphocyte turnover will eventually dilute micronucleus frequencies. Sampling should probably be done at various intervals so as not to miss peak elevations in micronucleus frequencies. For chronic exposures, determining sampling time is less of an issue. Lymphocytes of chronically exposed people, however, have heightened repair mechanisms (Natarajan and Obe, 1982).

Detecting Dose–Response Relationships

Several studies have noted dose–response relationships between lymphocyte exposure to radiation in culture (Pincu et al., 1984; Fenech and Morley, 1985, 1986; Kormos and Köteles, 1988) and the frequency of micronuclei. At doses above 400 rads, Pincu et al. (1984) found a decreased micronucleus frequency, probably from cell death. Erexson et al. (1987) noted a dose–response relationship with in vivo exposure of mice to the chemotherapeutic agent diaziquone, using the Fenech and Morley method to analyze micronucleus frequency. Högstedt et al. (1983b), however, found no dose–response relationship between levels of styrene exposure and frequency of micronuclei. Perhaps the range of styrene exposures (1–36 ppm time weighted average) was not sufficient to show an effect.

Assay Variability

There are two main sources of variability in lymphocyte assays. The length of time cells are cultured is one source of technique-induced variation in some lymphocyte assays. Högstedt et al. (1983b) found no statistically significant difference in micronucleus frequencies after exposure to styrene when they cultured cells for 72 hours; they did, however, find a significant difference when they cultured cells for 96 hours. Peak micronucleus frequencies occurred between 80 and 88 hours. The second source of variability arises from the observers who score the assay. Ideally, one observer who is blind to exposure status should score smears for both exposed and unexposed subjects. Högstedt et al. (1984) had two different technicians score cultures for micronuclei. Although there was a good correlation between the results of the two observers ($r=0.95$), there was a 30 percent difference in micronucleus frequencies.

Potential Confounders

Several investigators using different methods for the lymphocyte assay have found an increase in micronucleus frequency with increasing age (Högstedt, 1984; Norman et al., 1985; Fenech and Morley, 1986). Högstedt (1984) reported an increase in the frequency of micronuclei in association with smoking and Norman et al. (1985) noted a nonsignificant increase in micronuclei among women as compared with men.

Summary of Advantages and Disadvantages of the Micronucleus Assay Using Peripheral Blood Lymphocytes

Advantages

1. Lymphocyte sampling can be done in a fairly noninvasive manner.

2. Chromosome damage that has occurred in vivo in the presence of the host's activating and deactivating mechanisms can be assayed in vitro.

3. Because lymphocytes circulate throughout the body, exposures at various sites can be detected in the peripheral blood.

4. Because lymphocytes have a fairly long life span and relatively low repair rates, damage can accumulate over the years (Natarajan and Obe, 1982).

5. Dose–response relationships have been noted with the lymphocyte assay (Pincu et al., 1984; Fenech and Morley, 1985, 1986; Erexson et al., 1987; Kormos and Köteles, 1988).

6. The Fenech and Morley (1985) assay allows easy recognition of binucleate cells and, hence, easy scoring for micronuclei. The assay offers enhanced statistical power: (1) because of the low spontaneous frequency of micronuclei, 4.4 ± 2.6 micronuclei/500 cytokinesis-blocked cells, and (2) because one can score twice the number of micronuclei for a given effort in these binucleate cells (Fenech and Morley, 1985).

7. The lymphocyte assay is more rapid, less expensive, less labor-intensive, and more sensitive than techniques for analyzing chromosome aberrations (Fenech and Morley, 1986).

8. Lymphocytes can be stored in liquid nitrogen for future use.

Disadvantages

1. Lymphocytes may or may not be target cells of interest with respect to future cancer development.

2. Culture conditions, such as length of time in culture, may affect micronucleus frequencies (Högstedt et al., 1983b).

3. Culture conditions can affect the proportion of cells that divide, and therefore, the eligibility of cells to develop micronuclei. To minimize the variability of the assay, investigators should keep culture conditions as consistent as possible.

THE MICRONUCLEUS ASSAY AND EXFOLIATED CELLS

Many investigators, in particular, Stich and co-workers (Stich et al., 1982, 1984, 1985; Stich and Rosin, 1983a,b) have explored the benefits of performing the micronucleus assay in various exfoliated cell populations. Exfoliated cells are typically epithelial cells sloughed from the surface of a body cavity, such as the respiratory tract, the gastrointestinal tract, and the genitourinary tract. Because epithelial cells are derived from basal cells, damage induced by a genotoxic agent at the basal cell layer should be reflected in the frequency of micronuclei in exfoliated cells. The presence of micronuclei in exfoliated cells serves as an internal dosimeter (Stich and Rosin, 1983a), measuring the extent to which an environmental agent is associated with DNA damage to tissues in vivo and, hence, potentially providing a measure of the risk of cancer development.

Exfoliated cells have several positive features in the micronucleus assay: most of the cell populations can be sampled noninvasively; because they are naturally dividing cell populations, cell culture is not necessary; and they allow assessment of in vivo damage to such target cells of interest as cells of the mouth, nasopharynx, esophagus, stomach (Stich et al., 1983), colon (Heddle et al., 1982; Goldberg et al., 1983), bladder (Reali et al., 1987), lungs (Fontham et al., 1986), and cervix (Fontham et al., 1986; Rosin et al., 1987).

Assay Techniques

The most extensively studied exfoliated cells in micronucleus assays have been buccal mucosa cells. A description of one preparation technique for buccal mucosa smears follows (Stich et al., 1982).

1. Rinse the person's mouth to remove particles of food and other debris.
2. Scrape the buccal mucosa with a wooden tongue depressor.
3. Apply cells to microscope slide.
4. Within 24 hours, pretreat air-dried mucosa cell smears for 3 minutes with 50 percent glycerin.
5. Fix smears with ethanol/glacial acetic acid (3:1) and air dry again.
6. Stain with Feulgen reaction.
   a). pretreat in 1 N HCl for 2 minutes at room temperature and 6 minutes at 60°C
   b). transfer into 1 N HCl at room temperature for 2 minutes
   c). rinse in distilled water
   d). put into Schiff reagent for 90 minutes
   e). wash with three changes (2 minutes each) of freshly prepared sulfite solution
   f). rinse twice with running water
7. Counterstain for 5 to 10 seconds with fast green dissolved in 95 percent ethanol.
8. Mount dehydrated preparations (tertiary butanol, xylene) in permount.
9. Count micronuclei under light microscope.

Methodologic Issues

Much more work has been done in human populations with the micronucleus assay in exfoliated cells than with other cell types. To explore the use of the micronucleus assay in epidemiologic studies, the following sections discuss such relevant issues as when to sample exfoliated cells, the assay's ability to detect dose–response relationships, and its variability and cost. Epidemiologic field studies that employed the assay illustrate the discussion.

Specimen Sampling Schedule

In deciding when to sample exfoliated cells after an individual is exposed to a potentially genotoxic agent, one must take two factors into consideration: the length of time it takes for cells at the basal layer to migrate to the surface (time to appearance of the marker) and the length of time between exposure and complete sloughing of all potentially exposed cells (persistence of the marker). For acute exposures, the rate at which cells migrate to the surface affects the frequency of micronuclei (Stich and Rosin, 1984). Information relevant to the time course of cell migration from the basal cell layer to exfoliation can be derived from a study conducted by Stich et al. (1983) in which patients received radiation therapy. Patients who received radiotherapy to the head and pelvic regions experienced an increase in frequency of micronuclei among buccal mucosa cells and urinary tract cells, respectively. After radiation therapy ended, micronuclei began to disappear after 5 to 7 days and completely disappeared after 24 days. Five to 7 days is believed to be the time necessary for undamaged new cells to migrate from the basal cell layer to the surface of the epithelial cell lining (Stich et al., 1983). For chronic exposures, sampling can take place at any time. Sampling for acute exposures should take place between 5 and 24 days after exposure to the agent of interest as it takes about 5 to 7 days for new cells to arrive at the surface of the lumen and 24 days for all affected cells to be completely sloughed.

Depending on the the type of tissue, the exposure, and the severity of damage to the tissue caused by the exposure, one may have to alter sampling times. For example, cell turnover rates differ from one tissue to another. Because radiation slows mitosis (Countryman and Heddle, 1976), exposure to radiation may cause a delay in the migration of cells from the basal layer to exfoliation. On the other hand, injury to a tissue may increase cell proliferation rates as the tissue attempts to repair the damage.

Detecting Dose–Response Relationships

Several studies (Stich et al., 1982; Stich and Rosin, 1983a,b; Fontham et al., 1986; Reali et al., 1987; Sarto et al., 1987) provide evidence for the assay's ability to distinguish dose–response relationships. In a study performed in India, Stich et al. (1982) compared the frequency of micronuclei in buccal mucosa cells among three groups. Two groups chewed betel quids, a known risk factor for oral squamous cell carcinoma (IARC, 1985), and the third group (the controls) did not. The results of the study showed that chewers had significantly higher frequencies of micronuclei in their buccal mucosa cells than nonchewers ($p<.001$). There was also a higher frequency of micronuclei at the site where the quid touched the mucosa. Right-sided chewers had higher frequencies of micronuclei on the right side and left-sided chewers had higher frequencies on the left. Those who chewed on both sides showed no difference in frequency of micronuclei on one side of the mouth or the other. The investigators did not find a clear dose–response relationship between number of quids chewed per day and the frequency of micronuclei, but noted a significantly higher frequency of micronucleated cells among those who chewed more than 15 quids per day (average 7.05% micronucleated cells) compared with those who chewed less than four quids per day (average 1.50% micronucleated cells) (Stich et al., 1983).

Several other conclusions can be drawn from this study: (1) the assay detects recent, rather than cumulative damage over time, as the number of micronucleated cells did not increase with number of years the subject chewed, a variable often employed as a surrogate for dose; (2) the micronucleus assay reflects differences in seemingly similar exposures to genotoxic agents, as those who chewed betel quids consisting mainly of perfumed tobacco, dried betel nut, betel leaf, lime, and spices had a higher frequency of micronuclei than those who ate raw betel nuts with betel leaves and lime; and (3) the micronucleus assay does not indicate stage of disease, as leukoplakia cells showed no elevation in frequency of micronuclei (Stich et al., 1982). Leukoplakia, however, may be caused by factors other than those leading to the formation of micronuclei. Even if micronuclei are present, rapid proliferation of leukoplakia cells may make them nondetectable.

Stich and Rosin (1983b) investigated the separate and combined effects of cigarette smoking and alcohol consumption on the frequency of micronuclei in buccal mucosa cells. They sampled 500 cells per person. Only one exposure category showed a significant increase in micronucleus frequencies: the group of people who both consumed 150 ml of alcohol or more per day and smoked at least a pack of cigarettes per day. Smoking and alcohol together have been shown in epidemiologic studies to synergistically increase the risk of oral cancer (Schmidt and Popham, 1981). Stich and Rosin found a dose–response relationship, based primarily on the number of cigarettes smoked per day, in the group that used both alcohol and cigarettes. They found an eightfold increase in the number of micronucleated cells among those who consumed alcohol and smoked three or more packs of cigarettes per day and a 4.2-fold increase among those who smoked one to two packs per day. Smoking three packs of cigarettes per day without drinking or drinking 1.2 L of alcohol per day without smoking did not yield a detectable increase in frequency of micronuclei in buccal mucosa cells.

In contrast, Fontham et al. (1986) did not find a dose–response relationship between number of cigarettes smoked and the frequency of micronuclei in buccal mucosa cells, bladder, cervical, or bronchial cells. Nor did they find a synergistic increase in micronucleus frequencies in people who both smoked cigarettes and drank alcohol. In their study of 486 patients at Charity Hospital in New Orleans, however, they did find elevated frequencies of micronuclei in all four organ sites among smokers (of any amount) in comparison with nonsmokers. They saw no significant elevations in micronucleus frequencies among nonsmokers married to smokers. It is possible, the authors suggest, that there was too little heterogeneity in numbers of cigarettes smoked in this population to reveal a dose–response relationship.

Similar findings were reported by Reali et al. (1987) who did not find a correlation between numbers of cigarettes smoked and frequency of micronuclei in urothelial cells of 12 smokers and 12 nonsmokers. Small sample size and lack of heterogeneity in numbers of cigarettes smoked may account for these results.

Both Stich and Rosin (1983a) and Sarto and co-workers (1987) have noted increases in micronucleus frequencies in exfoliated cells upon exposure to increasing doses of radiation. At high doses, however, micronucleus frequencies decrease due to cell death.

Intervention Studies

Stich et al. (1984, 1985; Stich, 1987) and Muñoz et al. (1987) explored the utility of the micronucleus assay in assessing the efficacy of chemopreventive measures. Stich and co-workers (1984) supplemented the diet of 40 rural Filipino betel nut chewers with vitamin pills containing retinol (100,000 IU/week) and β-carotene (300,000 IU/week) twice weekly for three months. Eleven chewers who were not supplemented served as controls. β-carotene, a precursor of vitamin A (retinol), inhibits the action of tumor promoters and acts as a free radical scavenger. Retinol is important in maintaining the integrity of epithelial cells. The investigators sampled 300 buccal mucosa cells per person, both before and after the vitamin supplementation. The results of the study confirmed the hypothesis that retinol and β-carotene supplements decrease micronucleus frequency in buccal mucosa cells. Supplemented subjects experienced a three-fold decrease in the mean proportion of cells with micronuclei over the 3-month period (4.2–1.4%). The 11 nonsupplemented betel quid chewers experienced no decrease (4.3–4.8%). The spontaneous frequency among 17 nonchewing controls was 0.0 to 0.8 percent initially and 3 months later.

Thus, Stich et al. first showed that exposure to a mutagen increased the frequency of micronuclei (Stich et al., 1982) and then showed that exposure to a protective agent lowered the frequency of micronuclei. They found similar results when they supplemented the diets of Inuit snuff dippers with β-carotene (Stich et al., 1985). Supplementation, however, was not successful in reducing the number of micronucleated cells of the mucosa of the palate and tongue of inverted smokers (Stich, 1987). (Inverted smokers put the burning end of the cigar in their mouths.)

Muñoz et al. (1987) noted mixed results in a study of micronucleus frequency in exfoliated cells from the buccal mucosa and esophagus among citizens of the People's Republic of China known to have an elevated risk of esophageal cancer. They studied 610 subjects who were randomly assigned to receive either an active treatment (15 mg or 50,000 IU of retinol, 200 mg of riboflavin, and 50 mg of zinc) or a placebo once a week for 13.5 months. They saw no statistically significant difference in micronucleus frequencies in buccal mucosa cells after treatment. They did, however, observe a significant reduction in micronucleus frequencies in cells of the esophageal mucosa ($p = .04$).

Assay Variability

Several studies illustrate issues related to the variability of micronucleus assays in exfoliated cells (Stich et al., 1982; Rosin and German, 1985; Sarto et al., 1987). Rosin and German (1985) investigated micronucleus frequencies in exfoliated cells of people with Bloom's syndrome, a chromosome breakage syndrome that is associated with an increased risk of cancer. They found that people with Bloom's syndrome had significantly higher frequencies of micronuclei in buccal mucosa and urinary tract cells than heterozygotes or controls. Samples taken from eight sites within the same persons showed that people with this genetic syndrome have low intraindividual variability in micronucleus frequencies.

Both the vulnerability of particular tissues to a genotoxic agent and the presence of other genotoxic exposures will affect intraindividual variability. Variability across tissue sites will be high for site-specific exposures such as chewing tobacco on the right or left side of one's mouth, as Stich et al. (1982) suggested earlier. Therefore, in epidemiologic studies of such exposures one must carefully select the sampling sites.

Interindividual variability depends largely on the activation and detoxifying mechanisms of both the person and the tissue under investigation. Two individuals may receive the same exposure to an agent, but because of differences in metabolism, may differ in the frequency of micronuclei present; therefore, the biologically effective dose may be different. Stich and Dunn (in press) note that background frequencies of micronuclei in buccal cells of nonsmokers vary relatively little, whereas the bronchial cells of nonsmokers who have no known exposures to polycyclic aromatic hydrocarbons show a wide range of frequencies of micronuclei.

Differences in criteria for scoring micronuclei is another source of assay variability. In fact, differences in criteria have resulted in different laboratories reporting different background frequencies of micronuclei in buccal mucosa cells (Sarto et al., 1987). One difficulty in scoring micronuclei is that some exposures, for example, snuff, cause severe cytotoxicity. As exposed cells degenerate, fragments of DNA from the nucleus move into the cytoplasm where they resemble micronuclei, that is, these fragments result from cytotoxic rather than genotoxic mechanisms. To obtain more accurate micronucleus counts, Sarto and co-workers (1987) suggest excluding cells with degenerative characteristics and analyzing at least 3000 cells per subject.

Potential Confounders

Because the micronucleus assay is a nonspecific indicator of chromosome breakage and spindle dysfunction, increased frequencies of micronuclei appear after exposure to any chemical or agent that causes such damage. Viruses, chemicals, x-rays, and tobacco can elevate micronucleus frequencies (Stich and Rosin, 1983b; Stich and Rosin, 1984; Fontham et al., 1986).

Cost

The micronucleus assay in exfoliated cells is a relatively inexpensive and rapid assay. Stich and Rosin (1983b) note that an experienced cytotechnologist can examine 500 cells in 40 to 60 minutes. Eventually, automated scoring of micronuclei will reduce costs (Callisen et al., 1986; Fenech et al., 1988); Stich and Dunn (in press) claim that a microscope image processing scanner can be used to scan 10^5 cells per minute.

Summary of Advantages and Disadvantages of the Micronucleus Assay Using Exfoliated Cells

Advantages

1. The frequency of micronuclei in exfoliated cells provides evidence of a biological response to a genotoxic agent in a naturally dividing cell population.

2. The assay has successfully identified people at high risk of cancer: betel quid chewers (Stich et al., 1982), people who both smoke and drink alcohol (Stich and Rosin, 1983b), and snuff dippers (Stich et al., 1985).

3. The assay allows the detection of damage in vivo to a whole organism that is using its activating and deactivating metabolic machinery.

4. One can detect evidence of exposure to a genotoxic agent in a target cell population likely to develop cancerous lesions (Stich et al., 1982).

5. One can sample a variety of sites and cell types in a minimally invasive or noninvasive manner. Such sites include the buccal mucosa (cheek cells), bronchi (sputum cells), urinary bladder (cells in urine), nasopharynx, esophagus, cervix, and colon.

6. The low spontaneous frequency of micronuclei in buccal cells (0.0–0.8%) enhances the statistical power of the assay (Stich et al., 1984).

7. The study of cigarette smoking and alcohol consumption (Stich and Rosin, 1983a) suggests that the assay detects the damaging effects of two or more agents acting together.

8. The test can be applied to large groups of people.

9. Prepared buccal cell smears can be stored indefinitely for future use. Fixed tissues, such as biopsy specimens, can be evaluated for micronuclei (Stich, 1987).

10. The test is quick and inexpensive. An experienced cytolotechnologist can examine 500 cells in 40 to 60 minutes (Stich and Rosin, 1983b).

11. The scoring of micronuclei (percentage of micronucleated cells, number of micronuclei per cell, and amount of DNA per micronucleus) can be automated (Stich and Dunn, in press; Callisen et al., 1986; Fenech et al., 1988).

Disadvantages

1. The assay cannot identify cytogenetic damage by agents that neither break chromosomes nor damage the spindle apparatus. Based on micronucleus frequencies alone, one cannot distinguish between damage induced by clastogenic agents and damage induced by agents causing chromosomes to lag at anaphase (Heddle et al., 1983).

2. It is difficult to know whether the frequency of micronuclei in exfoliated cells is representative of damage induced in the basal layer. At high doses of radiation, for example, a decrease in micronucleus frequency may result from cell killing (Stich and Rosin, 1983a).

3. It is possible to miss very recent, short-term, or past exposures (Stich, 1986).

THE USE OF THE MICRONUCLEUS ASSAY IN EPIDEMIOLOGIC RESEARCH

Invasiveness

To be useful in large scale epidemiologic research, an assay should possess a low degree of invasiveness. Bone marrow sampling, for example, is highly invasive. For large populations, it is far more practical to use less invasive techniques, such as drawing blood, to obtain peripheral blood erythrocytes (PBEs) and peripheral blood lymphocytes (PBLs), and obtaining scrapings of exfoliated cells.

Specimen Sampling Schedule

The issue of when to sample cells in relation to the time of exposure depends both on the cells to be sampled and on the biology of the tissue from which they are derived.

One must keep in mind that micronuclei indicate recent damage, not the effects of cumulative damage from chronic exposures. For many of these assays, multiple sampling times will guard against missing peak or intermittent elevations in micronucleus frequencies. With chronic exposures, sampling time is less of an issue.

For peripheral blood erythrocytes, time to appearance of micronuclei is based on the time between exposure and the appearance of new erythrocytes in the blood, which is believed to be about 3 to 4 days (Schlegel et al., 1986). Because erythrocytes persist in the blood for about 120 days, sampling should be done 4 to 120 days after exposure. In individuals with normally functioning spleens, however, the spleen removes micronucleated cells from the circulation. Thus, this assay is likely to be limited to people who have been splenectomized.

In lymphocytes, damage should be detectable almost immediately (within a day). Lymphocytes vary in longevity from 3 days to over 20 years (Leavell and Thorup, 1976) and 90 percent are long-lived, with a half-life of about 3 years (Natarajan and Obe, 1982). Because lymphocyte turnover will dilute micronucleus frequencies, sampling should occur as soon as possible after exposure.

In exfoliated cells, the time to appearance of micronuclei depends on how long cells take to migrate from the basal layer, where the damage occurs, to the surface of the epithelium where they are exfoliated. In buccal cells, this is believed to be about 5 to 7 days. After about 24 days all potentially affected cells are sloughed (Stich et al., 1983). Therefore, sampling should occur between 5 and 24 days after exposure.

Detecting Dose–Response Relationships

Ideally, one would like to see a clear dose–response pattern between the frequency of micronuclei and the dose of a particular agent to quantitate the degree of exposure. Dose–response patterns depend on the cell type assayed as well as on the genotoxic agent (Schmid, 1976). Among splenectomized individuals, a dose–response relationship was noted between duration of chemotherapy treatment and frequency of micronuclei detected in peripheral blood erythrocytes (Schlegel et al., 1986). In studies of exfoliated buccal cells, Stich and Rosin (1983b) noted a dose–response relationship, based primarily on the number of cigarettes smoked per day, among people who both smoked cigarettes and drank alcohol. Fontham et al. (1984), on the other hand, did not find a dose–response relationship in buccal, bladder, or bronchial cells in association with numbers of cigarettes smoked, nor did Stich et al. (1982) find a clear dose–response relationship between the frequency of micronuclei and the number of betel quids chewed per day. They did, however, note a significantly higher frequency of micronucleated cells among those who chewed more than 15 quids per days versus those who chewed less than four quids per day (Stich and Rosin, 1983a). Decreased micronucleus frequencies have been observed in populations at high risk of cancer who were given vitamin supplements containing β-carotene (Stich et al.,1984, 1985; Muñoz et al., 1987).

Sensitivity, Specificity, and Positive Predictive Value

The micronucleus assay has been evaluated for sensitivity and specificity only in mouse bone marrow studies. Jenssen and Ramel (1980) evaluated the micronucleus assay as a short-term test for detecting carcinogenic damage. They compared the sensitivity and specificity of the mouse micronucleus assay and the Ames test against the known carcinogenic potential of a variety of chemicals, based on malignant tumor induction studies in experimental animals and epidemiologic studies in humans.

They analyzed 143 chemicals evaluated by the micronucleus assay and 115 assayed by the Ames test. Both the micronucleus assay and the Ames test had a specificity of about 80 percent. The two tests differed significantly with respect to sensitivity. The Ames assay had a sensitivity of 80 percent, whereas the micronucleus assay had a sensitivity of 58 percent. Together, the two tests had a sensitivity of 86 percent. Jenssen and Ramel (1980) suggest that increasing the number of cells sampled from 1,000 to 4,000 per animal would increase the sensitivity of the micronucleus assay. Studies of chromosome damage in *Drosophila*, however, indicate that the dose required to induce point mutations is lower than the dose needed to produce nondisjunctional events or chromosome aberrations. Thus, the sensitivity of the micronucleus assay may never reach that of the Ames test (Jenssen and Ramel, 1980).

From a literature search of mouse micronucleus assays performed on various chemicals, Heddle et al. (1983) determined that of 150 known clastogens tested, 50 percent produced an increased incidence of micronuclei. The 50 percent sensitivity in clastogen detection agrees fairly well with the 58 percent sensitivity found by Jenssen and Ramel (1980) in carcinogen detection.

Given this information, how should one interpret the results of the micronucleus assay? The interpretation of a positive result depends on the assay's specificity and the prevalence of micronuclei in the population under investigation. The positive predictive value of the assay depends on the prevalence of micronuclei in the population. Although the assay has a high specificity, the sensitivity is low. If the prevalence of micronuclei in the population is also low then the false-positive rate will be high lowering the positive predictive value of the assay. Given the assay's low sensitivity, a negative test may be interpreted several ways. It may be that the agent really does not cause DNA damage. On the other hand, the agent may cause DNA damage that is not detected for a variety of reasons. For example, the assay may not be sensitive enough to detect damage at low doses. Or, the power of the test may be too low. Power depends in part on the number of cells scored per subject and the number of subjects tested. Another explanation for a negative result may be that the agent does not cause DNA damage to the cells assayed, but does damage other target cells, such as those in the liver. Or again, the agent may cause damage that cannot be detected by the micronucleus assay.

Thus, the assay may not be a good discriminator of individual exposure, but by detecting population elevations in micronucleus frequencies, may be useful in distinguishing populations likely to develop cancer. Sensitivity and specificity estimates from human studies do not exist. Therefore, the implications of the mouse bone marrow studies with regard to humans are unclear.

Assay Variability and Intraindividual and Interindividual Variability

The variability of the assays depends on both the laboratory procedures used and the characteristics of the individuals assayed. In both the mouse bone marrow assay and the exfoliated cell assay, the test seems to yield reproducible results (Schmid, 1976;

Rosin and German, 1985). Control levels of micronuclei are consistently low in mice (Schmid, 1976) and in buccal mucosa cells (Stich et al., 1984), although different investigators report different baseline levels of micronuclei in exfoliated cells (Sarto et al., 1987). Establishing criteria for the identification of micronuclei, adequate training of personnel, running both positive and negative controls, and having the same individual—one who is blind to exposure status—read slides from both exposed and control subjects can reduce differential misclassification bias from laboratory errors.

Intraindividual variability depends both on the exposure of interest and the cell type assayed. Certain chemicals have an affinity for certain tissues, and within tissues, there may be site-specific elevations in micronucleus frequencies. If the same person is assayed over time, cell turnover and additional exposures may affect micronucleus frequencies. Interindividual variability is largely influenced by the metabolic functioning of the individuals assayed. The same dose of the same agent may elicit different responses from different individuals.

Cost, Time, Personnel

The micronucleus assay is a relatively quick, simple, and inexpensive way to detect chromosomal damage. Compared with classic methods of assessing chromosome aberrations, such as metaphase scoring, the micronucleus assay is less expensive to perform and an order of magnitude faster to score (Heddle, 1973). Because micronuclei are easily recognizable, the assay does not require highly trained personnel. The test has enhanced statistical power because a large number of cells are available and can be scored in a short period of time. Stich and Dunn (in press) claim that the assay lends itself to automated scoring; a microscope image processing scanner can scan 10^5 cells per minute.

Potential Confounders

In human studies, potential confounders of the effects of chromosome-damaging agents on micronucleus frequencies include age (Högstedt, 1984; Norman et al., 1985; Fenech and Morley, 1986), with the frequency of micronuclei increasing with advancing age, cigarette smoking (Högstedt et al. 1983a; Högstedt, 1984; Fontham et al., 1986), cigarette smoking combined with alcohol consumption (Stich and Rosin, 1983b), low levels of folic acid and vitamin B_{12} (Abe et al., 1984; Everson et al., 1988), and possibly gender (Norman et al., 1985), with women showing a slightly higher frequency of micronuclei than men. In addition, because the micronucleus assay is a nonspecific indicator of chromosome damage, exposures to chemicals, viruses, or x-rays other than the exposure of interest may increase the frequency of micronuclei.

Conclusion

The peripheral blood lymphocyte assay and exfoliated cell assay appear to be the most promising for future epidemiologic research. Each assay possesses a low level of invasiveness, is applicable to large human populations, and has been shown to indicate dose–response relationships. Although the exfoliated cell assay has been used in far more field applications than the lymphocyte assay, both need more field work to assess the characteristics of each assay more fully. In particular, the variability of the assays and dose–response relationships could use further characterization. More work needs to be done with the exfoliated cell assay on cells other than buccal and urinary tract cells.

Questions That Can Be Addressed With the Micronucleus Assay

Micronuclei are indicators of chromosome damage due to genotoxic agents that cause chromosome breaks or spindle dysfunction. Micronuclei can serve as markers of exposure as well as markers of biological response, as the effectiveness of activation and deactivation mechanisms determine whether micronuclei form. Micronuclei may also be used to predict the carcinogenic potential of environmental agents, given that most carcinogens are found to be mutagens and that chromosomal aberrations are believed to be initial steps in carcinogenesis. It is not known, however, how the presence of micronuclei relates to the risk of cancer, although both micronucleus formation and the development of cancer are associated with x-rays, tobacco and alcohol use, and betel quid chewing. Thus, the question of the relationship between the frequency of micronuclei and the risk of cancer remains unanswered. Perhaps future epidemiologic studies can establish this link.

Epidemiologists seek to understand causes of disease. Hence, they try to determine whether associations exist between exposures and disease outcomes. Determining the utility of biological markers in epidemiologic research appears to be a three-step process. First, one needs to establish whether the exposure of interest leads to a detectable increase in the marker (frequency of micronuclei). Next, one needs to determine what relevance elevated levels of the marker have in future development of disease. Finally, one needs to characterize the dose–response relationship between exposure status, level of the marker, and risk of disease.

The most direct way of answering these questions is to periodically assess micronucleus frequencies in a group of people with known exposures to a genotoxic agent (one that is capable of elevating micronucleus frequencies) and determine whether the people with the highest micronucleus frequencies develop cancer. Unfortunately, this costly and time-consuming endeavor would require thousands of subjects, many years, and much personnel time.

Short-term projects are far more practical. Studies by Stich and Rosin (1982) have already shown that populations known to be at high risk of cancer and exposed to carcinogenic agents also have higher micronucleus frequencies in buccal mucosa cells. Future studies using elevated micronucleus frequencies as measures of outcome may identify tissues particularly susceptible to the carcinogenic effects of certain agents (Stich, 1986). Furthermore, as the test may be performed in a variety of cells and species, studies with micronuclei may serve as a link in risk assessment studies of cell cultures in vitro and in studies with animals and humans in vivo (Stich, 1986).

Because micronucleus assays in short-lived cells detect recent damage, the assays can be used as a measure of exposure that can be related to current disease status. Case-control studies of cancer patients, for example, might include assessments of current micronucleus frequencies. The relevance of such analyses depends on the nature of the association between current micronucleus frequencies and current cancer status.

Possibly of more interest would be case-control studies of cancer patients assessing the relevance of past exposures. This could be accomplished with the use of cells stored for other purposes, assuming that a large number of cells were stored and that the people were exposed to some genotoxic agent. Given that lymphocytes are long-lived, perhaps using the micronucleus assay with peripheral blood lymphocytes can show the relevance of past exposures.

The micronucleus assay can also be used to ask questions associated with treatment efficacy. For example, Stich et al. (1984, 1985) and Muñoz et al. (1987) explored the utility of the micronucleus assay in assessing the efficacy of chemopreventive measures. These studies are particularly important because they show the effects of treatment in a relatively short period of time.

The micronucleus assay is a useful indicator of genotoxic damage from a number of environmental agents in a variety of cell types and populations. Improvements in the scoring of micronuclei through the standardization of criteria for their identification and through automation of the scoring process should enhance the usefulness of this promising assay. Applications of the micronucleus assay in population studies with different genotoxic exposures may augment our knowledge of the carcinogenic potential of environmental agents in humans, and may help elucidate mechanisms of carcinogenicity.

REFERENCES

Abe T, Isemura T, Kikuchi Y: Micronuclei in human bone-marrow cells: Evaluation of the micronucleus test using human leukemia patients treated with antileukemic drugs. *Mutat Res* 1984;130:113–120.

Boller K, Schmid W: *Humangenetik* 1970;11:35–54, as summarized in Heddle et al., 1983.

Boyes BG, Koval JJ: Technical note: A cautionary note on the use of BUdR when determining micronucleus frequencies. *Int J Radiat Biol* 1985;47:341–342.

Callisen HH, Pincu M, Norman A: Feasibility of automating the micronucleus assay. *Anal Quant Cytol Histol* 1986;8:219–223.

Countryman PI, Heddle JA: The production of micronuclei from chromosome aberrations in irradiated cultures of human lymphocytes. *Mutat Res* 1976;41:321–332.

Erexson GL, Kligerman AD, Allen JW: Diaziquone-induced micronuclei in cytochalasin B-blocked mouse peripheral blood lymphocytes. *Mutat Res* 1987;178:117–122.

Evans HJ, Neary GJ, Williamson FS: The relative biological efficiency of single doses of fast neutrons and gamma rays on *vicia faba* roots and the effect of oxygen. Part II chromosome damage: The production of micronuclei. *Int J Rad Biol* 1959;1:216–229.

Everson RB, Wehr CM, Erexson GL, MacGregor JT: Association of marginal folate depletion with increased human chromosomal damage *in vivo:* Demonstration by analysis of micronucleated erythrocytes. *JNCI* 1988;80:525–529.

Fenech M, Morley AA: Measurement of micronuclei in lymphocytes. *Mutat Res* 1985;147:29–36.

Fenech M, Morley AA: Cytokinesis-block micronucleus method in human lymphocytes: Effect of *in vivo* ageing and low dose X-irradiation. *Mutat Res* 1986;161:193–198.

Fenech M, Jarvis LR, Morley AA: Preliminary studies on scoring micronuclei by computerized image analysis. *Mutat Res* 1988;203:33–38.

Fontham E, Correa P, Rodriguez E, Lin Y: Validation of smoking history with the micronucleus test. In: Hoffmann D, ed.: *Mechanisms in Tobacco Carcinogenesis, Banbury Report 23.* 1986;113–119.

Goetz P, Srám RJ, Dohnalava J: Relationship between experimental results in mammals and man. I. Cytogenetic analysis of bone marrow injury induced by a single dose of cyclophosphamide. *Mutat Res* 1975;31:247–254.

Goldberg MT, Blakey DH, Bruce WR: Comparison of the effects of 1,2-dimethylhydrazine and cyclophosphamide on micronucleus incidence in bone marrow and colon. *Mutat Res* 1983;109:91–98.

Heddle JA: A rapid *in vivo* test for chromosomal damage. *Mutat Res* 1973;18:187–190.

Heddle JA, Blakey DH, Duncan AMV, Goldberg MT, Newmark H, Wargovich MJ, Bruce WR: Micronuclei and related anomalies as a short-term assay for colon carcinogens. In: Bridges B, Butterworth B, Weinstein IB, eds.: *Indicators of Genotoxic Exposure.* Cold Spring Harbor, Banbury Report #13, ISSN 0198-0068, 1982.

Heddle JA, Hite M, Kirkhart B, Mavournin K, MacGregor JT, Newell GW, Salamone MF: The induction of micronuclei as a measure of genotoxicity: A report of the US Environmental Protection Agency Gene-Tox Progam. *Mutat Res* 1983;123:61–118.

Högstedt B, Gullberg B, Mark-Vendel E, Mitelman F, Skerfving S: Micronuclei and chromosome aberrations in bone marrow cells and lymphocytes of humans exposed mainly to petroleum vapors. *Hereditas* 1981a;94:179–187.

Högstedt B, Nilsson PG, Mitelman F: Micronuclei in erythropoetic bone marrow cells: Relation to cytogenetic pattern and prognosis in acute nonlymphocytic leukemia. *Cancer Genet Cytogenet* 1981b;3:185–193.

Högstedt B, Gulberg B, Hedner K, Kolnig A, Mitelman F, Skerfving S, Widegren B: Chromosome aberrations and micronuclei in bone marrow cells and peripheral blood lymphocytes in humans exposed to ethylene oxide. *Hereditas* 1983a;98:105–113.

Högstedt B, Akesson B, Axell K, Gullberg B, Mitelman F, Pero R, Skerfving S, Welinder H: Increased frequency of lymphocyte micronuclei in workers producing reinforced polyester resin with low exposure to styrene. *Scand J Work Environ Health* 1983b;9:241–246.

Högstedt B: Micronuclei in lymphocytes with preserved cytoplasm—A method for assessment of cytogenetic damage in man. *Mutat Res* 1984;130:63–72.

Högstedt B, Karlsson A: The size of micronuclei in human lymphocytes varies according to inducing agent used. *Mutat Res* 1985;156:229–232.

International Agency for Research on Cancer (IARC): *IARC monographs on the evaluation of the carcinogenic risk of chemicals to humans: Tobacco habits other than smoking; betel quid and areca-nut chewing; and some related nitrosamines.* Vol 37, IARC, Lyon, France, 1985.

Jensen MK, Hüttel MS: Assessment of the effect of azathioprine on human bone marrow cells *in vivo*, combining chromosome studies and the micronucleus test. *Dan Med Bull* 1976;23:152–154.

Jensen MK, Nyfors A: Cytogenetic effect of methotrexate on human cells *in vivo*. Comparison between results obtained by chromosome studies on bone-marrow cells and blood lymphocytes and by the micronucleus test. *Mutat Res* 1979;64:339–343.

Jenssen D, Ramel C: The micronucleus test as a part of a short-term mutagenicity test program for the prediction of carcinogenicity evaluated by 143 agents tested. *Mutat Res* 1980;75:191–202.

Jenssen D: Chapter 4, The induction of micronuclei. In: Sandberg AA, ed.: *Sister Chromatid Exchange.* New York, Alan R. Liss, 1982, pp. 47–63.

Kormos C, Köteles GJ: Micronuclei in X-irradiated human lymphocytes. *Mutat Res* 1988;199:31–35.

Leavell BS, Thorup OA: *Fundamentals of Clinical Hematology,* ed. 4. Philadelphia, WB Saunders Co, 1976.

McCann J, Ames BN: Detection of carcinogens as mutagens in the *Salmonella*/microsome test: Assay of 300 chemicals: Discussion. *Proc Natl Acad Sci USA* 1976;73:950–954.

Muñoz N, Hayashi M, Bang LJ, Wahrendorf J, Crespi M, Bosch FX: Effect of riboflavin, retinol, and zinc on micronuclei of buccal mucosa and of esophagus: A randomized double-blind intervention study in China. *JNCI* 1987;79:687–691.

Natarajan AT, Obe G: Mutagenicity testing with cultured mammalian cells. In: *Mutagenicity-New Horizons in Genetic Toxicology.* New York, Academic Press, 1982, pp. 171–214.

Norman A, Adams FH, Riley RF: Cytogenetic effects of contrast media and triiodobenzoic acid derivatives in human lymphocytes. *Radiology* 1978;129:199–203.

Norman A, Bass D, Roe D: Screening human populations for chromosome aberrations. *Mutat Res* 1985;143:155–160.

Pincu M, Bass D, Norman A: An improved micronuclear assay in lymphocytes. *Mutat Res* 1984;139:61–65.

Reali D, Di Marino F, Bahramandpour S, Carducci A, Barale R, Loprieno N: Micronuclei in exfoliated urothelial cells and urine mutagenicity in smokers. *Mutat Res* 1987;192:145–149.

Rosin MP, German J: Evidence for chromosome instability *in vivo* in Bloom Syndrome: increased numbers of micronuclei in exfoliated cells. *Hum Genet* 1985;71:187–191.

Rosin MP, Dunn BP, Stich HF: Use of intermediate endpoints in quantitating the response of precancerous lesions to chemopreventive agents. *Can J Physiol Pharmacol* 1987;65:483–487.

Sarto F, Finotto S, Giacomelli L, Mazzotti D, Tomanin R, Lewis AG: The micronucleus assay in exfoliated cells of the human buccal mucosa. *Mutagenesis* 1987;2:11–17.

Schlegel R, MacGregor JT, Everson RB: Assessment of cytogenetic damage by quantification of micronuclei in human peripheral blood erythrocytes. *Cancer Res* 1986;46:3717–3721.

Schmid W: The micronucleus test. *Mutat Res* 1975;31:9–15.

Schmid W: The micronucleus test for cytogenetic analysis. Chapter 36. In: *Chemical Mutagens—Principles and Methods for Their Detection,* Vol. 4. New York, Plenum Press, 1976, pp. 31–53.

Schmidt W, Popham RE: The role of drinking and smoking in mortality from cancer and other causes in male alcoholics. *Cancer* 1981;47:1031–1041.

Schroeder TM: Cytogenetische und cytologische Befunde bei enzymopenischen Panmyelopathien und Pancytopenien: Familiäre Panmyelopathie Typ Fanconi, Glutathionreduktasemangel-Anämie und megaloblastäre Vitamin B_{12}-Mangel-Anämie. *Humangenetik* 1966;2:287–316, as summarized in Heddle et al., 1983.

Stich HF, Stich W, Parida BB: Elevated frequency of micronucleated cells in the buccal mucosa of individuals at high risk for oral cancer: betel quid chewers. *Cancer Lett* 1982;17:125–134.

Stich HF, Rosin MP: Micronuclei in exfoliated human cells as an internal dosimeter for exposures to carcinogens. In: Stich HF, eds.: *Carcinogens and Mutagens in the Environment,* Vol 2. Boca Raton, Florida, CRC Press, 1983a, pp. 17–25.

Stich HF, Rosin MP: Quantitating the synergistic effect of smoking and alcohol consumption with the micronucleus test on human buccal mucosa cells. *Int J Cancer* 1983b;31:305–308.

Stich HF, San RHC, Rosin MP: Adaptation of the DNA-repair and micronucleus tests to human cell suspensions and exfoliated cells. *Ann NY Acad Sci* 1983;407:93–105.

Stich HF, Rosin MP: Micronuclei in exfoliated human cells as a tool for studies in cancer risk and cancer intervention. *Cancer Lett* 1984;22:241–253.

Stich HF, Rosin MP, Vallejera MO: Reduction with vitamin A and β-carotene administration of proportion of micronucleated buccal mucosal cells in Asian quid nut and tobacco chewers. *Lancet* 1984;i:1204–1206.

Stich HF, Hornby AP, Dunn BP: A pilot beta-carotene intervention trial with Inuits using smokeless tobacco. *Int J Cancer* 1985;36:321–327.

Stich HF, Dunn BP: DNA adducts, micronuclei, and leukoplakias as intermediate endpoints in intervention trials. In: *Detection Methods for DNA-Damaging Agents in Man: Application in Cancer Epidemiology and Prevention.* Lyon, France, IARC Sci Publ. Ser. International Agency for Research on Cancer, in press.

Stich HF: The use of micronuclei in tracing the genotoxic damage in the oral mucosa of tobacco users. In: Hoffmann, D, ed.: *Mechanisms in Tobacco Carcinogenesis, Banbury Report 23,* 1986.

Stich HF: Micronucleated exfoliated cells as indicators for genotoxic damage and as markers in chemoprevention trials. *J Nutr Growth Cancer* 1987;4:9–18.

Williams WJ, Beutler E, Erslev AJ, Rundles RW: *Hematology* ed. 2. New York: McGraw-Hill Book Company, 1977, p. 104.

8

CHROMOSOME ABERRATIONS

GARY G. SCHWARTZ

INTRODUCTION

Chromosomal aberrations have been implicated in carcinogenesis since 1914, when Boveri proposed the somatic mutation theory of cancer. Boveri held that a "wrongly combined chromosomal complex" in a somatic cell was the heritable cause of abnormal cell proliferation.

We now know that structural changes in specific chromosomes may indeed be involved in the etiology of some malignant diseases. In most instances, however, the pathogenetic significance of chromosomal aberrations—if any—is yet unknown. Whatever their significance for an individual's ultimate risk of disease, aberrations in chromosome number or structure are increasingly being used in monitoring populations exposed to environmental hazards (Office of Technology Assessment, 1983, 1986). This chapter reviews the methodology of human chromosome analyses and explores their application in epidemiologic studies.

Although it is beyond the scope of this chapter, the history of cancer cytogenetics is itself a fascinating subject. Readers may want to consult any of several recent reviews (e.g., Hsu, 1979, 1987; Therman, 1986).

METHODOLOGY OF THE LYMPHOCYTE ASSAY

To analyze chromosomal aberrations, one needs to use cells that are capable of rapid division in culture. Because they are easy to obtain, white blood cells are the samples epidemiologists encounter most frequently. (Erythrocytes have no nucleus and, therefore, no chromosomes.)

In the preparation of a lymphocyte culture, a sample of peripheral blood is obtained and mixed with heparin to prevent clotting. The sample is centrifuged so that the white blood cells form a distinct layer that can be collected and placed in a tissue culture medium. The addition of a mitogen (mitosis-producing agent), usually phytohemagglutinin (PHA), will stimulate the cells to divide. The PHA, an extract of the kidney bean, is capable of stimulating cell division by an as yet unknown mechanism. The culture is then incubated for 48 to 72 hours. Although the optimal incubation time is a point of contention (see "Technical factors in aberration type and yield"), in general, most investigators prefer 48-hour incubation.

The steps just described are known collectively as *culturing*. A process called *harvesting* allows one to obtain cells for analyses from cultured cells. The first step in harvesting is the addition of a very dilute solution of colchicine, which binds specifically to the tubulin of spindle microtubules. Because colchicine arrests mitosis at metaphase, cells in metaphase accumulate in the culture. A hypotonic solution is then added to cause the cells to swell from the influx of water. This allows the chromosomes to disperse freely within the cell membrane, separating the paired chromatids but leaving them still attached at the centromere. The cells are then fixed, to harden the chromatin and enhance the morphology. The fixed cells are spread on slides and may be stained (discussed later). The goal of slide preparation is to disperse the chromosomes well, leaving little overlap between them.

Microscopic examination of the slides involves counting the number of chromosomes per cell in a specified number of cells. After observing the morphology of each chromosome, one may want to take photomicrographs for a permanent record. Chromosomes can be cut from photographs of individual cells to form a karyotype. The normal human karyotype contains 46 chromosomes, arranged and numbered by size and centromere position from largest (1) to smallest (22). There are 44 autosomes (22 pairs) and two sex chromosomes.

Similar procedures are used for specimens of bone marrow cells. Because a portion of the cells in the bone marrow are already in the cell cycle, however, PHA is not necessary to stimulate mitosis. Modifications of this methodology for use with bone marrow cells are described by Dale (1980).

This is a general outline of the methodology. For complete technical details of the peripheral blood lymphocyte technique consult Evans and O'Riordan (1975).

Shipping and Storage of Samples

It is often desirable to take blood samples in a field setting. Blood specimens taken far from the cytogenetics laboratory should be maintained at about 4°C during shipping and storage. Cultures prepared from freshly drawn blood samples have more favorable growth characteristics than cultures prepared from stored blood. In general, storage times longer than 5 to 7 days will probably result in poor growth.

Technical Factors in Aberration Yield and Type

The length of time cells are maintained in culture is the most important in vitro factor that can influence the chromosome aberration result. After 48 hours in culture at 37°C, most of the lymphocytes are undergoing their first mitosis. Thus, cultures incubated for longer periods, that is, 72 hours, will contain increasing numbers of cells in their second or even third divisions. An important issue is the differential survival and multiplication of healthy versus genetically damaged lymphocytes. For example, if lymphocytes with chromosome-type damage fail to undergo repeated mitoses in vitro because of genetic damage or mechanical difficulties, an examination of cells at 72 hours will underestimate the true aberration rate, as some aberrant cells could not enter their second division. Moreover, a proportion of the observed chromosome-type aberrations seen later may actually be "derived" aberrations, resulting from the duplication of aberrations that were initially of the chromatid-type (see "Types of chromosome damage"). For this reason, many investigators (e.g., Evans and O'Riordan, 1975) strongly recommend the 48-hour harvest time, and one consensus report of cytogeneticists deems fixation after 54 hours "unacceptable" (Bloom, 1981).

Efficiency, however, favors the 72-hour harvest time because it yields a considerably greater harvest of metaphase chromosomes. Several studies (reviewed in Gebhart, 1982) report that the observed chromosome aberration rates obtained in 48- and 72-hour samples show no significant difference. In some cases higher chromosome aberration rates were seen in the 48-hour samples, but in others, the reverse was observed. Thus, it would seem that the choice of sampling time per se, 48 versus 72 hours, may not be critical. The 72-hour period, however, is clearly advantageous in terms of cell yield (Gebhart, 1982).

The culture medium used to incubate the cells is also a relevant factor, particularly combined with sampling time. In 72-hour samples, the proportion of cells in their first, second, and third cycles varies with the culture medium (Gebhart, 1982). For example, when Obe et al. (1975) compared two media, TC medium 199 and Ham's F-10, they found that DNA synthesis and mitoses occurred much earlier and to a greater extent with Ham's F-10. These investigators reported that sufficient quantities of exclusively first mitoses were obtained in 48 hours using Ham's F-10. Because accurate determinations of aberration frequencies should include only cells in their first mitoses, culture techniques that provide adequate numbers of dividing cells using the 48-hour harvest time may be the procedure of choice.

A possible "compromise" method, which insures that only first division cells are analyzed, involves adding bromodeoxyuridine (BrdUrd) to the culture medium and then performing a staining procedure that detects first, second, and subsequent divisions. This technique has been widely used in radiation studies. The principal drawback of this method is the possibility that BrdUrd itself may alter the aberration frequency, either alone, or by interacting with DNA damage induced by a chemical agent. Advantages and disadvantages of the BrdUrd technique are briefly discussed by Preston (1984).

AN OVERVIEW OF CHROMOSOME STRUCTURE

Brief *user-friendly* overviews of chromosome nomenclature are available in Yunis (1981) and Larson (1983). Readers who want more detailed accounts of human chromosome structure can consult the recent volumes by Therman (1986) and by the International System for Cytogenetic Nomenclature (ISCN) (1985). For the present, however, here is a brief review. A metaphase chromosome is composed of two identical (sister) chromatids, attached at a constricted region, the centromere. The centromere divides the chromosome into two short arms, designated "p" (for petite), and two long arms, designated "q." The position of the centromere in human chromosomes can be in the middle of a chromosome (metacentric), near the middle (submetacentric), or very near the end (acrocentric).

At anaphase, each chromosome divides longitudinally at the centromere, and each sister chromatid is incorporated into one of the two daughter cells.

It should be noted that the term *chromosome* is potentially ambiguous, as it refers to different structures at different stages of the cell cycle. To preclude confusion, a brief outline of the cell cycle may be helpful.

The Mitotic Cycle

Mitotic division comprises only a small portion of a cell's life cycle (Fig. 8-1). After mitosis, the new daughter cells enter a postmitotic phase during which no DNA synthesis occurs. This is G_1 (Gap 1). *Resting cells,* those not preparing for cell division, are considered to be in a subphase of G_1 called G_0. The next stage is S, the period of DNA synthesis. During S, the DNA content of the cell doubles, as each DNA molecule acts as a template to make a complementary copy of itself. The S phase is followed by a second nonsynthetic period, G_2 (Gap 2). G_2 ends with the onset of mitosis (M). The complete cell cycle in cultured human cells may last 12 to 24 hours, only 1 hour of which involves mitosis (Thompson and Thompson, 1986).

The potential ambiguity of the term chromosome stems from the fact that the chromosomes of G_1 cells are made up of one chromatid, whereas those of G_2 cells are made up of two chromatids. Cells in S contain chromosomes made up of both one and two chromatids.

As we will see later, the stage of the cell cycle that cells are in when they are exposed to a clastogenic (chromosome-breaking) agent is a major determinant of the type of chromosome aberration observed.

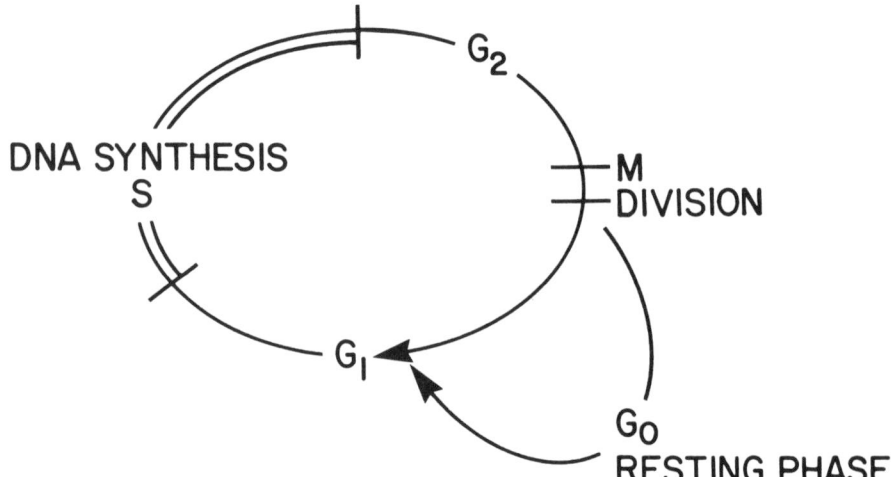

Figure 8-1.   The cell cycle. (Modified after Thompson and Thompson, 1986.)

Banding Techniques

Chromosomes are identified by their morphology and staining characteristics. Cytogenetic staining methods are known as *banding techniques*. Banding refers to the appearance of horizontal alternating light and dark areas along the length of a chromosome. The advent of banding techniques in the early 1970s revolutionized cytogenetics, because it permitted the identification of individual chromosomes, a feat previously possible for only a few chromosomes (Hsu, 1987).

Three types of banding are in general use: G-banding, Q-banding, and R-banding. Most laboratories generally use routinely one or another of these techniques in identifying chromosome abnormalities.

G-banding

G-banding is the most popular banding technique. The G stands for Giemsa, the dye generally used to visualize the bands. G-bands are produced by pretreating slides with trypsin, which denatures chromosomal protein, and then staining the slides with Giemsa. A simple method for G-banding is described by Sanchez et al. (1973).

The numbering of G-bands follows an internationally standardized system that permits precise definition of numerical and structural aberrations (ISCN, 1978). This convention is as follows. The centromere divides the chromosome into short and long arms. Each arm is divided into several regions by specific bands that serve as landmarks. Numbering begins at the centromere and proceeds outwards in each arm. To designate a specific band one lists the chromosome number, the arm symbol, the region number, and the band number in order, without spacing. Thus, band 1q42 indicates chromosome 1, long arm, region 4, band 2. Subbands may be described by placing a decimal point after the band designation, followed by the number assigned to the subband (ISCN, 1981).

Q-banding

Q-bands, the first bands described, are the reference bands for the standard classification. The Q stands for the dye quinacrine, which causes the bands to fluoresce under ultraviolet light. With a few minor exceptions, Q-bands are comparable to G-bands. Unlike G-bands, however, Q-bands are not permanent: after several photomicrographic exposures the fluorescence fades too much to be usable. For this reason, G-bands may be more suitable for routine work.

R-banding

The R in R-banding stands for reverse. Reverse-banding involves pretreatment with hot alkali and subsequent staining with Giemsa or with flurochromes. R-bands are the reverse of Giemsa bands, dark where G is light and light where G is dark. R-banding is not common in the United States, but is used extensively in European laboratories. Figure 8-2 illustrates G, Q, and R bands.

Several other banding techniques (e.g., high-resolution banding) may be used to study specific chromosomes or specific areas of certain chromosomes. These are rarely employed in epidemiologic studies unless some hypothesis predicts specific chromo-

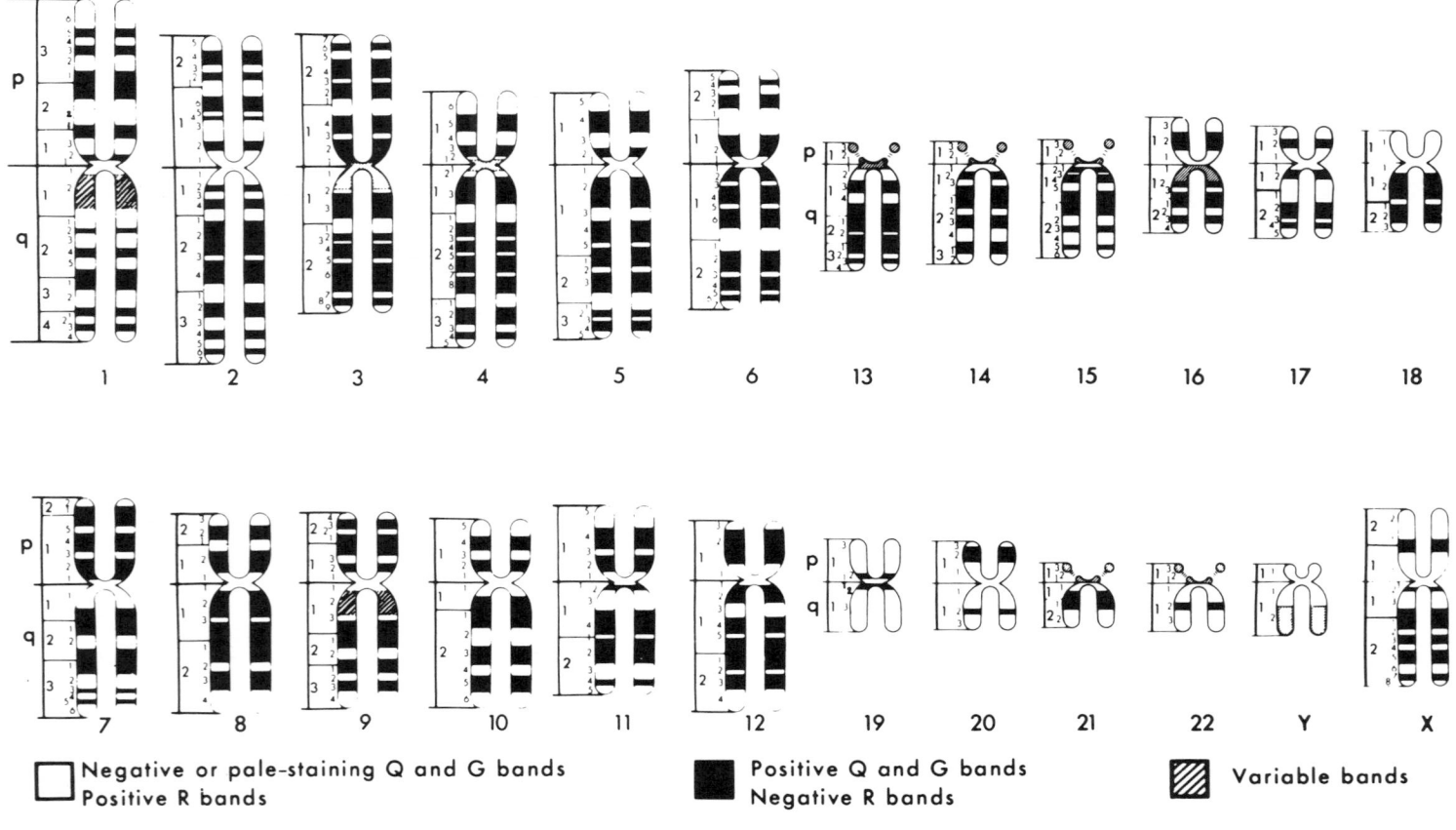

Figure 8-2. Diagrammatic representation of G, Q, and R banded chromosomes. Reprinted from Paris Conference (1971). Standardization in human cytogenetics. *Birth Defects:*1972;8(7).

some breaks. For technical details of these techniques, see Dale and Jurgens (1980), Yunis (1981), and Therman (1986).

From the standpoint of identifying chromosome aberrations, banded preparations are optional: most aberrations can be detected without banding (Preston, 1984). Banded preparations, however, increase the sensitivity of the lymphocyte assay for several common classes of structural aberrations: terminal deletions, inversions, and reciprocal translocations, as discussed later.

TYPES OF CHROMOSOME DAMAGE
Numerical Abnormalities

Chromosomal abnormalities may be either *numerical* or *structural*. Numerical aberrations denote any deviation from the normal human complement of 46 chromosomes. Numerical aberrations usually result from an error in division at metaphase, nondisjunction. When nondisjunction occurs during mitotic division, the sister chromatids fail to separate. As a result, one daughter cell receives an extra chromosome, and the other daughter cell receives none. An extra or whole missing chromosome is indicated by a "+" or "-" placed before the chromosome number. Probably the best known numerical anomaly is trisomy 21, which results in the phenotype of Down syndrome (Lejeune et al., 1959).

Structural Abnormalities

Two types of induced structural chromosome damage can be distinguished at metaphase: *chromosome-type* and *chromatid-type*. In chromosome-type damage, the unit of breakage and reunion is the whole chromosome (i.e., both chromatids at the same locus). Chromosome-type damage occurs when exposure to ionizing radiation or to other mutagens occurs during the G_0 or G_1 phase of mitosis. This may seem paradoxical, as chromosomes in the G_1 phase consist of only one chromatid. However, if a chromosome break occurs during G_1, the break will be duplicated during the S phase and, therefore, will affect both chromatids when they are observed in the following metaphase.

Chromatid-type damage takes place if exposure to these mutagens occurs during S or G_2. In this case, usually only a single chromatid is involved. Some agents, such as some alkylating agents, are exceptions in that they produce only chromatid-type aberrations even though the cells are exposed in G_0 or G_1 (Preston, 1984).

Chromosome-Type Aberrations

Numerous classification systems for structural chromosome aberrations abound (e.g., Evans and O'Riordan [1975], Savage [1975], and ISCN [1985]). Because they are essentially similar, any comprehensive classification system that permits clear and accurate identification of aberrations is acceptable. This chapter follows the classification of Evans and O'Riordan (1975).

This classification system distinguishes seven classes of chromosome-type aberrations. Types 1–5 involve only a single chromosome and are, therefore, called *intra-*

changes; types 6 and 7 exchange material between chromosomes and thus are *interchanges.*

1. *Terminal deletions* are paired acentric fragments that result from a simple break across the chromosome.

2. *Minutes* are pairs of acentric fragments that are smaller in size than terminal deletions. Minutes appear as small spheres of chromatin (hence their name) and probably represent intercalary, rather than terminal deletions. Synonyms are *interstitial, isodiametric* or *dot deletions.*

3. *Acentric rings* are paired segments of chromatid without a centromere, joined physically to form a ring.

4. *Centric rings* are ring structures containing a centromere. Centric rings are generally accompanied by an acentric fragment.

5. *Inversions* may be of two types: *paracentric,* in which both points of breakage and reunion lie on the same arm of the chromosome, and *pericentric,* in which the points of breakage and inversion lie on opposite sides of the centromere. That is, pericentric inversions are intrachromosome exchanges between the p and q arms.

The relative position of the centromere may not be altered in inversions and will appear to change only if the broken arms are of dissimilar size. As a result, inversions are generally detectable only in banded preparations.

6. *Reciprocal translocations* involve the breakage of two chromosomes and the reciprocal exchange of their broken segments. If reciprocal exchanges occur between segments of equal size, the translocations will not be detectable unless banded preparations are used (see inversions). Interchanges may occur in the centromere regions and thus result in whole arm exchanges. When these translocations involve acrocentric chromosomes, they are referred to as *Robertsonian translocations* or *centric fusions.*

7. *Dicentric or polycentric aberrations* involve exchanges between two or more chromosomes and result in a dicentric or polycentric chromosome, plus an associated acentric fragment.

When aberration types 1–3 (terminal deletions, minutes, and acentric rings) are not associated with a chromosome rearrangement, they are often lumped together as *acentric fragments.* Fragments associated with chromosomal exchange (e.g., a minute associated with a dicentric) are scored as part of that exchange, and not as aberrations in their own right. The seven classes of chromosome-type aberrations are illustrated in Figure 8-3.

Chromatid-Type Aberrations

Chromatid-type aberrations are induced by ionizing radiation and other mutagens during the S or G_2 stage of the cell cycle. Viruses and many chemical agents, however, will cause only chromatid-type aberrations even though cells are exposed in G_1 and are examined in their first mitosis. These chromatid-type aberrations result from errors in DNA replication that occur during the S phase. Thus, these chromatid-type aberrations are not primary genetic lesions (lesions arising from direct mutagenesis), but are secondary lesions resulting from defective DNA repair.

The nomenclature of chromatid-type aberrations parallels closely that of chromosome-type aberrations, as follows.

1. A *chromatid and isochromatid gap* (= *achromatic lesion*) appears as a nonstaining, constricted region in the chromatid arm. The apparently broken segments of the

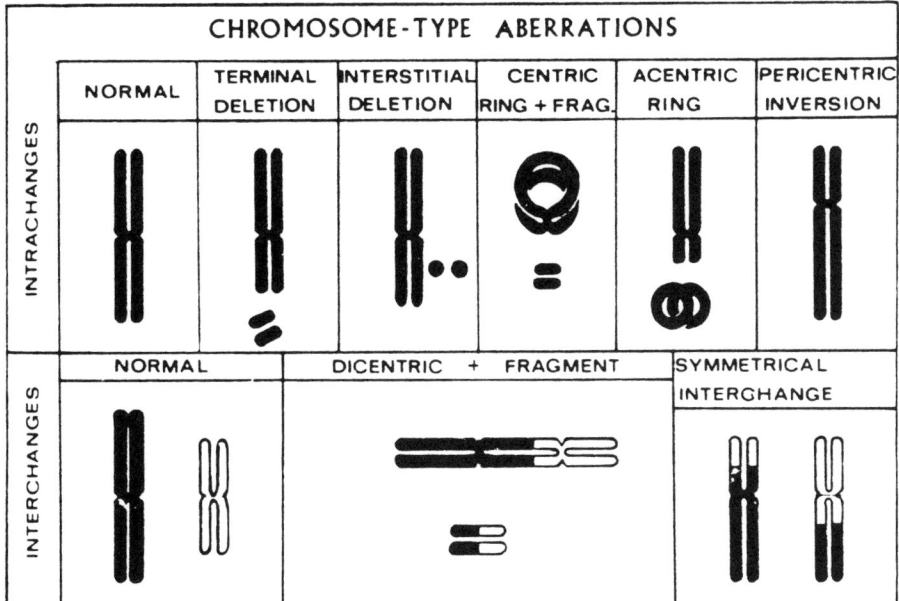

Figure 8-3. Seven classes of chromosome-type aberrations distinguishable at mitotic metaphase. (From Evans, 1984.)

chromatid are aligned. Gaps involving both chromatid arms at the same position are termed *isolocus* or *isochromatid gaps*.

2. A *chromatid break* is a discontinuity and displacement in the chromatid arm such that the broken chromatid ends are not aligned. *Simple* chromatid breaks result in a terminal deletion.

3. *Chromatid minutes* are unpaired intercalary fragments.

4. *Chromatid acentric* rings are intercalary fragments joined to produce ring structure.

5. *Centric rings* are intrachanges that result in rings that include a centromere.

6. *Inversions* can be *paracentric* or *pericentric*, as in *chromosome-type* inversions. Paracentric inversions are generally not scorable.

7. *Isochromatid aberrations* involve exchanges between paired chromatids (= *sister chromatid exchanges*). These can be confused with *chromosome-type* terminal deletions, but can be distinguished because isochromatid breaks usually involve a reunion of the broken chromatids.

8. *Symmetrical interchanges* involve an exchange(s) between two (or more) chromosomes. Exchanges between one chromatid in each of two chromosomes results in a four-arm structure termed a *quadri-radial*.

9. *Asymmetrical interchanges* are exchanges between two or more chromosomes resulting in one or more dicentric chromatids.

Unlike chromosome-type aberrations, chromatid breaks, and especially, chromatid gaps, are unreliable indicators of exposure-induced genetic damage. In part, this is because the scoring of gaps and breaks can be extremely subjective. Moreover, many gaps are technical artefacts—the results of poor culture conditions and drastic procedures during slide preparation (Evans and O'Riordan, 1975). For this reason, many investigators (e.g., Bloom, 1981; Therman, 1986) recommend that chromatid gaps not be counted in the total aberration score. If gaps are scored, it is important that control cell cultures be prepared at the same time as the exposed cultures to estimate the background rate of gap formation (Preston, 1984).

Other Chromosome Aberrations

1. *Shattering*. In shattering, chromosomes seem to have fractured into many small pieces. Shattering may affect all, or only a small number of the chromosomes in a cell. Shattered cells should be recorded separately and should not be included in the total number of cells analyzed (see Scoring of Aberrations).

2. *Pulverization*. Pulverization is similar to shattering, except that usually the entire cell is affected. As in shattering, pulverized cells should be recorded separately and should be excluded from the total cells analyzed.

3. *Polyploidy*. Cells with more than two full sets of chromosomes (polyploidy) may be observed. Aberrations observed in polyploid cells should be recorded separately (as above).

SCORING OF ABERRATIONS

It is important that each of the aberration types described be recorded separately. Results should be reported as frequency of aberration types per cell and frequency of aberrant cells per aberration type. The score "total breaks per cell" obscures valuable information and is no longer acceptable as state of the art (Bloom, 1981; Preston, 1984). For statistical analysis, however, it is often appropriate to combine frequencies of aberration types, such as chromatid-type exchanges and chromosome-type exchanges.

Much of the inconsistency observed in the results of chromosome aberration studies may reflect the fact that currently there is widespread variation in the way abnormalities are scored. The adoption of consistent rules might help avoid some of this cytogenetic information bias. Therman (1986) has suggested the following five rules for chromosome-breakage studies:

1. If the analysis is done on cultured cells, the control cells should be from the same individual and cultured at the same time. If this is not possible (for instance, in the study of whole-body irradiation), the control person should be of the same age and sex. In animal studies, the control should belong to the same inbred strain.
2. Diagrams or drawings should illustrate scored abnormalities, and particularly show what is scored as a gap or a break.
3. The chromosome slides of treated and control cells, made and stained at the same time, ought to be randomly coded to avoid investigator bias.
4. The investigator should establish clear rules about which metaphases are included in the study. Furthermore, published results should state whether the whole chromosome complement has been analyzed in all cells or only in those with obvious abnormalities.

5. The analysis should be done by a competent cytogeneticist, not by part-time, inexperienced laboratory helpers (Therman, 1986, p. 85).

Specific guidelines for scoring aberrations as well as a sample score sheet are available in Bloom (1981).

As Therman notes, it is essential that the cytotechnologist analyzing the slides be blind to the group (exposed or unexposed) to which they belong. Commonly several individuals and laboratories share the analysis. Thus, precautions must be taken so that possible bias caused by interindividual or interlaboratory variation will not influence the result. For example, control slides should not be scored exclusively by Laboratory A and exposed slides by Laboratory B. If possible, researchers (or laboratories) should keep photographic records of all aberrant and suspect cells. It is also desirable to produce and keep a permanent banded karyotype for each individual in the study, whether or not banded preparations are employed in the analysis of chromosomal aberrations themselves. (Banded preparations may be judged too time consuming to warrant the small added gain in sensitivity [see Preston, 1984, p. 132].) The banded karyotype ensures that any observed chromosomal abnormalities cannot be attributed, at some later date, to a congenital chromosome abnormality.

It is not possible to determine exactly the number of cells to be analyzed from any sample, as this number will depend on the expected aberration frequency, and hence, on the specific exposure under study. In general, however, 200 cells should be analyzed from each sample (Preston, 1984; see Sample Size and Power Considerations).

STATISTICAL ANALYSIS OF CHROMOSOME ABERRATIONS

The goal of analysis is to determine whether there is evidence of prior exposure to chemical mutagens, ionizing radiation, or both. Bloom (1981) provides an excellent discussion of the logic of data analysis on structural aberrations. Highlights of that discussion follow.

Analysis Strategies

The data of any individual studied consist of the number of aberrant cells identified from the total number of cells examined. In other words, the data are proportions. Thus, the number of cells with aberrations should conform to a binomial distribution with parameters n (sample size) and p (the true population of aberrant cells in the individual sampled). The basic statistical task is to compare the sets of proportions observed among the exposed and unexposed groups and to test the hypothesis that, on average, the proportions are greater in the exposed group.

The analysis that yields the greatest statistical power involves pooling data across individuals within exposure groups. The total number of cells examined in each group is used as the denominator for the estimate of the overall aberration rate. Because large aberration scores in a few individuals can influence the pooled analysis (e.g., 10 aberrations in a single individual is "equivalent" to one aberration in each of 10 individuals), it is important to ensure that the observed interindividual variability among the proportions does not exceed the variability expected from repeated sampling from a *single* binomial distribution. Fisher's variance test is recommended for this purpose (Cochran, 1954).

If one can assume a single aberration frequency within each group, one can analyze with statistical techniques for comparing two binomial frequencies. The data can be cast in the familiar 2 x 2 table, as follows:

	Exposed	Not Exposed	Total
Aberrant cells	a	b	a + b
Nonaberrant cells	c	d	c + d
Total cells	a + c	b/(b + d)	N
Proportion aberrant	a/(a + c)	b/(b + d)	

The question central to the analysis is whether the observed proportion in the exposed group, a/(a + c), is greater than the observed proportion in the unexposed group, b/(b + d), and whether this difference is sufficiently large to rule out chance as a competing explanation.

If there is an apparent difference between the exposed and control groups, either in terms of frequencies of cells with aberrations or frequencies of aberrations per cell, then further analysis is necessary to ascertain whether there is a dose–response relationship and whether interactions exist with potential confounding variables (Bloom, 1981).

Sample Size and Power Considerations

The number of cells examined can greatly influence a study's conclusions and is thus of particular importance in interpretating apparently negative findings. A valuable discussion of sample size and power as they pertain to human cytogenetic studies appears in papers by Whorton (1985) and Whorton et al. (1979).

To illustrate the importance of sample size, let us consider the following: If an aberration frequency of 1 percent is expected in the control group (as might occur if all aberrations were tallied), then it will be necessary to score 325 cells in each group to detect a fourfold increase in aberration frequency in an exposed group at the 5 percent significance level, with 80 percent power. Detecting a threefold increase would require some 600 cells, and detecting a relative risk of two would require nearly 2,000 cells per group. (These estimates assume equal numbers of exposed and unexposed in each group.)

If an exposed group as a whole shows an elevated frequency of aberrations, then the specificity with which an individual's aberration frequency can be ascertained becomes of interest. In general, it is necessary to have large quantities of data to estimate small frequencies accurately. For example, if no aberrations are detected in 100 cells from a given individual, that individual's aberration frequency can be determined only as less than 4 percent. To conclude that the true aberration rate is less than 1 percent at the 95 percent confidence level would require 375 normal cells. Of course, such precise determinations generally may not be cost effective. One feature of studies using chromosome aberrations, however, is that, given an adequate supply of stored blood, it is relatively easy to increase sample sizes.

Finally, it should be noted that there is considerable variation in frequency of chromosome breakage among cultures from different individuals and among consecutive cultures from the same individual (Littlefield et al., 1975; Galloway et al., 1986). This suggests that the frequency of chromosome aberrations in peripheral lymphocytes is influenced by many factors that are yet unidentified.

COST OF THE LYMPHOCYTE ASSAY

Analyzing metaphase chromosomes is a costly and labor-intensive process. Apart from the expense of obtaining blood samples, the processes of culture handling, slide preparation, and analysis of cells requires approximately 4.5 person-hours per culture of 100 cells (Evans and O'Riordan, 1975). Because most of this time—4 hours—is required for scoring aberrations, the lymphocyte assay requires a considerable expenditure of a trained cytogeneticist's time.

Attempts have been made to automate chromosome analysis (e.g., Philips and Lundsteen, 1985). But, although there are semiautomated techniques that can expedite the analysis of a relatively small number of cells (those needed for fetal chromosome diagnosis, for example), techniques for automated analysis of the large numbers of cells required for epidemiologic purposes are not currently practical.

ACCURACY OF THE LYMPHOCYTE ASSAY

To illustrate the limitations of the lymphocyte assay as a method of detecting aberrations and predicting possible exposure to chromosome damaging agents, we need to consider several aspects of the assay and of particular clastogens themselves. Discussions of the sensitivity of the lymphocyte assay appear in papers by Preston (1984), Buckton and Evans (1982), and Schinzel and Schmid (1976).

The accuracy of the lymphocyte assay varies according to the type of clastogenic exposure. In general, the assay is a sensitive tool for detecting exposure to radiation; it is much less sensitive for detecting exposure to chemicals.

Radiation Exposures

Radiation and a small number of chemical agents (the truly *radiomimetic* drugs, e.g., cytosine arabinoside, bleomycin, streptonigrin, and 8-methoxy caffeine) cause aberrations in all stages of the cell cycle: chromosome-type aberrations in G_1 and chromatid-type aberrations in S and G_2. In contrast, most chemical agents induce aberrations only when the cell is in the S phase or when it passes through the S phase between exposure and observation at mitosis. These aberrations occur either at the time of DNA replication or as a postreplication event, and are exclusively of the chromatid-type. This difference in the mode of aberration induction has important consequences for the ability of the assay to detect aberrations after radiation or chemical exposures.

Peripheral lymphocytes are in a noncycling stage of G_1 (generally referred to as G_0) until they are stimulated in vitro to reenter a cycling phase. If these noncycling cells are exposed to radiation, then chromosome-type aberrations will be induced directly. The frequency of aberrations observed at the first mitotic division in vitro will be the induced frequency, hence the importance of analyzing cells in their first in vitro division.

There is ample evidence, from studies that made physical estimates of exposure, that the frequency of observed chromosome aberrations is proportional to the radiation exposure (Awa, 1975). In individuals exposed to radiation, it is thus possible to use the chromosome aberration frequency to estimate exposure with a reasonable degree of accuracy (Preston, 1984). We must note, however, that this can be done reliably only in instances in which blood samples are taken relatively soon after exposure—within 6 weeks.

For samples taken at much longer intervals after acute radiation exposure (e.g., in the atom bomb survivors in Hiroshima and Nagasaki), attempts to infer exposure levels become more complex because of the importance of cell turnover in the lymphocyte population. Although no selective disadvantage has been ascribed to aberrant cells in G_0, repopulating cells tend to be those that do not contain cumbersome, cell-lethal aberrations such as rings, dicentrics, and acentric fragments. The selective death of aberrant cells means that the aberration frequency in samples taken at increasing intervals after exposure will contain fewer and fewer aberrant cells. The numbers of newly arising cells will dilute the numbers of aberrant cells. Because a portion of lymphocytes are very long-lived, however, a small proportion of aberrant lymphocytes can be detected in the circulating population 30 years or more after exposure.

Unlike the majority of observed chromosome-type aberrations (dicentrics, rings, and acentric fragments), reciprocal translocations and inversions usually are not cell-lethal. Because these can be transmitted with a high probability, the numbers of cells containing these aberrations will decline less after exposure. Although one might want to analyze these types of aberrations, the sensitivity of the assay for these aberrations is only about 50 percent, even with banded preparations (Preston, 1984).

In the case of long-term chronic exposure to radiation (e.g., in nuclear dockyard workers), some aberrations in the G_0 cells will accumulate in the population of the long-lived lymphocytes and can indicate that an exposure has occurred. Unlike samples taken after acute exposure, the observed aberration frequency will not be a direct measure of the actual amount of exposure.

In summary, the fact that chromosome aberrations induced by radiation occur at the same stage of the cell cycle as that in which exposure occurs means that, under appropriate circumstances, these aberrations can be reliable dosimeters of exposure. The lymphocyte assay is less sensitive in measuring chronic exposures, or if it is performed long after acute radiation exposure has occurred. Such exposures are detectable, however, in a long-lived subpopulation of lymphocytes.

Exposure Specificity and Marker Persistence

The lymphocyte assay is not a one-size-fits-all detector of exposure to all clastogenic agents, simply because the nature and longevity of the aberrations vary from one agent to another. For example, occupational exposures to some chemicals, such as arsenic and benzene, are associated with very long-lived chromosomal aberrations that probably reflect cumulative exposure (for a review of these exposures, see Office of Technology Assessment, 1983). Conversely, aberrations seen with exposure to vinyl chloride monomers are very short-lived, often disappearing within weeks or even days. In this instance, chromosomal aberrations could be used to document recent, but not chronic exposure. What mechanism underlies this difference is not known.

Such differences in the persistence of induced aberrations indicate the need to determine the appropriateness of chromosomal endpoints in occupational studies on a case by case basis. Ideally, meaningful use of the assay requires some prior information about the type and persistence of the aberrations expected. For an illustration of how to use the lymphocyte assay, see the case of ethylene oxide (under "Occupational Monitoring").

Chemical Exposures

The interpretation of the lymphocyte assay is less certain and its potential sensitivity is less well understood in cases of exposure to chemical agents. As described previously, most chemicals induce aberrations only when the cell passes through an S phase between exposure and observation. Because the peripheral lymphocyte is in G_0, the first S phase takes place in vitro after mitogenic stimulation. DNA damage induced in G_0 will be manifest in the S phase as chromatid-type damage, due in part to aberration-induced misrepair. That is, the frequency of chromatid-type aberrations will depend on the amount of chromosome damage, whose preservation and/or misrepair results in chromatid aberrations that remain at replication. Several factors influence these aberrations including the amount of initial damage and the amount and accuracy of repair that takes place in G_0 and G_1 after mitogenic stimulation.

The time between exposure to a chemical agent and sampling is a far more important consideration in the case of chemical agents than for radiation. This is because several factors operate to reduce the amount of DNA damage present at the time of replication and thus to reduce the aberration frequency. A striking illustration of the importance of time in diluting the frequency of observed chromatid-type aberrations can be seen in patients who have received cytostatic drug chemotherapy. Such people have very high aberration frequencies in lymphocyte samples taken during therapy, but virtually no induced aberrations in samples taken 2 months after therapy ends (Schinzel and Schmid, 1976).

Furthermore, because chromosomes have complex mechanisms of repair, the frequency of aberrations observed in a cell population exposed to a chemical agent is not likely to be directly related to exposure. However, one might find a proportional relationship. Unlike exposure to radiation, in which an observed aberration frequency that is not significantly elevated above background can be used to rule out exposure of a given magnitude, it is impossible to estimate a maximum possible exposure to chemical agents. Again, study of patients exposed to cytostatic drugs shows that, even after exposure to massive doses of clastogens, a normal frequency of aberrations can be found after enough time has passed (Schinzel and Schmid, 1976).

As with acute chemical exposures, the lymphocyte assay is also an unreliable tool to indicate chronic chemical exposures because of the repair that constantly occurs in the G_0 lymphocyte. This constant repair is reflected in less damage observable in the S phase. As a result, the chromosome aberration frequency observed will be very low, and the probability of detecting a frequency significantly above background will be small (Preston, 1984).

Table 8-1 Radiation Versus Chemically Induced Chromosome Aberrations in Peripheral Lymphocytes

	Radiation	Chemicals
Aberration type	Chromosome	Chromatid
Reliability	Good	Uncertain/poor
Dose-response	Yes	Variable
Persistence of marker	Long duration	Short/variable duration

In conclusion, because aberrations caused by nonradiomimetic chemicals are not induced at the time of exposure to the clastogenic agent, and as several time-dependent repair processes reduce the induced aberration frequency, the lymphocyte assay is much less sensitive as a measure of exposure to chemicals than of exposure to radiation. Table 8-1 presents a comparison of different properties of the lymphocyte assay for chemical and for radiation exposures.

CONTROL GROUPS AND THE ISSUE OF "BACKGROUND" FREQUENCY

To gauge whether the frequency of chromosome aberrations is elevated in a human population exposed to some factor, it is necessary to compare this frequency with the frequency of aberrations in an unexposed, or control, group. How one selects an appropriate reference group will depend on the type of exposure: whether to radiation or to chemicals.

In the case of suspected exposure to radiation, determining background frequencies of chromosome aberrations is fairly straightforward. Radiation-induced aberrations are of the chromosome-type. Because they can be scored easily and reliably, dicentric chromosomes are generally used to estimate exposure. Because the frequency of dicentrics in unexposed populations is low (about 1/1000 cells), it is easy to detect the effect of even small radiation doses. Moreover, because most other environmental agents that influence the background rate of aberrations are expected to induce chromatid-type aberrations, these factors should not be important confounders in comparing radiation-exposed and nonexposed groups. In general, the factors that induce chromosome-type aberrations are very well studied (Awa, 1975), and Lloyd et al. (1980) have assembled a compendium of data on the frequencies of chromosome-type aberrations in numerous groups occupationally exposed to radiation.

As discussed, most chemical agents induce chromatid-type aberrations. Thus, factors that influence the frequency of these aberrations in exposed and nonexposed populations are important. The Office of Technology Assessment (1983) has compiled background frequencies for chromosomal aberrations in unexposed populations from several reported studies. Although diverse laboratory methodologies make accurate comparisons among these studies difficult, the range of reported frequencies of individual aberrations per cell was:

Chromosome breaks	0.11–6.72%
Chromatid breaks	0.1–3.0%
Exchange aberrations	0–0.34%
Cells containing any aberrations	0.2–8.5%
Sister chromatid exchanges	5.8–16.2 per cell

The wide variations in the range of normal values for chromosomal endpoints emphasize the potential importance of individual differences in laboratory methodology and illustrate the difficulty in making quantitative comparisons of aberration frequencies across studies. It is especially noteworthy that the 40-fold differences reported for normal values of chromosome aberrations are far in excess of those reported in individual studies between occupationally exposed and unexposed groups (Office of Technology Assessment, 1983).

"Matched" Controls

Most investigators recommend comparing the aberration frequency observed in an exposed group with that of a matched control group. The matching variables, such as gender, age, socioeconomic status, geographic location, and others, are attempts to ensure that the aberration frequency observed in a control population is, save for the exposure, similar to the background frequency of the exposed population. Because it is not clear what factors actually influence the background frequency of chromatid-type aberrations, attempts to provide a matched control group should be viewed as attempts to control for unmeasured confounders.

In occupational exposures, the ideal controls clearly would be the individuals themselves. That is, blood samples could be taken from individuals before they began work in a potentially hazardous environment. Although this has been done rarely, it certainly should be considered in planning studies. Further discussions on selecting control populations appear in Preston (1984).

Potential Confounders

Many factors have been reported to influence the background rate of chromosome aberrations, including recent viral infections, age, gender, smoking habits, oral contraceptive use, and season of the year (see Office of Technology Assessment, 1983, for complete citations). Of these, only viral infection is an undisputed and strong independent risk factor. Age and smoking status probably are risk factors, albeit moderate ones.

Acute viral infections, particularly with measles virus, are potent clastogens. Chromosome damage caused by viral infection varies from single chromatid breaks to pulverization of the entire chromosome complement (Therman, 1986). The mechanism(s) of virus-induced chromosome breaks are poorly understood. For a review of the role of viruses in clastogenesis, see Nichols (1983).

There are many conflicting reports on the role of age. Some studies report an increase in background aberration frequency with age, and others report no effect. One study with a large sample size ($> 4,000$ cells) supports the hypothesis that aberration frequency does increase with age. Kuhn and Therman (1979) report that an analysis of

2,324 cells from subjects under 40 years of age yielded an average of 0.8 percent of cells with chromosome aberrations (excluding gaps). A sample of about the same size from individuals with a mean age of 55.8 years gave an average of 2.4 percent abnormal cells. Galloway et al. (1986) also found an increase in chromosome aberrations with age. Similarly, Bochov and Kuleshov (1972) reported that the frequency of chromosome aberrations induced in vitro by alkylating agents increased sequentially in lymphocytes from newborns, young adults (mean age 23), and elderly persons (mean age 70). In this much smaller study, however, these authors found no increase with age in the background aberration rate.

There has been considerable controversy about the clastogenic effects of cigarette smoke. Many positive and negative studies have been reported (see Littlefield and Joiner, 1986, for citations). Few have used comparable methodologies. In a recent carefully conducted study, Littlefield and Joiner (1986) compared the incidence of chromosome aberrations in 500 first-division metaphases from 48-hour lymphocyte cultures from six nonsmokers and from six people who had smoked at least one pack of cigarettes per day for at least 20 years. The subjects were similar in age and in their consumption of beverages containing caffeine, a potent co-clastogen. Analysis of coded slides revealed a total of three aberrations in the 3,000 slides from the nonsmokers (an aberration rate of 0.1%) versus 22 aberrations in the 3,000 slides from the smokers (an aberration rate of 0.7%). Thus, these data support the hypothesis that cigarette smoke is clastogenic. Therefore, in epidemiologic studies, it is important to ensure that smokers are not distributed disproportionately between the unexposed and the exposed groups under study. It is also possible that smoking may modify the clastogenic effects of other exposures.

In conclusion, established potential confounders of an exposure-chromosome aberration association include current viral infections, age, and heavy smoking. Thus, it is necessary to obtain smoking histories on all participants in a planned study. Potential subjects with exposures to ionizing radiation, chemotherapy, and recent vaccinations should be excluded.

BIOLOGICAL SIGNIFICANCE OF CHROMOSOME ABERRATIONS

An empirical association between chromosome damage and carcinogenesis has been established in animal studies. We must emphasize, however, that the lymphocyte assay is a marker of exposure or biological response to exposure. Except in rare cases, such as the Philadelphia chromosome described later, it is not a general marker of disease or of an individual's susceptibility to disease.

An important issue that needs to be clarified is the difference between the epidemiologic significance of an increased aberration frequency in populations, and the clinical significance of an elevated aberration frequency in a given individual.

Ongoing epidemiologic studies of the Japanese survivors of the atomic bomb have established that these populations have an increased risk for many types of cancer, particularly leukemias, cancers of the thyroid, female breast, and lung (Awa, 1975). All of these cancers have shown a dose-dependence for radiation, although the shape of the dose–response curve differs for the different cancers. Extensive cytogenetic investigations of the survivors have also revealed a dose-dependent increase in chromosomal aberrations. Evidence of chromosomal aberrations, malignancy, and other clinical findings studied among individuals in the Hiroshima population, however, seemed not to show correlations among these factors (King et al., 1975). Thus, although chromosome aberrations can serve as dosimeters of exposure to known carcinogens, they appear to be predictive of an increased disease frequency at the ecological level only.

A notable exception to the generalization that chromosomal aberrations are not predictive of disease is the case of the Philadelphia chromosome—a translocation of the long arm of chromosome 22, usually to the long arm terminus of chromosome 9. This translocation correlates highly with chronic myelogenous leukemia: about 90 percent of patients having this marker chromosome later develop the disease (see Sandberg et al., 1986, for a review of the Philadelphia chromosome). Specific aberrations, such as the Philadelphia chromosome, which carry a probable prognosis of serious disease raise ethical questions for investigators who discover them during cytogenetic analysis. Has the investigator a responsibility to inform an individual that that he or she is at risk? As yet, the epidemiologic literature has rarely addressed such questions.

CHROMSOME ABERRATIONS VERSUS SISTER CHROMATID EXCHANGES

Sister chromatid exchange (SCE) was first described by Taylor in 1958. In the 1970s, SCE analysis was shown to be applicable to both in vivo and in vitro mutagenicity testing (for a review, see Latt et al. (1980)). Chapter 6 presents a detailed discussion of the SCE assay. In the context of the present review, however, several points bear repetition.

In the late 1970s, cytogenetics witnessed a period of "SCE-euphoria" during which many investigators substituted the comparatively simple and less costly SCE test for classic cytogenetic analyses (Gebhart, 1981). Two major developments have since tempered this euphoria: the realization that the biological consequences of SCEs are unknown and the recognition that the results of SCE and chromosome aberration tests often do not agree.

Gebhart (1981) has summarized the world literature on the concordance between chromosomal aberrations and SCEs. He found a 30 percent qualitative disagreement between chromosome aberrations and SCEs in both in vivo and in vitro tests of the same chemical. Ionizing radiation offers a clear illustration of the disparity between aberrations and SCEs. Radiation doses of about 400 R, which can cause a 100-fold increase in the rate of chromosome breaks, raise the baseline rate of SCEs only twofold. This suggests that the mechanism(s) through which particular agents interact with DNA to produce SCEs may differ from the mechanism(s) that produces chromosomal aberrations.

Compared with SCEs, chromosome breakage in untreated cells is very rare. In one laboratory (Gebhart, 1981), the average baseline frequency of SCEs is 5.6 per metaphase. In contrast, the average breakage rate is 0.02 per metaphase, yielding a SCE-to-break ratio of 280:1. This large disparity between the baseline frequencies of SCEs and chromosome breaks should be remembered when one compares results from both systems.

OCCUPATIONAL MONITORING: ETHYLENE OXIDE

Having set out the basic methodology for using the lymphocyte assay in epidemiologic studies, we can now compare several recent investigations that have examined occupational exposure to the same chemical agent, ethylene oxide.

Ethylene oxide, an alkylating agent, has been produced commercially since 1921 and is used worldwide as a chemical intermediate in the production of manufactured goods and in sterilizing medical supplies.

Ethylene oxide has been shown to induce mutations in bacterial, plant, and animal test systems (see Glazer, 1979, for a review). Several investigators (e.g., Embree et al., 1977) estimate that the genetic risk from exposure to ethylene oxide may be as high as that from exposure to ionizing radiation. Because of the compound's high volatility, the opportunities for human exposure are great, especially among industrial workers, medical staff, and patients.

The current Occupational Safety and Health Administration (OSHA) standard for ethylene oxide is 50 ppm, time-weighted average. There are two reports of increased leukemia among people industrially exposed to this chemical (Högstedt et al., 1979a, 1979b).

In 1967, Kalling reported an increased chromosome aberration rate in exposed workers' lymphocytes 18 months after an accident involving ethylene oxide. He also reported that 2 hours of acute exposure to the chemical produced a significant increase in the number of cells with chromosome aberrations. The report, however, gave no details about the actual study methods used.

The first completely reported work of chromosome aberrations in workers exposed to ethylene oxide was a study by Thiess et al. (1981). They studied 43 men (average age 47.1 years) who were exposed to the chemical in a German plant. The men were divided into four groups: group 1, long-term exposure of 20 years or more; group 2, exposure less than 20 years; group 3, long-term plus accidental exposure, and group 4, accidental acute high exposure only. Thiess and colleagues were not able to make accurate measurements of past exposure levels to ethylene oxide, but they estimated that the accidental exposure caused acute exposure levels as high as 1,900 ppm.

The control group of 25 men (average age 38.6 years) was composed mostly of office workers from the West German Occupational Medicine and Health Protection Department (the authors' institution).

The investigators carried out chromosome analyses using a 70- to 72-hour culture period, but did not use BrdUrd. They coded and examined 100 metaphases from each exposed man and each control.

The results indicated that the mean frequency of aberrant metaphases 6.4 percent (excluding gaps) in the long-term exposure group (group 1) was significantly higher that the mean frequency of aberrations in the control group, 4 percent. Aberration frequencies for groups 2 through 4 had slightly, but not significantly increased aberration frequencies (6.0, 4.7, and 5.2%, respectively). On resampling group 1 and the control group 1 year later, there was still a significantly elevated aberration frequency. The authors concluded that the increased chromosome aberration rate in group 1 reflected a mutagenic exposure. But, as the workers had been exposed to many other agents (e.g., benzene), the authors noted that the results did not support the assumption that the risk is specific to ethylene oxide.

This study can be criticized on several grounds. First, the culturing period, 70 to 72 hours, was too long. No attempts were made to ensure the analysis of only first division cells. Other criticisms apply to the selection of the controls, who were roughly 10 years younger than the exposed groups (thus creating a potential bias away from the null), and largely drawn from a population, health professionals, probably unlike the factory population. It is, thus, possible that other exposures, such as smoking, could be partly responsible for the observed effect.

Sarto and colleagues (1984) investigated cytogenetic damage (SCEs and chromosome aberrations) in sanitary workers exposed to ethylene oxide in eight hospitals in Venice. They studied two exposure groups: one was exposed to 10.7 ± 4.9 ppm ethylene oxide (19 individuals), and the other to 0.35 ± 0.12 ppm (22 individuals). Each exposed worker was matched to a control of similar age and smoking habits. The controls also were sanitary engineers from the same hospitals who were not occupationally exposed to ethylene oxide, cytostatic drugs, anesthetic gases, or ionizing radiation.

The authors cultured lymphocytes for 48 to 52 hours, analyzed 100 metaphases for each person, and scored them blind to exposure status.

The results revealed a significant elevation of SCEs for both the low- and high-exposure groups (i.e., a dose-response). Similarly, in the higher exposure group, the number of both chromatid- and chromosome-type aberrations was significantly increased. In the lower exposure group, the frequency of chromosome-type aberrations only was significantly higher than in controls. A reexamination of 10 individuals 18 months after exposure was ended or lowered indicated that the elevated frequencies of both SCEs and chromosome-type and chromatid-type aberrations had changed little. Of the cytogenetic changes, the chromosome aberrations were more stable. The frequency of cells with chromosome aberrations was found to be weakly but significantly correlated with ethylene oxide exposure, but not correlated with smoking, age, or SCE frequency.

The work by Sarto and colleagues represents a large methodologic advance over the earlier work by Thiess et al. (1981). The Sarto study took particular care to ensure the comparability of exposed and unexposed persons (matching by job title and hospital) and to minimize confounding (matching on age and smoking status). As in the previous study, Sarto and colleagues noted chromosome aberrations of apparently long duration. Because the aberrations in the Sarto study were seen in individuals not occupationally exposed to other known clastogens (e.g., benzene), this result suggests that ethylene oxide may indeed be the cause of the long-lived aberrations.

Van Sittert and colleagues (1985) examined the occurrence of chromosome abnormalities and other hematologic parameters in workers in an ethylene oxide manufacturing plant. They studied 36 individuals (mean age 32 years) who had been employed up to 14 years in ethylene oxide manufacture. They studied two exposure groups: one with exposure of more than 5 years duration (17 workers), the other with exposure of less than 5 years (19 workers). The exposed workers were matched to individuals who had no exposure to ethylene oxide manufacturing or to other known or suspected clastogens. They obtained information on smoking habits and previous occupational history for all groups.

For the cytogenetic analysis, they incubated cells either 48 hours or 72 hours using Ham's F-10 medium. The percent of cultures left for 72 hours was unspecified.

The results indicated no statistically significant differences between the plant workers and the control group with respect to chromosome aberrations or any of the other hematologic parameters investigated. The duration of employment in the ethylene oxide industry, however, was correlated positively with the frequency of chromosome breaks. This effect could not be attributed to the older age of the workers with longer work histories.

Although the Van Sittert study did not find an increased aberration frequency in ethylene oxide-exposed workers compared with nonexposed workers, there are several reasons why the study might not have detected such exposure effects. Most salient among these is the type of manufacturing plant. Unlike the workers in previous studies, these workers were employed in a modern, open-air manufacturing plant. The work site had the lowest exposures of any in the previous studies. Furthermore, the exposure durations (years worked) were lower than in the Thiess et al. study. The fact that the duration of work exposure correlated significantly with the frequency of chromosome breaks is consistent with previous findings and suggests that the otherwise negative findings may be due to the low level and relatively short duration of exposure.

The most recent study of chromosome aberrations in workers exposed to ethylene oxide was reported by Galloway et al. (1986), who studied the aberration frequencies of 61 employees potentially exposed to ethylene oxide. They studied three different worksites. For each potentially exposed worker, a randomly selected control matched for sex and age was identified in the same plant. They also selected a second control group of age-matched and sex-matched individuals who lived in the same community and were not exposed to ethylene oxide. They obtained a smoking history from all study participants.

The authors processed blood samples from potentially exposed and unexposed individuals concurrently. They processed lymphocytes from community controls on separate occasions from the other groups. Cells were incubated for 48 to 51 hours.

The results indicated an elevated chromosome aberration rate in exposed workers in worksite III, the site with the greatest historical exposure to ethylene oxide. Worksite III was subdivided a priori into high and low exposure categories. The frequency of cells with aberrations was 5.6 percent in the two workers in the high exposure category and 2.6 percent in the 23 individuals in the low exposure category. The overall frequency of aberrations in the 304 matched control individuals was 1.4 percent.

Within the 304 control individuals, the authors found significant increases in aberrations with smoking and with increasing age. The authors also compared the frequency of chromosome aberrations with data they had previously reported on SCEs (Stolley et al., 1984). There was only a weak overall association between SCEs and chromosome aberrations. The correlation was found in potentially exposed but not in control groups. For a given individual, they found that they could not use data on SCE frequency to predict the frequency of chromosome aberrations.

The study by Galloway and colleagues represents the best in state of the art epidemiology using cytologic endpoints. The study is distinguished by its large sample sizes, use of multiple worksites, and of community and worksite controls, and complete reporting of aberration subtypes and frequencies.

SUMMARY: ADVANTAGES AND DISADVANTAGES OF THE PERIPHERAL LYMPHOCYTE ASSAY

Advantages

1. Peripheral blood lymphoctyes are readily available. A few milliliters of peripheral blood can be easily and repeatably obtained from an individual. Each milliliter of blood contains $1-3 \times 10^6$ lymphoctyes.

2. The lymphocytes circulate through all tissues in the body. A portion of them are long-lived.

3. Blood lymphocytes are a synchronized population; virtually all the cells are in the same G_0 or G_1 stage of mitotic interphase.

4. A proportion of the lymphocytes can be stimulated to undergo mitosis in culture and provide a supply of dividing cells for the study of chromosome abnormalities.

5. Lymphocytes from unexposed people have a low spontaneous aberration frequency.

6. Exposures to ionizing radiation produce persistent aberrations that permit estimations of received dose.

Disadvantages

1. Although lymphocytes are a synchronized population, there are different subpopulations of cells within the same individual. These may have varying responses to mitogenic and clastogenic agents.

2. It is probable that less heavily damaged cells will grow preferentially in culture; in Thilly's (1985) words, "dead cells don't form mutant colonies." This will underestimate the true clastogenic effect of any agent under study.

3. In humans, only the T or thymus-derived lymphocytes can be stimulated to undergo mitosis in culture. Because T lymphocytes are involved in immune responses, any previous immunologic stimulus may positively or negatively alter the number of cells with chromosome aberrations, depending on when the cells are drawn from the individual.

4. Although the spontaneous aberration frequency is low, the assay's interlaboratory and even interculture variation is large. This can confound real associations of interest.

5. In general, the lymphocyte assay is an uncertain indicator of exposure to chemicals. The need to consider exposures on a case-to-case basis complicates matters when individuals are exposed to more than one chemical.

6. The assay is expensive, time intensive, and requires trained personnel.

REFERENCES

Awa AA: Review of thirty years study of Hiroshima and Nagasaki atomic bomb survivors. *J Radiat Res [Suppl]*, 1975.

Bloom AD (ed.): *Guidelines for studies of human populations exposed to mutagenic and re-*

productive hazards. Report of Panel 1. March of Dimes Birth Defects Foundation, New York, 1981.

Bochov NP, Kuleshov NP: Age sensitivity of human chromosomes to alkylating agents. *Mutat Res* 1972;14:345–353.

Boveri T: *Zur Frage der Erstehung Maligner Tumoren.* Jena, Fischer, 1914.

Buckton KE, Evans HJ: Human peripheral blood lymphocyte cultures: An *in vitro* assay for the cytogenetic effects of environmental mutagens. In: Hsu TC, ed.: *Cytogenetic Assays of Environmental Mutagens.* Osmun, Allanheld, 1982, pp. 183–202.

Cochran WG: Some methods of strengthening the common 2x2 tests. *Biometrics* 1954;10:417.

Dale K: Cytogenetic review couse: III. Bone marrow culture. *Karyogram* 1980;6:33–53.

Dale K, Juergens L: Cytogenetic review course: V. Straining techniques. *Karyogram* 1980;6:49–55.

Ehrenberg L, Hallstrom T: Hematologic studies on persons occupationally exposed to ethylene oxide. (communicated by LO Kalling) In: *Radiosterilization of Medical Products.* Vienna: International Atomic Energy Agency SM 92/26, 1967, pp. 327–334.

Embree JW, Lyon JP, Hine CH: The mutagenic potential of ethylene oxide using the dominant lethal assay in rats. *Toxicol Appl Pharmacol* 1977;40:261–267.

Evans HJ, O'Riordan ML: Human peripheral blood lymphocytes for the analysis of chromosome aberrations in mutagen tests. *Mutat Res* 1975;31:135–148.

Evans HJ: Human peripheral blood lymphocytes for the analysis of chromosome aberrations in mutagen tests. In: Kilbey BJ, Legator M, Nichols W, Ramel C, eds.: *Handbook of Mutagenicity Test Procedures.* Amsterdam, Elsevier, 1984, pp. 405–428.

Galloway SM, Berry PK, Nichols WW, Wolman SR, Soper KA, Stolley PD, Archer P: Chromosome aberrations in individuals occupationally exposed to ethylene oxide, and in a large control population. *Mutat Res* 1986;170:55–74.

Gebhart E: Sister Chromatid Exchange (SCE) and structural chromosome aberration in mutagenicity testing. *Humangenetik* 1981;58:235–254.

Gebhart E: The epidemiologic approach: Chromosome aberrations in persons exposed to chemical mutagens. In: Hsu TC, ed.: *Cytogenetic Assays of Environmental Mutagens.* Osmun, Allanheld, 1982, pp. 385–408.

Glazer ZR: Ethylene oxide: Toxicology review and field study results of hospital use. *J Environ Pathol Toxicol* 1979;2:172–207.

Högstedt C, et al.: A cohort study of mortality and cancer incidence in ethylene oxide production workers. *Br J Ind Med* 1979a;36:276–280.

Högstedt C, et al.: Leukemia in workers exposed to ethylene oxide. *JAMA* 1979b;241:1132–1133.

Hsu TC: Human and mammalian cytogenetics: A historical perspective. New York, Springer-Verlag, 1979.

Hsu TC: A historical outline of the development of cancer cytogenetics. *Cancer Genet Cytogenet* 1987;28:5–26.

Hungerford DA: Leukocytes cultured from small inocula of whole blood and the preparation of metaphase chromosomes by treatment with hypotonic KC1. *Stain Technol* 1965;40:333–338.

ISCN: An international system for human cytogenetic nomenclature (1978). *Cytogenet Cell Genet* 1978;21:309–404.

ISCN: An international system for human cytogenetic nomenclature—high resolution banding (1981). *Cytogenet Cell Genet* 1981;31:1–23.

ISCN: An international system for human cytogenetic nomenclature (1985). *Birth Defects* 1985;21.

King RA, et al.: Chromosome abnormalities in A-bomb survivors. *Atomic Bomb Casualty Commission Technical Report,* 1972; pp. 15–72.

Kuhn EM, Therman E: No increased chromosome breakage in three Bloom's syndrome hetero-zygotes. *J Med Genet* 1979;16:219–222.

Larson L: Human chromosome analysis: Methodology and applications. *Am J Med Technol* 1983;10:687–698.

Latt SA, Schreck RR, Loveday KS, Dougherty CP, Shuler CF: Sister chromatid exchanges. *Adv Hum Genet* 1980;10:267–331.

Lejeune JC, Gautier M, Turpin R: Etude des chromosomes somatiques de neuf enfant mongloiens. *Comptes Rendus* 1959;248:1721–1722.

Littlefield LG, Joiner EE: Analysis of chromosome aberrations in lymphocytes of long-term heavy smokers. *Mutat Res* 1986;170:145–150.

Littlefield LG, Lever WE, Miller FL, Goh K: Chromosomal breakage studies in lymphocytes from normal women, pregnant women, and women taking oral contraceptives. *Am J Obstet Gynecol* 1975;121:976–980.

Lloyd DC, Purrott RJ, Reeder EJ: The incidence of unstable chromosome aberrations in pe-ripheral blood lymphocytes from unirradiated and occupationally exposed people. *Mutat Res* 1980;72:523–532.

Miller OJ: Structure and organization of mammalian chromosomes: Normal and abnormal. *Birth Defects* 1987;23:19–63.

Nichols WW: Viral interactions with the mammalian genome relevant to neoplasia. In: German J, ed.: *Chromosome Mutation and Neoplasia*. New York, Liss, 1983, pp. 317–332.

Obe G, Beek B, Dudin G: The human leukocyte test system. V.DNA synthesis and mitoses in PHA-stimulated 3-day cultures. *Hum Genet* 1975;28:295–302.

Office of Technology Assessment. *Technologies for Detecting Heritable Mutations in Human Beings* (1986). U.S. Government Printing Office, Washington, D.C.

Office of Technology Assessment. *The Role of Genetic Testing in the Prevention of Occupational Disease* (1983). Congress of the United States, Office of Technology Assessment, Wash-ington, D.C.

Philip J, Lundsteen C: Semiautomated chromosome analysis: A clinical test. *Clin Genet* 1985;27:140–146.

Preston JR: Cytogenetic abnormalities as an indicator of mutagenic exposure. In: Ansari A, De Serres F, eds.: *Single-Cell Mutation Monitoring Systems*. New York, Plenum, 1984, pp. 127–143.

Ruddon RW: *Cancer Biology*. New York, Oxford University Press, 1981.

Sandberg AA, Gemmill RM, Hecht BK, Hecht F: The Philadelphia Chromosome: A model of cancer and molecular cytogenetics. *Cancer Genet Cytogenet* 1986;21:129–146.

Sanchez O, Escobar JI, Yunis JJ: A simple G-banding technique. *Lancet* 1973;ii:269.

Sarto F, Cominato I, Pinton AM, Brovedani PG, Faccioli CM, Bianchi V, Levis AG: Cytogene-tic damage in workers exposed to ethylene oxide. *Mutat Res* 1984;138:185–195.

Savage JRK: Classification and relationships of induced chromosomal structural changes. *J Med Genet* 1975;12:103–122.

Schinzel A, Schmid W: Lymphocyte chromosome studies in humans exposed to chemical mutagens: The validity of the method in 67 patients under cytostatic therapy. *Mutat Res* 1976;40:139–166.

Stolley PD, Soper KA, Galloway SM, Nichols WW, Norman SA, Wolman: Sister-chromatid exchanges in association with occupational exposure to ethylene oxide. *Mutat Res* 1984;129:89–102.

Taylor JH: Sister chromatid exchanges in tritium-labelled chromosomes. *Genet* 1958;43:515–529.

Therman E. *Human Chromosomes*, New York, Springer-Verlag, 1986.

Thiess AM, Schwegler H, Fleig I, Stocker WG: Mutagenicity study of workers exposed to alkylene oxides (Ethylene oxide/Propylene oxide) and derivatives. *J Occup Med* 1981;23:343–347.

Thilly WG: Dead cells don't form mutant colonies: A serious source of bias in mutation assays. *Environ Mutagen* 1985;7:255–258.

Van Sittert NJ, De Jong G, Clare MG, Davies R, Dean BJ, Wren LJ, Wright AS: Cytogenetic, immunological, and haematological effects in workers in an ethylene oxide manufacturing plant. *Br J Ind Med* 1985;42:19–26.

Whorton EB Jr: Some experimental design and analysis considerations for cytogenetics studies. *Environ Mutagen* 1985;4(suppl):9–15.

Whorton EB Jr, Bee DB, Kilian J: Variations in the proportion of abnormal cells and required sample sizes for human cytogenetic studies. *Mutat Res* 1979;64:79–86.

Yunis JJ: New chromosome techniques in the study of human neoplasia. *Hum Pathol* 1981;12:540–549.

9

ONCOGENES:
A PRIMER FOR EPIDEMIOLOGISTS

GARY G. SCHWARTZ

INTRODUCTION

Oncogenes are genes that cause cancer (Bishop, 1987). They represent altered versions of normal genes, protooncogenes, that exist in every cell. Protooncogenes code for proteins that involve cell growth and differentiation. When a protooncogene is altered to become an oncogene, it may produce an abnormal product, produce an excess of a normal product, or express a normal product at an abnormal time. These changes confer transforming properties leading to neoplasia. Like the legendary Dr. Jekyll, protooncogenes can turn into malefactors, called oncogenes.

Recent explosions of information in virology, tumor biology, and cytogenetics have done much to increase our understanding of oncogenes. Although this new information promises in turn to extend the scope of cancer epidemiology, the literature on oncogenes can, unfortunately, be a daunting and inaccessible one for many epidemiologists. This chapter seeks to introduce the nonspecialist epidemiologist to oncogenes and to several of the new genetic techniques. The review begins at the beginning, with the discovery of oncogenes.

DISCOVERY OF ONCOGENES

The discovery of oncogenes follows two lines of investigation. The first of these involves RNA viruses, that is, retroviruses, and their ability to cause cancer.

In the early 1900s, a farmer discovered a tumor in one of his hens, which he brought to Dr. Peyton Rous at the Rockefeller Institute in New York. Rouse demonstrated that a cell-free isolate from this tumor, a sarcoma, could induce sarcomas in healthy chickens (1910). Reports of this research were not well received, and eventually Rous abandoned his work on tumor viruses because of the disapproval of his peers.

Nearly a half century later the reality of the virus first identified by Rous was established beyond doubt, as it and other tumor viruses were purified by physical techniques and visualized with the electron microscope. Tumor viruses soon became everyday agents in cancer research. In 1966, the 85-year-old Rous was awarded a Nobel prize.

In the next decade, the advent of recombinant DNA technology spawned an era of enormous activity in the retrovirus field. In the early 1970s investigators learned that the tumorigenic properties of the Rous sarcoma virus were due to the expression of only a single gene from among the virus's regular complement of genes (Anderson et al., 1975). This gene was named *src* for sarcoma. The protein it encoded was dubbed *pp60 src, "pp"* for phosphoprotein and *"60"* for its molecular weight, 60,000 daltons.

In 1976, the group led by Harold Varmus and J. Michael Bishop discovered that *src* was not really a viral gene. Instead, it was almost an exact copy of a normal gene found in all chicken cells. For lack of a more informative name, the normal gene was called a *protooncogene*. The authors hypothesized that the viral oncogene originated when RNA coded for by the protooncogene (i.e., the normal cellular gene) was accidentally picked up by a retrovirus during the course of a vertebrate infection. Somehow in the process, the *src* protooncogene became a cancer gene.

The discovery of protooncogenes was extremely important—it implied that the normal cell contains genes that can induce malignant transformation after its DNA is altered appropriately. Moreover, virus-mediated activation of the *src* protooncogene suggested to scientists that nonviral mutations might produce oncogenes as well. In 1989, Bishop and Varmus received a Nobel Prize.

Soon after the *src* protooncogene gene was discovered in the normal cells of chickens, the same protooncogene was found in mammalian cells, and a vigorous search began for other *transforming* (i.e., tumor-forming) sequences. To date, about 30 sequences homologous to retroviral oncogenes have been identified in the *genomes,* that is, the total genetic complement, of normal human cells. In addition, some 20 genes *not* homologous to retroviral gene sequences have been identified in mammalian cells as having transforming properties. The functions of most of these genes are as yet unknown.

The Heubner–Todaro Hypothesis

The second line of investigation leading to the discovery of oncogenes concerns the virogene–oncogene hypothesis proposed by Huebner and Todaro in 1969. This hypothesis held that covert retroviral oncogenes were a part of the genetic baggage of all vertebrate cells. These retroviral sequences would be innocuous as long as they remained quiescent. When activated by carcinogens, or by such mutagens as radiation, or by invading viruses, these sequences could convert cells to neoplastic growth. Although this hypothesis turned out to be incorrect in detail, because the genes involved in tumorigenesis are cellular and not viral in origin, the Heubner–Todaro hypothesis has nevertheless had a productive influence on both virology and tumor biology.

Retroviruses and Cancer Genes

Cellular genes involved in tumorigenesis were first identified through studies of retroviruses. The molecular events involved are best understood against the backdrop of the central dogma of molecular biology.

The central dogma states that genetic information resides in DNA and is expressed by means of RNA. Active genes in the cell nucleus are *transcribed* into messenger RNA, which carries the genetic blueprint into the cytoplasm, where it then directs the synthesis of protein. This latter process is called *translation* (Fig. 9-1).

When retroviruses infect cells, the RNA of their genome is copied into DNA (*cDNA*) by the viral enzyme, reverse transcriptase. This reverse flow of information, from RNA to DNA, is the distinguishing feature that gives rise to the name *retrovirus*. The retroviral cDNA insinuates itself into the host's chromosomal DNA in a process known as *integration*. The integrated double-stranded cDNA is now called a *provirus*. The viral genes are then expressed through the use of the host cell's machinery. This scenario offers two mechanisms for uncovering cancer genes.

First, integration of viral DNA into the host's DNA is potentially mutagenic. Integration may disrupt vital cellular genes, and it can influence the expression of cellular genes by bringing them under the control of regulatory elements in the viral genome (Bishop, 1987). These events, called *insertional mutagenesis,* have been implicated in the tumorigenic properties of many retroviruses.

Second, recombination may occur between cellular and viral genomes in such a way that cellular genes are implanted into the virus. This is the converse of insertional mutagenesis, in which viral genes are implanted in the cellular genome. If the retrovirus infects an animal, the transplanted cellular genes may become oncogenic in their new setting, or they may be damaged in transit, leading to altered functions and possibly to tumorigenic forms of their encoded proteins. The genesis of retroviral oncogenes from cellular protooncogenes is called *transduction;* although strictly speaking, the term applies only after a gene has been transmitted from one cell to another by viral infection. Transduction explains how retroviruses like the Rous sarcoma virus can contain cellular oncogenes among their endogenous viral genes.

Many protooncogenes have been highly conserved during evolution. For example, there is only a 1 percent divergence in the protein sequence of the *c-ras* protooncogene between mouse and humans. By contrast, there is an 18 percent divergence in beta-globin gene sequences between these species. Protooncogenes have been identified in all vertebrates species, as well as in *Drosophila* and in yeast. The ubiquity of these genes throughout the animal kingdom strongly suggests that they perform essential biological functions.

Protooncogenes and Cancer

Retroviruses appear not to be a major cause of human cancer (Duesberg, 1985; Stubblefield and Sanford, 1987). Nevertheless, studies of these agents have identified

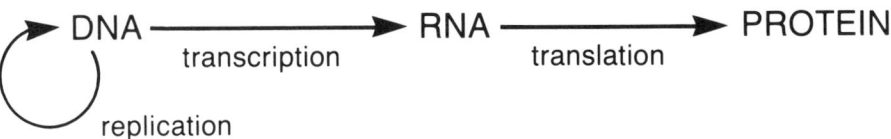

Figure 9-1. The central dogma of molecular biology. Genetic information is stored in DNA. Replication is the process by which DNA is duplicated before each cell division. The information stored in DNA is transcribed into mRNA (messenger RNA), which carries these instructions from the cell nucleus to the cytolplasm. Each mRNA contains the genetic instructions to synthesize a protein in a process called translation. (After Rothberg, 1987.)

mechanisms through which many cancers may arise. It is now generally accepted that protooncogenes are the substrates for diverse carcinogenic influences: "a keyboard on which various carcinogens can play" (Bishop, 1985). Abnormal *alleles* of protooncogenes are found both in retroviruses, where they first came to scientific attention, and in tumors, where they can arise without the intervention of viruses. (An allele is an alternate form of a gene.) That is, protooncogenes may give rise to oncogenes by "conventional" somatic mutations that are caused by chemicals, radiation, and nononcogenic viruses.

Figure 9-2 depicts a current view of the activation of cellular and retroviral oncogenes culminating in cancer.

Abbreviations for Cellular and Viral Oncogenes

The nomenclature of protooncogenes and oncogenes has yet to be fully standardized and can at times be confusing. One source of confusion is that some protooncogenes become oncogenic not by an alteration in their gene sequence per se, but by an increase in the number of copies of the gene sequences, a phenomenon known as *amplification*. In these instances, the protooncogene is structurally indistinguishable from the oncogene. Terminology is further complicated by the fact that protooncogenes and oncogenes may exist in both cellular and viral forms.

The abbreviation *c-onc*, which stands for a cellular oncogene, as in *c-ras*, designates an oncogene present in tumor cells. Its normal counterpart, that is, its protooncogene, is

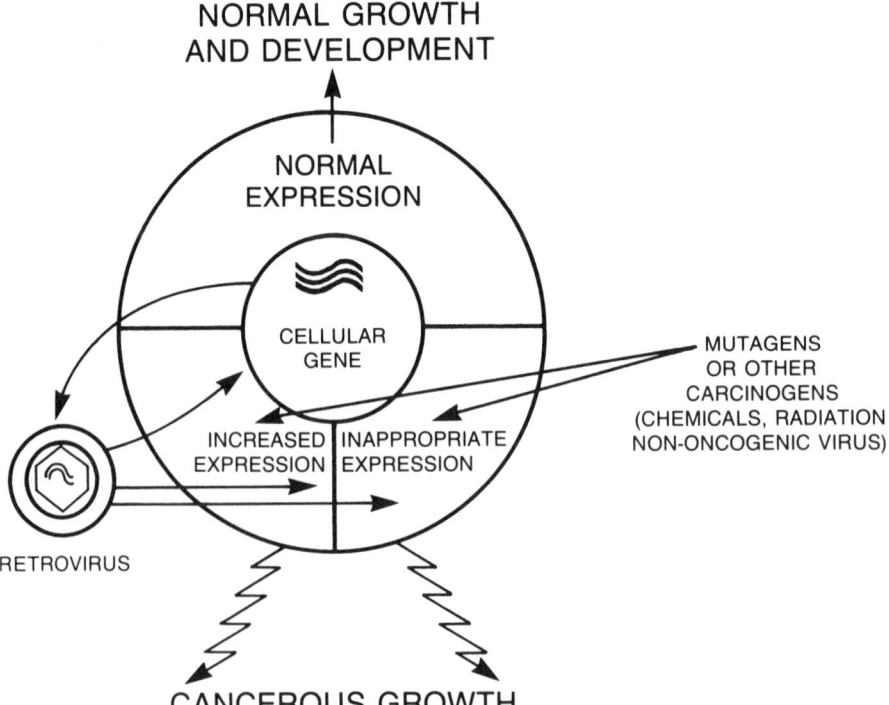

Figure 9-2. The oncogene concept. (After Bishop, 1982.)

referred to as the corresponding *c-onc* protooncogene (e.g., the *c-ras* protooncogene). Similarly, *v-onc* designates a viral oncogene (e.g., *v-src*), and its protooncogene is referred to as a *v-onc* protooncogene (e.g., the *v-src* protooncogene) (Murray et al., 1988).

MECHANISMS OF ONCOGENE FORMATION

At least four mechanisms alter the expression or structure of protooncogenes and thus contribute to their metamorphosis into oncogenes. These mechanisms are: promoter/enhancer insertion, chromosomal translocations, gene amplification, and single point mutations. But before we describe them, we need to introduce some terms. The first is *activation*, the process by which the transcription of a gene increases from zero or a relatively low level. *Upstream* and *downstream* are two other terms that need introduction. Upstream refers to gene sequences located in the opposite direction to transcription. Similarly, downstream refers to sequences further along in the direction of transcription (Murray et al., 1988).

Promoter/Enhancer Insertion

When the RNA of a retrovirus is copied into cDNA, the cDNA copies of the viral genome are flanked by sequences at both ends called *long terminal repeats*. These long terminal repeats assist in proviral integration. They also act as promoters of transcription, that is, they increase the quantity of messenger RNA. For example, when the B lymphocytes of chickens are infected by certain avian leukemia viruses, the leukemia provirus becomes integrated near the *myc* protooncogene. The presence of an upstream long terminal repeat acts as a promoter and activates the *myc* gene. As a result, transcription of both the corresponding *myc* mRNA and translation of its protein product increase. The result is a B-cell tumor.

In some instances, the provirus is inserted downstream from the *myc* protooncogene, which nevertheless becomes activated. In these instances, sequences in the long terminal repeats that are similar to promoters and are called enhancers appear to be involved.

Promoter and enhancer insertion may be common mechanisms of retroviral carcinogenesis (Fig. 9-3) and are also models for nonviral activation of protooncogenes, such as chromosomal translocations (Tereba, 1985).

Chromosomal Translocations

The fact that cancer cells often show aberrations in chromosome structure has been recognized at least since the time of Boveri (1914). One type of chromosomal aberration frequently seen in cancer cells is *translocation* in which one piece of a chromosome breaks off and joins onto another. Translocations in which two chromosomes exchange fragments are said to be *reciprocal* (see Chapter 8).

Perhaps the best known reciprocal translocation is that involved in Burkitt's lymphoma, an especially fast-growing cancer of human B lymphocytes. In Burkitt's lymphoma, an arm of chromosome 8 that contains the *myc* gene is translocated to chromo-

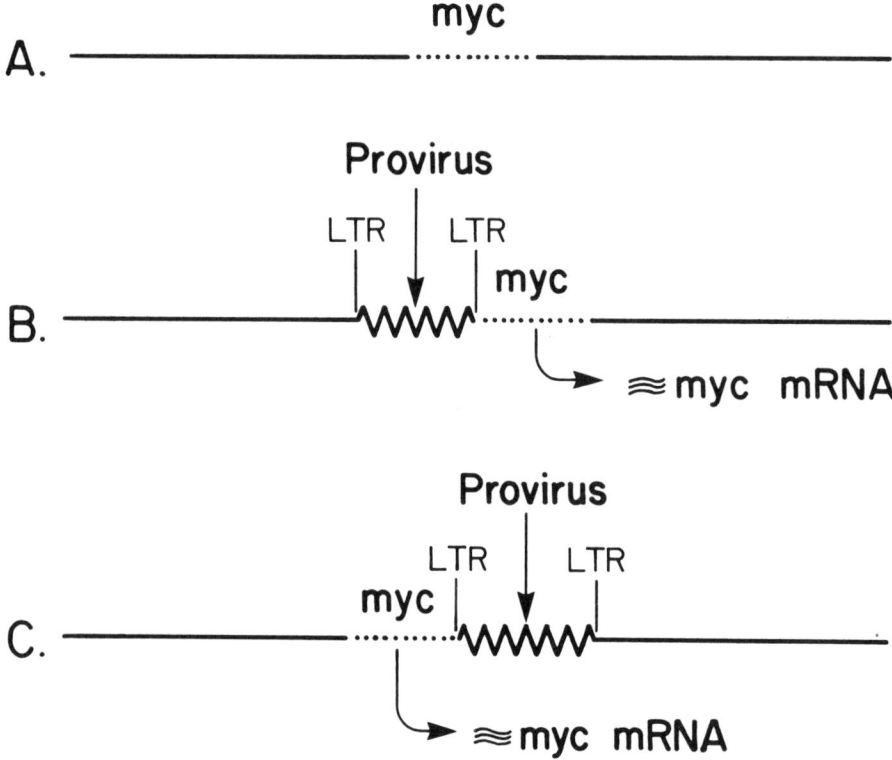

Figure 9-3. Schematic representation of how promoter insertion and enhancer insertion may activate a protooncogene. **A.** Normal chicken chromosome showing an inactive *myc* gene. **B.** An avian leukemia virus has integrated itself into the chromosome in its proviral form, adjacent to the *myc* gene. Its right-hand long terminal repeat (LTR) contains a strong promoter. The promoter lies upstream of the *myc* gene and activates it. **C.** Here an avian leukemia virus has integrated itself into the chromosome adjacent to the *myc* gene. The site of integration, however, is just downstream of the gene. In this case, a proviral sequence acts as an enhancer and activates the *myc* gene. For simplicity, only one strand of DNA is depicted. (Modified from Murrary et al., 1988.)

some 14. This translocation places the previously quiescent *myc* gene under the influence of strong enhancer sequences in the genes coding for the heavy chain of immunoglobulins. Activation of *c-myc* results in greatly increased amounts of the *myc* gene product, an as yet poorly understood protein that binds DNA. Excessive production of this protein appears to "force" the cell to malignancy by creating an incessant stimulus for cell proliferation. The mechanism of *myc* activation in Burkitt's lymphoma is in principle similar to that observed during enhancer insertion, except that a translocation of human DNA takes the place of integration of the provirus. The result is that the *c-myc* protooncogene is placed under the influence of an enhancer.

A similar translocation occurs in chronic myelogenous leukemia and in other types of leukemia. In chronic myelogenous leukemia, a reciprocal exchange takes place between chromosomes 9 and 22. This relocates a portion of the protooncogene *c-abl* and fuses it with a newly recognized genetic locus called the *breakpoint cluster region* (*bcr*). The genetic fusion creates a gene that codes for a new protein with far greater enzymatic activity than the normal protein (Konopka et al., 1984). Thus, this transloca-tion produces a mutation that affects the biochemical function, rather than the level of expression of a gene.

In addition to *bcr,* there are specific sites on several chromosomes that are known as fragile sites and are particularly prone to breakage. Many of these fragile sites are near cellular protooncogenes, and are thus thought to play roles either in the initiation or the maintenance of tumors (Tereba, 1985; Helm and Mitelman, 1987).

Gene Amplification

In addition to structural chromosomal changes, *gene amplification*—an increase in the number of copies of a gene—has been found in a number of tumors. A well-known example of gene amplification occurs after administration of the anticancer drug, methotrexate, which is an inhibitor of the enzyme dihydrofolate reductase. Some tumor cells that become resistant to this drug do so by increasing the number of copies of the dihydrofolate reductase gene. Amplified copies of genes may be observed karyologically in *double minute chromosomes* (small supernumerary chromosomes) and in *homogeneously staining regions* (areas that do not appear to be banded on a G-banded karyotype) on specific chromosomes. An increase in the number of copies of genes has been reported in several neoplasms, for example, amplification of *N-myc* in neuroblastoma and of *HER-2/Neu* in breast carcinoma, and is associated with aggres-sive tumor behavior (Seeger et al., 1985; Slamon et al., 1987).

Single Point Mutations

Some protooncogenes may be activated by a change in only a single base pair. This was first reported in 1982 for the oncogene *c-H-ras* in human bladder carcinoma cell lines (Reddy et al., 1982; Tabin et al., 1982). These investigators discovered that the *c-H-ras* oncogene had a point mutation at the twelfth *codon* in which the nucleotide thymidine replaced guanine. (A codon is a sequence of three adjacent nucleotides that codes for one amino acid. *Stop* or *termination* codons code for the termination of protein synthesis. One gene is composed of many codons.) Unlike the case in which the *myc* oncogene was activated, this change did not result in overproduction of gene product. Instead, the change in only one base pair resulted in a change in the structure of the protein. How this mutation leads to tumorigenesis is unclear; however, confor-mational changes in the protein's *tertiary structure* (its three-dimensional shape) proba-bly affect protein function.

Several carcinogens produce mutations in the *ras* gene. These include nitrosomethyl-urea, which produces point mutations at codon 12, and dimethylbenzanthrene, which causes a mutation at codon 61. Similar mutations have been produced by other hydro-carbons and nitrosamines (Brosman and Liu, 1987).

FUNCTIONS OF ONCOGENES

Whatever the means of activation, oncogenes wreak their damage by means of their encoded proteins. At present, the precise functions of these protein products are poorly understood. In the normal cell, protooncogenes function in a well-controlled manner. They are probably active during embryogenesis and in normal tissue repair. At least some protooncogenes are also involved in cellular processes other than growth. For example, *c-src* is expressed at high levels in nerve cells, cells that, under normal conditions, never undergo cell division (Brugge et al., 1985).

The known functions of the protein products of viral and cellular oncogenes fall into three general classes based on their biochemical mechanisms and sites of action: (1) modified phosphorlyation of proteins, (2) metabolic regulation by guanosine triphosphate binding, and (3) altered control of gene expression by DNA-binding proteins. A fourth group includes oncogenes whose functions have not yet been determined. For details of known mechanisms that are considered only briefly here, readers can consult several reviews (Stubblefield and Sanford, 1987; Brosman and Liu, 1987).

Protein Phosphorylation

Members of the tyrosine kinase family all code for proteins that are either membrane-bound receptors for growth factors, or are associated with the *plasma membrane* (the membrane separating the cytoplasm from the extracellular environment).

Protein kinases are enzymes that act at the inner surface of the plasma membrane, where they catalyze the addition of a phosphate molecule to the amino acids serine, threonine, and tyrosine. Prominent members of this group are *abl,* the gene associated with chronic myelogenous leukemia, and *src.* How abnormal phosphorylation leads to cell transformation is not well understood. It is possible, however, that the normal transmission of exogenous signals across the plasma membrane may be altered.

Other oncogenes of this general class act by coding for *growth factors* or their receptors. Growth factors are small hormonelike peptides that stimulate mitosis in target cells (see Goustin et al., 1986). For example, the *sis* oncogene encodes a protein that is virtually identical to the B chain of platelet-derived growth factor (PDGF), a powerful mitogen. Although PDGF delivers its signal only during appropriate occasions (e.g., wound healing), the *sis*-encoded protein does so continually, causing unregulated cell division.

Regulation of Proteins by GTP-Binding

The second known function of oncogenes, protein regulation by GTP-binding, involves the *ras* family of viral oncogenes. These oncogenes, *H-ras, K-ras,* and *N-ras,* code for a 21 kilodalton protein associated with the plasma membrane. *V-ras* products are thought to stimulate and regulate cyclic AMP. *V-ras* genes, which transform virally infected cells, have point mutations resulting in a lowered GPTase activity compared with normal cellular *ras* proteins. Precisely how this lowered GTPase activity leads to tumorigenesis, however, is not clear.

DNA-Binding

Unlike the oncogenes previously described, which encode proteins that operate at the level of the plasma membrane, oncogenes of the DNA-binding class act within the cell nucleus. These oncogenes produce proteins that bind to DNA and the nuclear matrix and participate in DNA replication. The best studied of these oncogenes belong to the *myc* family of genes, which are commonly amplified in several human tumors, notably small cell lung cancer and neuroblastoma. Of the oncogenes found in human tumors, those belonging to the *myc* family are among those most frequently represented (Table 9-1). The chromosomal location and function of many known human oncogenes will be given in Table 9-3.

There is evidence that *c-myc* may act cooperatively with other oncogenes. That is, cellular transformation may be the result of a complex cascade of cellular events involving the actions of several oncogenes (Brosman and Liu, 1987).

Tumor-Suppressor Genes (Antioncogenes)

It is important to recognize a class of genes involved in tumorigenesis that operates on biological principles that are very different from those of oncogenes. These genes are commonly called *antioncogenes* or, more appropriately, *tumor-suppressor genes* (Knudson, 1978; Sager, 1986).

The existence of tumor-suppressor genes has been well illustrated by research on several rare tumors, particularly retinoblastoma and Wilm's tumor. These tumors are of

Table 9-1   Human Oncogenes[a]

Oncogene	Mechanism of Activation	Type of Tumor	Proportion of tumors containing activated oncogene (%)
H-ras-1	Single point mutation	Several carcinomas, melanomas	1–10
K-ras-2	Single point mutation Amplification	Several carcinomas, rhabdo-myosarcoma, ALL Lung and bladder carcinomas	1–15 1
N-ras	Single point mutation	Several leukemias, some carcinomas, melanomas and sarcomas	1–25
c-myc	Chromosomal translocation Amplification	Burkitt's lymphoma SCLC, breast and colon carcinomas, PML	100 1–25
N-myc	Amplification	Neuroblastoma, SCLC, retinoblastoma	20–50
L-myc	Amplification	SCLC	25
HER-2/Neu	Amplification	Breast carcinoma	20–40
c-abl	Chromosomal translocation	CML	100
bc1-1	Chromosomal translocation	B-cell lymphomas	80–100[b]
bc1-2	Chromosomal translocation	Follicular lymphoma	80–100

[a]Only includes those oncogenes frequently found in human malignancies. SCLC, small cell lung cancer, ALL, acute lymphocytic leukemia, PML, granulocytic leukemias, CML, chronic myelogenous leukemia.

[b]100% refers to B-cell lymphomas with t(11 : 14) translocation.

From Barbacid, 1986, with additional material.

special interest because they exist in both a familial and a nonfamilial, or "sporadic" form.

Retinoblastomas are often the result of loss of genetic material that maps to the q14 band of chromosome 13 (see Chapter 8 for a discussion of chromosome banding). Genetic analyses indicate that this tumor can result when both copies of a normal gene mapping to this region are lost. Individuals with a hereditary predisposition to retinoblastoma are born with one normal and one defective "Rb" gene (Knudson, 1971). If the normal allele in a retinal cell is lost during retinal development, these cells will grow into tumors. The sporadic cases of retinoblastoma appear to be due to the somatic loss of both alleles in a single retinal cell during retinal development (Cavenee et al., 1983).

Study of another childhood cancer, Wilm's tumor, has yielded data of a similar type. A portion of these cases are inherited, and some of these cases have a constitutional deletion on the 11p band of chromosome 13. In the sporadic cases, some patients show a deletion at the identical locus. The initial event in both types of Wilm's tumor patients is the same: deletion or inactivation of a locus on chromosome 13p11 (Kaneko et al., 1981).

Antioncogenes, such as the ones involved in the genesis of retinoblastoma and Wilm's tumor, function in ways that are diametrically opposed to those of oncogenes. Protooncogenes contribute to tumorigenesis through their hyperactive alleles, the oncogenes. The role of protooncogenes in carcinogenesis takes place only through somatic mutation. Tumors develop if one protooncogene of a pair becomes an oncogene; that is, the expression of oncogenes is dominant. Conversely, antioncogenes contribute to cancer when their functions are *eliminated* through mutations. Tumor-producing alleles of the antioncogenes are heritable and thus influence congenital tumor predisposition. Tumors develop only when both copies of antioncogenes are inactivated; that is, the expression of antioncogenes is recessive. Oncogenes and antioncogenes also differ from an epidemiologic standpoint; whereas oncogenes are markers of disease, antioncogenes, when present in a single copy, are markers of susceptibility. Table 9-2 summarizes these differences.

Because a myriad of mutational events is capable of inactivating a gene, although only a specific few can precisely reactivate one, it is likely that antioncogenes contribute even more frequently to tumorigenesis than oncogenes (Weinberg, 1988). The inactivation of antioncogenes has recently been implicated in the cause of common tumors of the colon and the lung (Solomon et al., 1978; Naylor et al., 1987).

The preceding brief introduction presents the basic cast of oncogenic characters. To understand how these characters perform in the laboratory, the next section provides some basic familiarity with laboratory methodologies to detect oncogenes.

Table 9-2   Contrasting Properties of Oncogenes and Antioncogenes

	Mode of Activation	Mode of Expression	Heritable	Type of Marker
Oncogenes	Somatic mutation	Dominant	No	Disease
Antioncogenes	Inactivation	Recessive	Yes	Susceptibility

Table 9-3 Human Oncogene Function and Location

Function	Oncogene	Chromosomal location
1. Protein phosphorylation	src	1
(protein kinases)	abl	9
	fes	15
	arg	1
	yes	18
	met	7
Protein kinases acting as	sis (PDGF)	22
growth factor and growth factor	erb-B(EGF)	7
receptor	fms (CSF-1)	5
	HER-2/Neu	17
	mos	8
2. Guanosine triphosphate binding	H-ras-1	11
	H-ras-2	X
	K-ras-1	6
	K-ras-2	12
	N-ras	1
3. DNA binding	myc	8
(replication and transcription)		
	N-myc	2
	myb	6
	ets	11
	ski	1
	fos	16
	L-myc	1
4. Unknown	erb-A	17
	rel	2
	B-lym	1
	raf-1	3
	raf-2	4
	PKS-1	X
	PKS-2	7
	fgr	1
	bcl-1	11
	bcl-2	18

After Brosman and Liu, 1987, with additions.

RECOMBINANT DNA TECHNOLOGY

To the uninitiated, the laboratory literature on oncogenes can seem a dizzying array of genetic techniques. Readers interested in details of these new techniques can consult several excellent reviews and handbooks (e.g., Emery, 1984; Rodriquez and Tait, 1983; Murray et al., 1988). For the present, however, it may be helpful to review the biological basis for the most important of these tools.

Restriction Endonucleases

The most fundamental tools of recombinant DNA technology are a group of enzymes that occur in microorganisms. These enzymes, first discovered in 1970 and now called *class II restriction endonucleases,* cleave DNA at specific sites. Restriction enzymes make it possible to produce DNA fragments of reproducible size. For example, DNA fragments containing a particular gene can be excised from the rest of the DNA molecule.

After the discovery of methods for joining (recombining) the DNA fragments produced by restriction enzymes, later research found *plasmid vectors* that can carry fragments of foreign DNA. Plasmids are naturally occurring pieces of circular DNA in the cytoplasm of bacteria. Plasmids are extrachromosomal and replicate independently of the bacterial DNA of their host. Suitable restriction endonucleases allow investigators to open up a plasmid and insert a piece of foreign (e.g., human) DNA. This is the actual recombinant part of *recombinant DNA* technology.

Plasmids are very useful vehicles, or vectors, for ferrying DNA fragments. When recombinant plasmids are taken up by a bacterium (usually *Escherichia coli*), the bacteria can be grown in culture to produce *clones* that have multiple copies of the DNA fragment. A clone is a large population of identical molecules, bacteria, or cells that arise from a single ancestor. Other cloning vectors include *bacteriophages* (viruses that infect bacteria), and *cosmids* (an artificial construction composed of plasmid DNA packaged in a phage particle).

As researchers gained more experience in cloning DNA sequences, they began to entertain the possibility of cloning DNA sequences from the entire human genome. DNA fragments produced by restriction endonucleases and cloned in appropriate vectors can be stored. A collection of such recombinant clones is called a *library*. A *genomic library* is one prepared from the total DNA of a cell line or tissue. Similarly, a *cDNA library* represents a library constructed using complementary DNA copies of the population of messenger RNAs in a tissue.

Gel Electrophoresis

A now ubiquitous technique in molecular genetic research was pioneered by E.M. Southern in 1975. If DNA is extracted from a tissue, say a breast carcinoma, this DNA contains all the thousands of genes of the host organism. In any one tissue, of course, most of these genes are "switched off" or repressed. How, then, can one identify any particular gene? The first step is to cleave the DNA with a restriction endonuclease. The DNA can then be subjected to electrophoresis on an agarose gel. In this technique, the fragments separate under an electric current according to size—smaller fragments moving farther than larger fragments. One of these fragments contains the gene or sequence of interest. To find it, one first denatures the DNA fragments on the gel with alkali. Denaturing renders the normally double-stranded fragments single-stranded so that they subsequently can *hybridize* with complementary pieces of DNA. (In hybridization, two single-stranded DNA molecules, or a single-stranded DNA molecule and an RNA molecule join to form a double-stranded molecule. Such hybridization can take place, however, only if the hybridizing DNA or RNA strands contain bases complementary to the base sequence on the denatured DNA fragment.)

Next, the single-stranded fragments are transferred to a nitrocellulose filter by blotting, that is, a filter is placed directly over the gel, and the denatured DNA binds firmly to the filter. This technique, in which DNA fragments bind to a nitrocellulose filter in the same position they occupied on an agarose gel, is universally referred to as a *Southern blot* (Southern, 1975). Because the DNA fragments are single-stranded, they will hybridize to a *probe* containing DNA complementary to the sequence of interest. When the *probe* is made radioactive (usually with a ^{32}P-containing nucleotide), the fragment can be identified and localized on the filter by *autoradiography*, that is, by exposing the filter to an x-ray film in the dark.

RNA fragments can be separated by electrophoresis in a similar manner. Because RNA does not bind to nitrocellulose, however, a modification of the procedure has been developed. The RNA procedure is commonly referred to as a *Northern blot*. A different procedure, used for fractionating proteins is called a *Western blot*. (These latter terms, originally begun as laboratory jargon, are now accepted terms [Murray et al., 1988]).

Southern analyses and other gel electrophoretic techniques are useful methods for detecting the presence of specific gene sequences. Sequences present in large amounts (e.g., amplified copies of a gene) appear as more densely staining blots on a gel. The intensity of staining can be quantified by various techniques and used to estimate the number of copies of a gene in a cell, the *copy number*. For example, a 50-fold amplification is indicated if a 1 : 50 dilution of the DNA is required to achieve a signal of single-copy intensity. This procedure is often called *dilution analysis*.

DNA Polymorphisms

Human genes are separated by large stretches of DNA with as yet no known function. These *intergenic regions,* or *spacers,* may constitute as much as 90 percent of the genome. Within this noncoding DNA, as elsewhere in the genome, there are variations in nucleotide sequence that have no recognized phenotypic effect on the host. Changes in base sequences mean that the restriction sites for a particular enzyme may be altered or missing. Thus, when one uses a restriction endonuclease to fragment the DNA for electrophoresis, one finds that the DNA fragments produced by the enzyme are of different lengths in different people. These genotypic changes, which can be identified by different mobilities of the restriction fragments on gel electrophoresis, are relatively frequent in human populations and are referred to as *polymorphisms*. Because they are recognized by differences in the lengths of restriction fragments, they are called *restriction fragment length polymorphisms,* or RFLPs. The RFLPs can be used to measure mutations and have proven useful tools in the detection of recessive genes involved in tumorigenesis (e.g., Naylor et al., 1987).

Transfection Assay

Experiments using DNA extracted from tumors have also demonstrated the existence of oncogenes. By far the most common technique used to detect mutations in cellular oncogenes is called *gene transfer* or *DNA transfection*. The technique consists of isolating DNA from tumor cells and adding it (in the presence of calcium phosphate, which facilitates its uptake) to recipient cells, usually a line of cultured mouse fibroblasts called NIH/3T3 cells. The NIH/3T3 cells ingest the foreign DNA, which then becomes part of the host's genome. The technique is sometimes called *transfection* to emphasize that DNA added in this manner is infectious. The tissue cultures of transfected cells are observed microscopically for a period of 1 to 2 weeks. If transformation occurs, the NIH/3T3 cells change their morphology from flat to rounded cells that grow in characteristic foci. DNA can then be extracted from the transformed cells and the procedure repeated, thus producing secondary transformants. This procedure is again repeated several times using DNA extracted from the transformed cells. These serial passages reduce the amount of transfected DNA that is not involved in transformation and facilitate identification of the actual transforming DNA sequence (e.g., by Southern blotting and a suitable probe).

Gene transfer techniques have been used to identify several different cellular oncogenes. These are either identical to normal cellular genes or show minute structural differences from their protooncogene counterparts. Figure 9-4 outlines the methodology for identifying human oncogenes by gene transfer.

The use of gene transfer techniques has proved a valuable tool to identify genetic lesions in cancer cells. The method, however, is not without idiosyncracy. For example, NIH/3T3 cells are much less sensitive to point mutations that occur in the *ras* gene at some codons than at others. Although the reasons for this are unknown, it does suggest that some oncogenes may go undetected. Moreover, only about 20 percent of transfected human tumor DNAs will transform NIH/3T3 cells (Weinberg, 1988). This may be because oncogenes are not present in all tumors, or it may be because present transfection assays can not detect them.

The transfection assay used to detect activated *ras* oncogenes has recently been supplanted by more powerful techniques that look for structural changes in the genes of

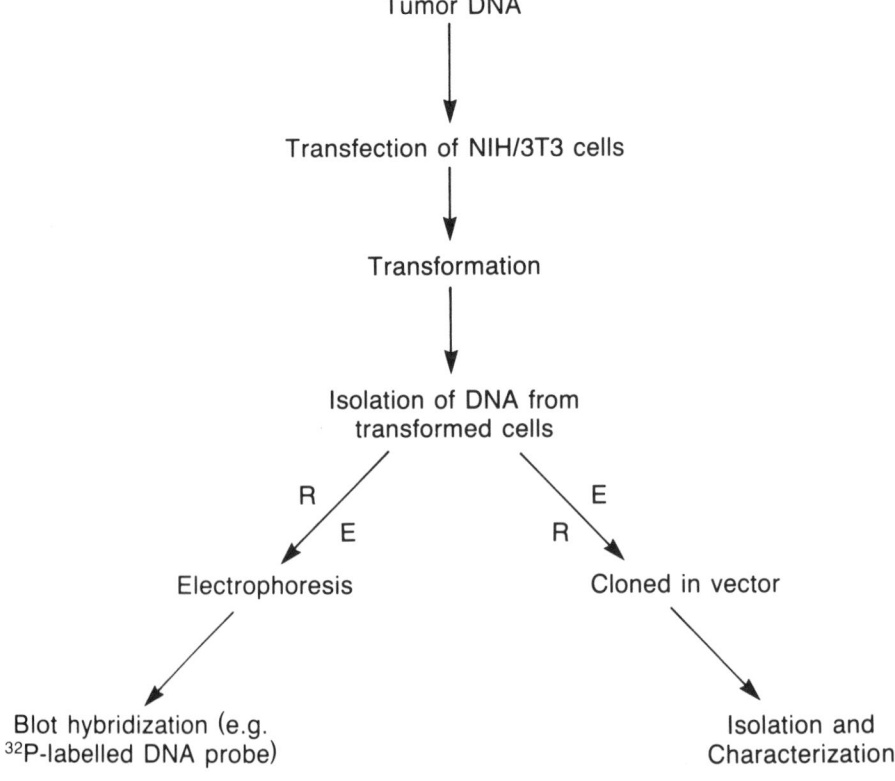

Figure 9-4. Methodology used to identify, isolate, and characterize human transforming DNA sequences. RE, restriction endonucleases. (Modified after Emery, 1984.)

a tumor DNA sample. The most promising of such techniques is called the *polymerase chain reaction.*

Polymerase Chain Reaction

The polymerase chain reaction (PCR) is an in vitro technique for the enzymatic amplification of specific DNA sequences (Erlich et al., 1988). The technique is capable of synthesizing over a million copies of a target DNA sequence in a few hours, thus greatly facilitating subsequent analytic procedures. The technique employs two *oligonucleotide primers,* short sequences of nucleotides that provide a start for the synthesis of a DNA chain. These primers flank the DNA fragment to be amplified and hybridize to opposite strands. The procedure entails repeated cycles of first denaturing DNA with heat and then annealing the primers to their complementary sequences. The primers are then joined with a *DNA polymerase* (an enzyme for linking DNA fragments). The products of one primer serve as a template for the other, so each successive cycle doubles the quantity of DNA in the previous cycle. The result is an exponential accumulation of the target molecule. This technique can generate unique fragments from both DNA and RNA templates in yields comparable to those obtained from clonally isolated recombinants. Indeed, PCR is a form of in vitro molecular cloning. It can accomplish in a 3- to 4-hour reaction what might otherwise take days of biological growth and biochemical purification (Erlich et al., 1988).

After a sequence has been amplified, a number of techniques, such as specific oligonucleotide probes and gel electrophoresis, can be used to distinguish allelic variants. The technique has recently been used successfully to study the presence of *ras* mutations in colorectal tumors (Bos et al., 1987).

One exceptionally promising application of PCR is its use in identifying specific DNA sequences in preserved tissues, human archival specimens in particular. The most common human archival materials are tissues fixed in formalin and embedded in paraffin, a storage technique used by pathologists since the turn of the century. Specimens preserved this way can be washed in xylene to remove the paraffin and then subjected to PCR (Shibata et al., 1988). In one study, Shibata et al. (1988) used the technique to detect human papilloma viruses 16 and 18 in archival material from patients who had died from cervical carcinoma 40 years before. The technique thus offers a rare opportunity to use the world's collections of paraffin-embedded tissues for retrospective studies of the associations of particular DNA sequences with disease.

ONCOGENES AND EPIDEMIOLOGIC STUDIES

"A rose," observed Gertrude Stein, "is a rose is a rose is a rose." Sadly, such horticultural uniformity does not extend to oncogenes, which can be quite variable in their biochemical structure, their means of activation, and the methods used in their detection. In this sense the epidemiology of oncogenes is more akin to the epidemiology of "accidents" (cancer being an accident of genes), than it is to the epidemiology of some *particular* mishap, say, boating accidents. This heterogeneity compounds the difficulty of proposing general guidelines for employing oncogenes as biological markers in epidemiologic studies. Nevertheless, we can make some general observations. The first of these pertains to the question of appropriate study design, and the second to basic analytic strategy. Last, a few remarks are made about bias and confounding.

Study Designs

An obvious limitation on epidemiologic studies of oncogenes is imposed by the nature of oncogenes themselves. In general, oncogenes are expressed at high levels in tumors; they are not expressed constitutively. The requirement for tumor tissue means that epidemiologic studies will principally be of two types: case series and case-control.

In the case series, the data consist of tumor tissue and medical records from a series of patients. The patients need not be living; one can easily use frozen ("banked") tissue, or banked DNA and medical records. In the case-control designs, the cases are organs from cancer patients, and the controls are the same organs from noncancer patients. In either case the question of interest is whether a correlation exists between measures of oncogene activation and the presence and/or severity of disease.

Whatever their specifics, both types of study address the null hypothesis that the evidence of oncogene activation is the same in two (or more) populations, versus the alternative, directional hypothesis that the level of oncogene activation is greater in a specified population. The "evidence" may take any of several forms, including increased copies of a gene, increased frequency of point mutations, increased quantity of a normal protein product, increased quantity of an abnormal product, and so on.

Analytic Strategies

The particular oncogene that is to be assayed and its means of activation dictate the technological approaches used to detect oncogenes. Genes that are activated by amplification, for example, such as *N-myc* and *HER-2/Neu,* generally are assayed by blotting, dilution, and densitometric techniques. Conversely, genes that are activated by mutation, such as members of the *ras* gene family, are commonly assayed by transfection, PCR, or by immunologic assays and probes specially constructed to recognize the specific alteration in the protein product. Similarly, oncogenes activated by chromosomal translocations are most appropriately analyzed by study of banded karyotypes (see Chapter 8) and by RFLPs. In other words, *there is no generic laboratory test for oncogenes.* The successful epidemiologic study is one that tests a focused hypothesis about the presence of particular oncogene or oncogenes and its relationship to a particular tumor and/or exposure.

Bias

The brief discussion of recombinant DNA technologies should reveal that these technologies are imperfect. For example, present techniques are unlikely to falsely detect oncogenes when they are not present. Under exacting or stringent experimental conditions, a specific DNA probe generally will not hybridize to unrelated DNA, and NIH/3T3 cells rarely transform spontaneously. Conversely, it is likely that transforming sequences in tumors that are, or were once, present may go undetected.

In solid tumors, two factors may prevent the detection of mutationally activated genes when these are tested in standard transfection assays. First, the DNA from primary human tumors is often slightly degraded, both because of necrosis in vivo, and because of degradation during surgery and subsequent tissue handling. This is especially problematic for large genes (>45,000 base pairs) such as *K-ras*. Statistical analyses indicate that even for DNA samples with an average fragment length of 100,000 base pairs, the *c-K-ras* gene will be intact in only one third of the fragments containing this gene (Bos et al., 1987).

Second, solid tumor specimens usually contain significant numbers of nonneoplastic cells (e.g., stromal and inflammatory cells) that will dilute any positive signal from neoplastic cells in the transfection assay. For these reasons, the standard assay may soon give way to more powerful new techniques, notably the polymerase chain reaction. The important conclusion here is that because of these technical limitations, *epidemiologic studies of oncogenes are inherently biased toward the null.*

Confounding

Until more definitive information is obtained about factors that modify the expression of oncogenes and protooncogenes, little can be said about potential confounding factors. One variable that clearly can influence oncogenes is chemotherapy. For example, methotrexate administration induces amplification of the dihydrofolate reductase gene. Similarly, in animal studies, radiation can contribute to oncogene activation (Emery, 1984). Thus, studies that seek to determine whether oncogenes are present in human tumors should either be restricted to untreated patients, or should stratify their statistical analyses into groups of treated and untreated individuals.

Selected Examples

Having introduced the basic tools of recombinant DNA, let us see how these are employed in epidemiologic studies of oncogenes. Thus, the rest of this chapter describes several examples of case series and case-control studies. These examples, although by no means exhaustive, illustrate many of the technologies that are fast becoming important additions to the armamentarium of cancer epidemiology.

In an important illustration of the case series epidemiologic approach, Seeger et al. (1985) studied the relation between the number of copies of the *N-myc* oncogene and the progression of neuroblastoma. Neuroblastoma is a rare nerve cell tumor with an incidence of 1 per 125,000 children. The disease is traditionally classified into four stages ranging from Stage I, a tumor confined to the organ or structure of origin, to Stage IV, a large primary tumor with multiple metastases.

The authors studied 89 children with this disease and obtained tumor samples surgically at diagnosis, before therapy. They then used Southern analyses and a radiolabeled plasmid probe to determine the number of copies of the *N-myc* gene. DNA from normal leukocytes or fibroblasts served as reference values for determining the hybridization intensity of a single copy of *N-myc*. Progression-free survival was analyzed with lifetable techniques.

The results indicated that genomic amplification of *N-myc* (3 to 300 copies) occurred in 38 percent of all tumors, but was most frequent in tumors at an advanced stage at diagnosis. Amplification was detected in 2 of 16 tumors in Stage II, 13 of 20 tumors at Stage III, and 19 of 40 tumors in Stage IV. Analyses of progression-free survival indicated that amplification of *N-myc* was associated with the worst prognosis. This was true despite the fact that patients received conventional therapy appropriate for their stage of disease. The association between gene amplification and tumor progression was observed in all tumor stages.

The Seeger study represents one of the first clinical applications of oncogene research. The observation that *N-myc* amplification was a better predictor of survival time than conventional staging of this tumor suggests that gene amplification may be a major pathway in disease progression.

Slamon et al. (1987) used a similar case series approach in their study of amplification of the *HER-2/Neu* oncogene and survival from breast cancer. The *HER-2/Neu* gene is a member of the tyrosine kinase gene family and is closely related to the gene that codes for epidermal growth factor receptor.

Slamon's study, conducted in two parts, involved the evaluation of breast tissue from 189 separate breast tumors that were part of an ongoing study at the University of Texas. This cohort of tumors was especially valuable because considerable information was available on prognostic factors known to influence disease progression. These included estrogen and progesterone receptor status, patient age, disease stage, tumor size, and status of the axillary lymph nodes.

In the initial study, Slamon and colleagues evaluated tissue from 103 primary untreated breast cancers for alterations in the *HER-2/Neu* gene. DNA was digested with restriction endonucleases and subjected to Southern blot analysis using a ^{32}P-labeled *HER-2/Neu* probe. Of the 103 samples examined, 19 (18%) showed evidence of *HER-2/Neu* amplification. The degree of amplification was determined by densitometry and dilution analysis. Individual tumors were assigned to groups containing a single gene copy, two to five copies, 5 to 20 copies, and greater than 20 copies. Individuals blind to the patients' disease status assigned the tumors to these groups. These 103 tumors showed no correlation between gene amplification and hormone receptor status, tumor size, or age at diagnosis. Gene amplification, however, was positively correlated with the number of affected lymph nodes, a variable widely known to predict disease recurrence.

To examine whether gene amplification gave any clinical information in women whose cancer had already spread, Slamon and colleagues next looked at data for 86 women in the Texas data bank who had positive nodes and for whom data on relapse and survival were available. DNA analyses were performed on this second sample. The data indicated that the *HER-2/Neu* gene was amplified in 40 percent of these patients. To test the hypothesis that gene amplification may be correlated with tumor behavior, time to relapse and survival time were correlated with number of gene copies. Univariate analyses found a strong correlation between the degree of oncogene amplification, time to relapse, and time of survival. Most of these women (83%) had received some form of therapy after mastectomy. Multivariate analyses of the data showed that amplification of the *HER-2/Neu* gene was superior to all other prognostic factors, with the exception of the number of positive nodes (which it equalled), in predicting time to relapse and survival in this sample of patients.

This finding, that greater gene copy number correlates with a worse prognosis, is similar to that observed by Seeger et al. (1985) in their study of *N-myc* and neuroblastoma. Both studies also indicate that, in addition to their importance as markers of disease severity, oncogenes hold a prominent place in the biostatistical analysis of tumor behavior.

A very different approach to the study of oncogenes appears in a study by Stock and colleagues (1987). These authors identified a *ras* oncogene-related product in the urine of patients with transitional cell carcinoma of the bladder. The product is a 55-kilodalton protein that is immunologically related to the *ras* oncogene product, p21. Stock et al. compared the concentration of this protein in the urine of bladder cancer patients with its concentration in noncancer controls.

They collected urine specimens from 29 bladder cancer patients, eight patients with benign prostatic hyperplasia, and 15 healthy individuals. The authors used an immunoblot procedure in which processed urine samples were incubated with antibody to a synthetic polypeptide corresponding to a fragment of the *K-ras* and *H-ras* p21 protein. Sixteen patients (55%) with transitional cell carcinoma showed high levels of expression of the p55 protein (levels at least three times the background level). Ten patients (35%) had levels that were elevated at least twice the background level, and three patients (10%) showed no elevations. None of the control patients showed high (threefold) levels of this protein. The levels of expression of the p55 marker also tended to correlate with tumor stage and grade, which were determined without knowledge of the immunoblot results. The authors concluded that the p55 gene product may be useful as a marker for transitional cell carcinoma.

One criticism of this interesting urologic study from an epidemiologic standpoint is that it lacks descriptive information on the cancer patients' prior therapeutic treatment. Because virtually half (14) of the cancer patients had extensive (Stage III) disease, presumably some of these patients had been treated. Because both radiation and chemotherapy are mutagenic, it is at least conceivable that some of the oncogene activation was iatrogenic.

The Stock et al. (1987) study also demonstrates that not all studies of oncogenes require tumor tissue. Their study raises the possibility that noninvasive procedures could be developed for sampling fluids from other organs, such as the prostate. This would be particularly valuable as both *c-ras* and *c-myc* show increased expression in individuals with prostatic cancer (Fleming et al., 1986; Phillips et al., 1987).

The *ras* oncogene family has been implicated in other solid tumors as well, notably tumors of the colon and rectum. Bos et al. (1987) studied colorectal tumors in 27 patients. They selected tumors that showed large areas of neoplastic cells with relatively little evidence of inflammatory or stromal proliferation, extracted DNA from the tumors, and used oligonucleotide probes to analyze for the presence of *ras* mutations. Before using the probes, Bos et al. used the polymerase chain reaction to amplify short genomic segments of the tumor DNA containing the coding sequence for *ras* gene.

Nine tumors were identified with mutations at codon 12 of the *c-K-ras* gene. In addition, one tumor was found with a mutation in codon 12 of *H-ras* and one tumor was found to have a mutation of the *N-ras* gene. No mutations were found in normal fibroblasts from each individual, indicating that the mutations had occurred somatically.

The authors repeated their procedures using adenomatous tissue from six individuals. (Adenomas are benign polyps that are widely believed to be precancerous.) In five of the six carcinomas with *ras* mutations, the same mutation was found in the adenomas, suggesting that the mutation preceded the development of malignancy.

Table 9-4   Study by Naylor et al. (1987) Seen as a Case-Control Study. Exposure Variable Is Loss of Alleles on the Short Arm of Chromosome 3

		Alleles absent	Alleles present
		E	Ē
Tumor DNA	D	9	0
Nontumor DNA	D̄	0	9

The Bos et al. study is one of the first in a new generation of studies in which biochemical methods, rather than transfection assays, are used to detect mutations. As in the Stock study, however, information about prior medical treatment and appropriate stratification of the data would have been desirable.

Deactivated antioncogenes as well as activated oncogenes may contribute to tumorigenesis. An unusual example of a case-control study used tumor DNA as the cases and nontumor DNA from the same individuals as the controls (Naylor et al., 1987). The "exposure" in this study was a loss of alleles on the short arm of chromosome 3, an event associated with small cell lung cancer (SCLC).

Naylor and colleagues (1987) prepared DNA samples from tumor and normal lung tissue from nine patients with histologically confirmed SCLC. Restriction endonucleases were used to digest DNA samples and generate restriction fragment length polymorphisms (RFLPs). Eight different probes detecting DNA polymorphisms on chromosome 3 were used to study individual chromosome 3s in SCLC tumors and in nontumor lung tissue from each patient. Two of these probes lie within 3p14–23, the region commonly missing in SCLC, as detected by karyotypic analyses.

The results indicated a loss of alleles on chromosome 3p in tumor tissue from all nine patients. This loss was not observed in the normal lung DNA. The authors concluded that loss of specific genetic sequences on chromosome 3p contributes to tumorigenesis in SCLC.

This study represents molecular epidemiology at its finest level of resolution. Although this investigation may not be immediately recognizable as a case-control study, construction of a familiar 2 x 2 table shows that it fits this rubric nicely (Table 9-4). One could also criticize this study on epidemiologic grounds: six of the nine patients had received chemotherapy, an exposure that renders interpretation of the data more difficult. An earlier study, however, had found a deletion of 3p in all of 16 SCLC patients studied, regardless of whether they had received chemotherapy (Whang-Peng et al., 1982), and other investigators have obtained similar results.

SUMMARY

1. Oncogenes are genes that cause cancer. They represent altered versions of normal genes, protooncogenes, that exist in every cell.

2. Whereas oncogenes are activated by somatic mutation and influence tumorigenesis in a dominant fashion, tumor-suppressor genes (antioncogenes) are deactivated by mutation and influence tumorigenesis in a recessive mode. Oncogenes are markers of disease; tumor-suppressor genes, when present in only a single copy, are markers of susceptibility.

3. There is no generic laboratory technique to detect oncogenes. Instead, laboratory techniques are selected to suit the means of activation of a particular gene. In general, oncogenes activated by amplification (e.g., *c-myc*) are assayed by Southern analysis. Oncogenes activated by mutation (e.g., *c-ras*) are assayed by transfection, or preferably, by the polymerase chain reaction.

4. Because of laboratory biases, most studies of oncogenes and human cancers are biased toward the null. As the techniques mature, the evidence implicating oncogenes as a "final common pathway" for the evolution of many malignancies is likely to increase.

5. Epidemiologic studies of oncogenes are both feasible and clinically important. By necessity, most studies will be case series or case-control designs. The availability of archival human specimens offers the opportunity to perform case-control studies in cohorts defined by samples of stored tissue.

REFERENCES

Anderson P, Goldfarb MP, Weinberg RA. A defined subgenomic fragment of in vitro synthesized Moloney sarcoma virus DNA can induce cell transformation upon transfection. *Cell* 1975;16:63–75.

Barbacid M: Mutagens, oncogenes and cancer. *Trends in Genet* 1986;2:188–192.

Bishop JM: Oncogenes. *Sci Am* 1982;246:80–92.

Bishop JM: Trends in oncogenes. *Trends in Genet* 1985;1:245–249.

Bishop JM: The molecular genetics of cancer. *Science* 1987;235:305–311.

Bos JL, Fearon ER, Hamilton SR, Verlaan-de Vries M, van Boom JH, van der EB AJ, Vogelstein B: Prevalence of *ras* gene mutations in human colorectal cancers. *Nature* 1987;327:293–297.

Boveri T: Zur frage der erstehung maligner tumoren. *Jena,* Fisher, 1914.

Brosman SA, Liu BC-S: Oncogenes: Their role in neoplasia. *Urology* 1987;30:1–10.

Brugge JS, Cotton PC, Queral AE, Barrett JN, Nonner D, Keane RW: Neurones express high levels of a structurally modified form of pp60$^{c\text{-}src}$. *Nature* 1985;316:554–557.

Cavanee WK, Dryja TP, Phillips RA, Benedict WF, Godhout R, Gallie BK, et al.: Expression of recessive alleles by chromosomal mechanisms in retinoblastoma. *Nature* 1983;305:779–784.

Cole MD: The *myc* oncogene: Its role in transformation and differentiation. *Annu Rev Genet* 1986;20:361–384.

Duesberg PH: Activated proto-onc genes: Sufficient or necessary for cancer? *Science* 1985;228:669–677.

Emery AEH: *An Introduction to Recombinant DNA.* New York, John Wiley and Sons, 1984.

Erlich HA, Gelfand DH, Saiki RK: Specific DNA amplification. *Nature* 1988;331:461–462.

Fleming WH, Hamel A, MacDonald R, Ramsey E, Pettigrew NM, Johnston B, et al.: Expression of the *c-myc* proto-oncogene in human prostatic carcinoma and benign prostatic hyperplasia. *Cancer Res* 1986; 46:1535–1538.

Goustin AS, Leof EB, Shipley GD, Moses HL: Growth factors and cancer. *Cancer Res* 1986;46:1015–1029.

Helm S, Mitelman F: Nineteen of 26 cellular oncogenes precisely localized in the human genomic map to one of the 83 bands involved in primary cancer-rearrangements. *Hum Genet* 1987;75:70–72.

Heubner RJ, Todaro GJ: Oncogenes of RNA tumor viruses as determinants of cancer. *Proc Natl Acad Sci USA* 1969;64:1087–1094.

Kaneko Y, Egues MC, Rowley JD: Interstitial deletion of short arm of chromosome 11 limited to Wilms' tumor cells in a patient without aniridia. *Cancer Res* 1981;41:4577–4578.

Knudson AG: Mutation and cancer: Statistical study of retinoblastoma. *Proc Natl Acad Sci* 1971;68:820–823.

Knudson AG: Retinoblastoma: A prototype hereditary neoplasm. *Semin Oncol* 1978;5:57–60.

Konopka JB, Watanabe SM, Witte ON: An alteration of the human *c-abl* protein in K562 leukemia cells unmasks associated protein kinase activity. *Cell* 1984;37:1035–1042.

Maniatis T, Fritsch EF, Sambrook J: *Molecular Cloning: A Laboratory Manual.* Cold Spring Harbor, 1982.

Murray RK, Granner DK, Mayes PA, Rodwell VW: *Harper's Biochemistry,* 21 ed. Norwalk, CT, Appleton and Lange, 1988.

Naylor SL, Johnson BE, Minna JD, Sakaguchi AY: Loss of heterozygosity of chromosome 3p markers in small-cell lung cancer. *Nature* 1987;329:451–454.

Phillips ME, Ferro MA, Smith PJ, Davies P: Intranuclear androgen receptor deployment and oncogene expression in human diseased prostate. *Urol Int* 1987;42:115–119.

Rabbitts TH: The *c-myc* proto-oncogene: Involvement in chromosomal abnormalities. *Trends Genet* 1985;1:331–427.

Reddy EP, Reynolds RK, Santos E, Barbacid M: A point mutation is responsible for the acquisition of transforming properties by the T24 bladder carcinoma oncogene. *Nature* 1982;300:147–152.

Rodriquez RL, Tait RC: *Recombinant DNA Techniques—An Introduction.* Reading, Massachusetts, Addison-Wesley, 1983.

Rothberg PG: The role of the oncogene *c-myc* in sporadic large bowel cancer and familial polyposis coli. *Semin Surg Oncol* 1987;3:152–158.

Rous P: A sarcoma of the fowl transmissible by an agent separable from the tumor cells. *J Exp Med* 1911;13:397–411.

Sager R: Genetic suppression of tumor formation: A new frontier in cancer research. *Cancer Res* 1986;46:1573–1580.

Seeger RC, Brodeuk GM, Sather H, Dalton A, Siegal S, Wong KY, Hammond D: Association of multiple copies of the *N-myc* oncogene with rapid progression of neuroblastomas. *N Engl J Med* 1985;313:1111–1116.

Shibata D, Martin JW, Arnheim N: Analysis of DNA sequences in forty-year-old paraffin-embedded thin-tissue sections: A bridge between molecular biology and classical histology. *Cancer Res* 1988;48:4564–4566.

Slamon DJ, Clark GM, Wong SG, Levin WJ, Ullrich A, McGurie WL: Human breast cancer: Correlation of relapse and survival with amplification of the *HER-2/Neu* oncogene. *Science* 1987;235:177–182.

Solomon E, Voss R, Hall V, et al.: Chromosome 5 allele loss in human colorectal carcinomas. *Nature* 1978;328:616–619.

Southern EM: Detection of specific sequences among DNA fragments separated by gel electrophoresis. *J Mol Biol* 1975;98:303–308.

Stehelin D, Varmus HE, Bishop JM, Vogt PK: DNA related to the transforming gene(s) of avian sarcoma viruses is present in normal avian DNA. *Nature* 1976;260:170–173.

Stock LM, Brosman SA, Fehey JL, Liu BC-S: *Ras* related oncogenic protein as a tumor marker in transitional cell carcinoma of the bladder. *J Urol* 1987;137:7889–7892.

Stubblefield E, Sanford J: A general survey of genetics and cancer. *Anticancer Res* 1987;7:1085–1104.

Tabin DH, Bradley SM, Bargmann CI, Weinberg RA, Papageorge AG, Scolnick EM, et al.: Mechanism of activation of a human oncogene. *Nature* 1982;300:143–149.

Tereba A: Chromosomal localization of proto-oncogenes. *Int Rev Cytol* 1985;95:1–43.

Varmus HE: The molecular genetics of cellular oncogenes. *Annu Rev Genet* 1984;18:553–612.

Whang-Peng J, Kao-Shan CS, Lee EC: Specific chromosome defect associated with human small-cell lung cancer: Deletion 3p(14-23). *Science* 1982;215:181–182.

Weinberg RA: The genetic origins of human cancer. *Cancer* 1988;61:1963–1968.

Weissman SM: Molecular genetic techniques for mapping the human genome. *Mol Biol Med* 1987;4:133–143.

10

MARKERS OF SUSCEPTIBILITY

MARILYN F. VINE AND LISA T. MCFARLAND

INTRODUCTION

Individual members of any human population show considerable variation in susceptibility to a number of adverse health outcomes, including heart disease (Rao et al., 1984), cancer (Littlefield, 1984), birth defects (Manchester and Jacoby, 1984; Chudley, 1985), and infectious diseases (Petersen et al., 1985). If exposed to similar toxins, irritants, or other agents, some people may become seriously ill, whereas others are hardly affected. For example, cigarette smoking is known to be strongly associated with lung cancer (USDHEW, 1982), yet the incidence of lung cancer among male smokers of one or more packs of cigarettes per day is low (about five cases per 1000 person-years) (Fontana, 1986).

In any epidemiologic study, then, it will be helpful to be able to identify individuals or population subgroups who have different susceptibility to disease. Markers of susceptibility may help epidemiologists identify such subgroups. These markers measure, or are associated with, factors that increase an individual's risk of developing a disease after exposure to some exogenous agent. They are independent of exposure and may be genetically determined or acquired.

To some extent susceptibility must be defined in the context of a particular environment or exposure. For example, the sickle cell trait predisposes individuals to anemia and altitude sickness yet protects them from childhood malaria (Omenn, 1982). Therefore, a trait that may make a person susceptible to one disease may actually be protective for some other outcome.

Genetically Determined Susceptibility

Genetically determined susceptibility factors produce an increase in disease frequency through variations in the DNA that codes for specific proteins. As a result, genetically susceptible individuals may produce proteins that are structurally different, or produce them in greater or lesser amounts than individuals who are not at increased risk of disease. The syndrome, xeroderma pigmentosum, is a classic example of a genetically determined susceptibility. Individuals who have this syndrome are at increased risk of developing skin cancer after exposure to ultraviolet light because of defects in DNA-repair proteins (Cleaver, 1968).

The study of genetically determined differences in susceptibility to disease is part of the broad field of ecogenetics, the study of genetically determined differences in response to environmental agents (Khoury et al., 1987). It grew out of pharmacogenetics, the study of differences in reactions to drugs and is based on the observation that individuals respond to drug therapy in different ways. For example, there are two major phenotypes of the liver enzyme, N-acetyltransferase. Investigators can use the rate of activity of this enzyme to divide the population into two groups: those who are slow acetylators and those who are fast acetylators. Adverse reactions to the antituberculosis drug, isoniazid, occur more often or at lower doses in people who are slow acetylators (Omenn, 1984).

Acquired Susceptibility

Acquired susceptibility factors may include age, diet, life-style, exposure to environmental agents, and previous infections or other diseases. Although genetically determined susceptibilities, for the most part, remain constant, acquired factors may change over time, leading to changes in degree of susceptibility. An example of an acquired susceptibility factor is alcohol consumption. Heavy alcohol consumption increases the risk of smoking-related deaths from cancers of the head and the neck (Schmidt and Popham, 1981). Table 10-1 lists examples of other susceptibility factors suspected of affecting the risk of cancer associated with an environmental exposure.

Mechanisms

Susceptibility factors may increase the toxic effect of environmental agents at any point along the route from entry into the body to the development of overt disease (see Fig. 1-2). One way that increased susceptibility may operate is by increasing an agent's internal dose. Cuts and other skin lesions, for example, can increase permeability to solvents, thereby raising the amount of these agents that are absorbed by the body. Heightened susceptibility may also operate by increasing the biologically effective dose, the amount of reactive agent that reaches the target tissue. Skin color, for example, is a genetically determined susceptibility factor for certain types of skin cancer (Harnden, 1984). Melanin in the skin protects against DNA damage by preventing absorption of ultraviolet light. Light-skinned people, therefore, receive a greater dose of ultraviolet light to their DNA than do dark-skinned individuals. Furthermore, some agents must be activated, or converted to a biologically active form, before they cause damage. Differing rates of activity of enzymes that control the activation (or detoxification) of foreign compounds can lead to differences in susceptibility by increasing or decreasing an agent's biologically effective dose.

Alternatively, susceptibility factors may influence a tissue's biological response to environmental agents. For example, although a chemical may reach a target tissue and produce chromosome breakage, the persistence of breakage will depend on the effi-

Table 10-1 Selected Genetic and Acquired Factors Suspected of Being Associated with Increased Susceptibility to Cancer

Susceptibility factor	Environmental agent	Disease
Genetic		
Debrisoquine hydroxylation phenotype	Cigarette smoke	Lung cancer (Ayesh et al., 1984)
	Aflatoxin	Liver cancer (Idle et al., 1981)
Acetylation phenotype	N-substituted aryl compounds	Bladder cancer (Cartwright et al., 1982)
Heterozygous for ataxia-telangiectasia gene	Ionizing radiation	Cancer of the breast, ovary, and gastrointestinal tract, as well as lymphoma, and leukemia (Swift et al., 1976)
Skin color	Ultraviolet light	Skin cancer (Harnden, 1984)
Xeroderma pigmentosum	Ultraviolet light	Skin cancer (Cleaver, 1968)
Aryl hydrocarbon hydroxylase (AHH) inducibility	Polycyclic aromatic hydrocarbons	Lung cancer (Kellerman et al., 1977)
Acquired		
Low vitamin A intake	Cigarette smoke	Lung cancer (Colditz et al., 1987)
Alcohol consumption	Cigarette smoke	Laryngeal cancer (Schmidt and Popham, 1981)

ciency of an individual's DNA repair mechanisms. Any indicator of variations in metabolic rate, absorption, distribution or excretion of exogenous materials, physiologic function, hormonal balance, DNA repair, immune response, cell proliferation, or nutritional status may be a potentially useful marker of susceptibility.

Significance of Susceptibility Markers

The ultimate goal of studying increased susceptibility to the effects of environmental agents is the prevention of disease. One way to prevent disease is to understand its causes and to use this knowledge to intervene in the disease process. For instance, because of a genetically determined defect in the ability to metabolize phenylalanine, individuals with phenylketonuria (PKU) develop mental retardation if they eat food containing this amino acid. Because PKU can be detected at birth and because we understand the mechanism by which the disorder operates, we can lessen the adverse effects of this metabolic defect by providing susceptible individuals with a diet low in phenylalanine (Thompson and Thompson, 1986).

To be useful, markers of susceptibility do not have to directly identify mechanistic factors that increase susceptibility. If one assumes that genetic mutations can lead to the development of cancer, it might be possible to determine an individual's susceptibility to cancer by determining the probability that his or her cells will mutate upon exposure to toxic chemicals. For example, Albertini et al. (1982) have developed an assay to detect mutations of the gene on the X chromosome that codes for the enzyme, hypoxanthine–guanine phosphoribosyl transferase (HGPRT). If the HGPRT gene of a person's white blood cells mutates when the cells are cultured in the presence of toxic chemicals in vitro, then the individual may be at greater risk of developing cancer than someone whose HGPRT gene does not mutate as readily. It is not clear that HGPRT itself is involved in the carcinogenic process. Mutations of the HGPRT gene, however, can be used as indicators of the potential for genetic damage from exposure to carcinogenic chemicals (Kolata, 1980). Thus, once individuals at high risk of disease have been identified, it becomes possible to protect them from harmful exposures, although the exact mechanism of disease causation is still unknown.

Factors that influence susceptibility to disease are especially important in epidemiologic research as potential effect modifiers in studies of the relationship between exposure and disease. The magnitude and direction of associations between exposures and diseases may differ according to the level of a susceptibility marker. For example, the risk of lung cancer among smokers and nonsmokers differs depending on the level of β-carotene intake. High β-carotene intake is protective against lung cancer. Low β-carotene intake is associated with an increased risk of lung cancer (Colditz et al., 1987).

As we emphasize in this chapter, there is considerable heterogeneity within human populations with respect to disease risk associated with exposure to exogenous agents. In epidemiologic studies that do not consider differences in susceptibility, overall risk estimates depend on the distribution of people in the study who have differing susceptibilities to disease. Ideally, one would like to stratify study subjects by degree of susceptibility to quantify the risk of disease given exposure to some exogenous agent more accurately. Markers of susceptibility can help identify individuals with different disease risk. For example, suppose one wanted to calculate the attack rate (proportion of people at risk of disease who develop the disease) of an infectious agent that conferred permanent immunity. For an accurate determination of the rate, one would want to eliminate all persons already immune to the disease as the result of prior infection from the denominator of the rate. In this example, the presence or absence of antibodies to the infectious agent could serve as a marker of susceptibility.

In summary, the goal of epidemiologic research is to prevent disease by identifying determinants of disease. Because the use of susceptibility markers in epidemiologic research is likely to enhance the identification of high-risk individuals, these markers should help clarify relationships between exposures and disease and may even aid in preventing future disease.

EVALUATION OF A POTENTIALLY USEFUL SUSCEPTIBILITY MARKER

Before using a potential marker of susceptibility in an epidemiologic field study, an investigator should be well acquainted with the marker's properties and measurement. In the following section, we illustrate how to evaluate susceptibility markers of potential use in epidemiologic research. The example we use is the genetically determined enzyme marker, N-acetyltransferase (NAT). NAT is a good example of a marker of susceptibility, as it serves as an indicator of elevated risk to a disease with known genetic and environmental components. Individuals with low N-acetyltransferase activity have been found to be at increased risk of bladder cancer in association with arylamine exposure (Wolf et al., 1980).

In this section, we pose questions that investigators should ask before they use a marker. The answers provided apply to the enzyme marker NAT, the example under discussion.

Basic Background Information

Does the marker have a normal function in the body, and if so, how does the marker function? For example, what is NAT and what does it do?

NAT is a noninducible enzyme group found primarily in the liver. The NAT enzyme group is species-specific and substrate-specific (Wolf et al., 1980). NAT is involved in a variety of activation and detoxification pathways. Its primary role is the detoxification by acetylation of N-substituted aryl compounds (arylamines), such as benzidine, 4-aminobiphenyl, and 2-aminonaphthalene (Lower et al., 1979). Acetylation of arylamines is a two-step process: (1) an acetyl group, CH_3CO, from acetyl coenzyme (cofactor) A is transferred to NAT, producing an acetyl-NAT intermediate (acetyl-N-acetyltransferase); and (2) the intermediate combines with the arylamine, yielding an acetylated arylamine and regenerating NAT (La Du, 1972).

Acetylator phenotype (fast or slow) determines the rate at which arylamine carcinogens are detoxified. People who are slow acetylators are believed to be at increased risk of bladder cancer as they cannot detoxify carcinogenic arylamines as readily as fast acetylators (Lower, 1982).

Acquisition of the Marker

Is the marker genetically determined or acquired? If the marker is genetically controlled, what is the genetic nature of the trait? If the marker is acquired, how is it acquired?

With respect to NAT phenotype, differences in acetylation status are generally considered to be genetically determined by two alternative alleles at one autosomal locus (Cartwright et al., 1982). One of the alleles is dominant and the other recessive, a situation that results in two distinct human NAT phenotypes. The "fast" or "rapid" acetylator phenotype usually includes both homozygous dominant and heterozygous genotypes, whereas the "slow" phenotype results from the homozygous recessive genotype. Chapron et al. (1980) as well as Lee and Lee (1982) have suggested that there may be a trimodal phenotype pattern that results in a separate heterozygous phenotype of intermediate acetylator activity.

Although the rate of NAT activity varies little within individuals over time (Weber and Hein, 1979), there can be 100-fold differences in the rate of NAT activity between individuals (Cartwright, 1984). Evidence from animal studies suggests that structural differences in the enzymes of fast and slow acetylators account for the variation in NAT activity (Weber and Hein, 1979).

Prevalence of the Marker

What is the frequency of the trait in the population under investigation?

The frequency of the trait under investigation determines the type of epidemiologic field study that can be conducted, the sample sizes required, and helps determine whether screening on a population basis is worthwhile. By genetic standards, common traits are those in which the least common allele is present in at least 1 percent of the population (Murray, 1986). Traits with this characteristic are known as polymorphisms. Genetic traits with a frequency of between 1/100 and 1/10,000 population are considered uncommon. Rare traits are those with a frequency of 1/10,000 or less (Murray, 1986).

NAT phenotype, for example, is considered a polymorphic trait. The frequency of NAT phenotypes (fast vs. slow) does not vary by age or gender (Lange et al., 1986), but does vary among ethnic groups. The frequency of slow acetylators ranges from 5 percent in Canadian Eskimos (Armstrong and Peart, 1960) to about 90 percent in Moroccans (Weber and Hein, 1985). For the most part, caucasians and blacks of African origin have an approximately equal ratio of slow to fast acetylators (Drayer and Reidenberg, 1977; Karim et al., 1981). Oriental populations have a lower proportion of slow acetylators than most other ethnic groups (Weber and Hein, 1979; Kukongviriyapan et al., 1984).

Susceptibility factors are usually investigated as modifiers of associations between exposures and diseases. Unless a trait exists with a reasonable frequency, it may be difficult to study. The difficulty increases if the disease or the exposure of interest is also rare. Thus, if the susceptibility factor, the exposure, and the disease are rare, studies may be impractical unless one can target groups exposed to the agent of interest in, for example, occupational settings.

With some traits, heterozygous individuals are also at increased risk of disease, but may be less susceptible than the homozygous individuals. For example, persons homozygous for ataxia telangiectasia (AT), an autosomal recessive syndrome characterized by the impaired ability to repair DNA damaged by ionizing radiation (Thompson and Thompson, 1986), are at increased risk of cancer (Swift et al., 1976). Swift and co-workers (1976) found that relatives of patients with AT, some of whom carry the gene for AT, are also at increased risk of developing certain cancers including carcinomas, lymphomas, and leukemias. Findings of elevated risks for heterozygous individuals are important as the heterozygous phenotype is often more prevalent than either of the homozygous phenotypes.

Laboratory Methods to Assess Marker Presence

Does the test used to measure the genetic trait or condition identify individuals reliably? Is the test cheap, quick, safe, and simple? How invasive is it? What are the sources of variability in the test procedures?

The example of NAT phenotyping, for the most part, provides satisfactory answers to these questions. Current laboratory techniques can clearly distinguish NAT phenotypes (Weber and Hein, 1985). The assessment of NAT phenotype is usually done with samples of blood or urine. The standard method for collecting biological specimens to determine NAT phenotype involves giving study subjects an oral dose of an arylamine or hydrazine test drug after they have fasted overnight and then drawing a venous blood sample or obtaining a urine specimen after drug absorption. Because an individual's NAT phenotype determines the rate of aromatic amine and hydrazine metabolism, there are several drugs with an arylamine or hydrazine group that can be used as test substrates to measure NAT activity including isoniazid, sulfamethazine (sulfadimidine), procainamide, sulphasalazine, and dapsone (4,4′diaminodiphenylsulfone) (Weber and Hein, 1985).

There are several laboratory techniques to determine NAT activity levels (Weber and Hein, 1985). The object of each technique is to quantify the ratio of acetylated to nonacetylated test drug after a given period of time. This ratio determines whether a person can be classified as either a fast or slow acetylator.

One of the simplest methods of evaluating NAT phenotype is a modified version of the Bratton–Marshall procedure (Weber and Brenner, 1974) (Fig. 10-1). With this method, 10 mg of sulfamethazine, an antibiotic, is administered orally to the study subjects. After 4.5 to 6 hours, blood or urine is obtained from the subjects and 0.1 ml of the sample is placed on filter paper and allowed to dry. The ratio of acetylated to nonacetylated test substrate is assessed with spectrophotometry. According to Weber and Brenner (1974), blood samples provide a better indication of acetylator status than urine, but using both blood and urine samples from the same individual yields the best

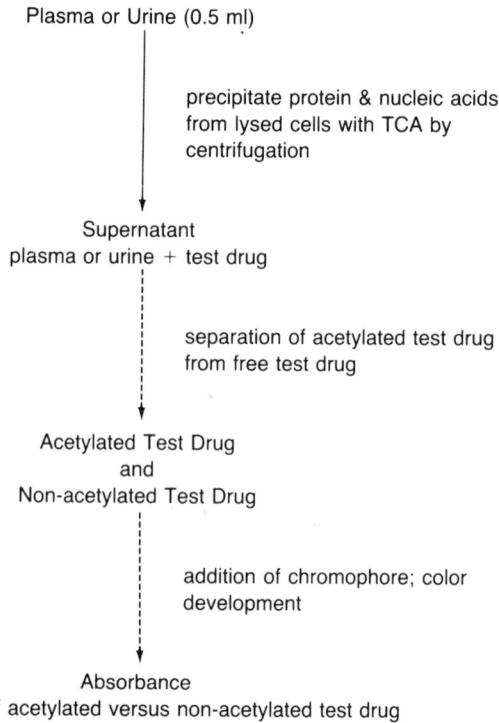

Preparation

• Subjects undergo an overnight fast
• Subjects are given an oral dose of test drug, e.g. 10 mg/kg body wt. of sulfamethazine or sulfadimidine in 1–2 oz. of water
• 4.5 hours after administration of test drug, samples of venous blood and urine are collected

Plasma or Urine (0.5 ml)

precipitate protein & nucleic acids from lysed cells with TCA by centrifugation

Supernatant
plasma or urine + test drug

separation of acetylated test drug from free test drug

Acetylated Test Drug
and
Non-acetylated Test Drug

addition of chromophore; color development

Absorbance
quantitation of acetylated versus non-acetylated test drug in a spectrophotometer at 540 nm

Figure 10-1. Method for determining acetylator phenotype using spectrophotometric analysis. (Weber & Brenner, 1974.)

assessment of acetylator status. One advantage of the modified Bratton–Marshall technique is its use of small amounts of the biological specimen on dried filter paper. The approach makes the technique good for field studies, as it avoids the need to transport liquid specimens (Weber and Brenner, 1974). Many of the studies assessing NAT as a susceptibility factor for bladder cancer have used this method.

Sulfamethazine has been the test drug of choice in many studies of acetylator status because of its heat stability and its ability to withstand long-term storage (Weber and Brenner, 1974). In addition, the dose necessary to determine acetylator phenotype is lower than the therapeutic dose and the incidence of side effects is low (Lang et al., 1986). One drawback to using sulfamethazine as the test drug is that it can sometimes be difficult to obtain approval to use it in the United States (Weber and Hein, 1985).

Grant and co-workers (1984) have developed a method of measuring NAT activity using caffeine as the substrate. Subjects ingest 1 to 1.5 mg/kg body weight caffeine in either coffee, tea, or a soft drink, and their urine is collected after 2 to 6 hours. The urine is analyzed with high performance liquid chromatography (HPLC) for the ratio of two caffeine metabolites: 5–acetylamino-6-formylamino-3-methyluracil (AFMU) and 1-methylxanthine (1X). This ratio is used as an indicator of NAT phenotype. The advantages of this method are (1) caffeine is safe and readily obtainable, (2) sampling time does not need to be precise, and (3) the ratio AFMU/1X is independent of urine flow and kidney function (Grant et al., 1984).

The laboratory methods (for example, HPLC and spectrophotometry) used to determine acetylator phenotype are relatively common. Because NAT phenotyping is not a routine clinical test, however, it is necessary to make special arrangements with a laboratory that does the testing.

Laboratory procedures to assess NAT phenotype are inexpensive (Cartwright, 1984) and reliable in healthy individuals (Weber and Hein, 1985). Both the test drug and certain characteristics of the subjects tested, however, can affect the reliability of the laboratory techniques. For example, using sulfamethazine as the test substrate gives better separation of fast and slow acetylators than using procainamide (Weber and Hein, 1985). Furthermore, using procainamide to ascertain NAT phenotype produces unreliable results in subjects with impaired renal function. When isoniazid is used as the test drug, the age and gender of the subjects affects acetylation ratios (Iselius and Evans, 1983).

Although NAT phenotyping may be a reasonable procedure for healthy adults, using this test on children, the elderly, or the sick may require some consideration (Weber and Hein, 1985). The test involves administering a drug and then waiting 4.5 to 6 hours (or longer for some test drugs) before obtaining the biological specimen. These procedures may be too demanding for some subgroups of the population. The use of caffeine as the test substrate may alleviate some of these concerns.

NAT activity can also be measured in studies of liver specimens in vitro. Unfortunately, NAT activity is unstable in autopsy specimens. To ascertain NAT phenotype in cadavers, one must freeze the liver within 2 hours of death to prevent enzyme inactivation (Hein et al., 1981). Even then, some degradation is likely. One possible marker of NAT inactivation after death may be p-aminobenzoic acid (PABA) (Hein et al., 1981). The PABA is an endogenous arylamine. There is little difference in the N-acetylation capacity of slow and fast acetylators to acetylate this compound. The PABA acetylation is high regardless of NAT phenotype. Low PABA NAT activity would indicate

NAT inactivation. High PABA NAT activity would indicate a lack of significant NAT inactivation. If PABA NAT activity can be shown to be an accurate indicator of NAT inactivation, then this assay may prove to be an indicator of the reliability of postmortem measurements of NAT activity in vitro (Hein et al., 1981).

Assessing a Marker's Association with an Exposure–Disease Relationship

Is the susceptibility marker clearly linked to an association between an exposure and a disease? Do different levels of the susceptibility marker indicate a difference in the association between the exposure and the disease? Is the susceptibility marker an independent risk factor for the disease in the absence of exposure?

Arylamines and Bladder Cancer

One association of interest in the NAT example is the relationship between exposure to N-substituted aryl compounds and the risk of bladder cancer. Several investigators have found that exposure to N-substituted aryl compounds is a risk factor for bladder cancer in humans (Rehn, 1895; Lower, 1982), and several arylamines have been shown to be carcinogenic in experimental animals (Hueper et al., 1938; Walpole et al., 1954; Lower, 1982). Aryl compound exposure occurs in such occupational settings as the dye, textile, rubber, and cable industries and workers in these industries have exhibited an increased risk of bladder cancer (Case et al., 1954; Davies, 1965). As many as 20 percent of bladder cancer cases in the United States are thought to be due to occupational exposure to arylamines (Wolf et al., 1980). Arylamines are also present in tobacco smoke and cigarette smoking is a known risk factor for bladder cancer (USDHEW, 1982). As many as 40 percent of bladder cancer cases in the United States are believed to stem from arylamine exposure from cigarette smoke (Wolf et al., 1980).

At least 10 case-control studies have examined the association between acetylator phenotype and urinary bladder cancer. Table 10-2 summarizes the study designs and results of these investigations.

In three of these studies (Wolf et al., 1980; Hanssen et al., 1985; Ladero et al., 1985), the investigators reported a statistically significant excess of slow acetylators among the bladder cancer cases as compared with controls. In three studies (Cartwright et al., 1982; Hanssen et al., 1985; Ladero et al., 1985), the researchers noted a statistically significant association among bladder cancer patients who were occupationally exposed to bladder carcinogens. Cartwright et al. (1982) found that 22 of 23 (96%) bladder cancer cases among workers exposed to chemicals were slow acetylators, whereas only 59 percent of bladder cancer cases that developed in nonchemical workers and 57 percent of controls were slow acetylators. In addition, Cartwright et al. (1982) found a greater proportion of slow acetylators among individuals with more severe stages of bladder cancer (tumor stages T3/T4 and carcinoma in situ vs. T1/T2). Wolf et al. (1980) attributed the excess of slow acetylators among bladder cancer cases in their study to exposure to bladder carcinogens in an urban environment.

Six studies (Lower et al., 1979; Woodhouse et al., 1982; Miller and Cosgriff, 1983; Evans et al., 1983; Mommsen et al., 1985; Karakaya et al., 1986) reported no statistically significant association between acetylator phenotype and bladder cancer, although four of them (Lower et al., 1979; Woodhouse et al., 1982; Evans et al., 1983; Mommsen et al., 1985) noted a slight excess of slow acetylators among the cases. In the other two studies, controls showed an excess of slow acetylators, and in the study by Karakaya et al. (1986), these results were nearly statistically significant. If acetylator status is a factor in bladder cancer development only after exposure to environmental bladder carcinogens, then the absence of exposure to arylamines may explain why several of these studies found no significant association between acetylator status and bladder cancer. Two studies (Woodhouse et al., 1985; Karakaya et al., 1986) did not include people with known exposures to occupational bladder carcinogens. Mommsen et al. (1985) and Lower et al. (1979) studied populations at low risk of bladder cancer, groups that had low exposures to bladder carcinogens. Miller and Cosgriff (1982) did not find a statistically significant excess of slow acetylators among cases occupationally exposed to bladder carcinogens, but small numbers may have been a problem. Only six of 15 cases (40%), who were occupationally exposed to bladder carcinogens, were slow acetylators.

From the results of these studies, it would seem that NAT phenotype is probably not an independent risk factor for bladder cancer. Acetylator phenotype appears to be a significant factor only in association with exposure to arylamine carcinogens. In epidemiologic investigations, acetylator status most likely functions as a modifier of the effects of arylamine carcinogen exposure. One would, therefore, expect the risk of bladder cancer development to be higher among slow acetylators who are exposed to arylamine bladder carcinogens than among fast acetylators who are exposed to bladder carcinogens. One would also expect acetylator status to be important in the development of bladder cancer among individuals occupationally exposed to bladder carcinogens, as Cartwright et al. (1982), Hanssen et al. (1985), and Ladero et al. (1985) found. The strength of the association among acetylator phenotypes still needs to be characterized accurately.

The role of NAT as an effect modifier in the association between arylamine exposure and bladder cancer is analogous to its role in drug metabolism. Individuals with different acetylator phenotypes react differently to certain drugs, and side effects of drugs have been related to both NAT phenotypes (fast and slow). For example, the most well known pharmacologic problem is the association between acetylation status and isoniazid (INH) toxicity. INH is an antibiotic agent used principally in treating tuberculosis. Because slow acetylators do not readily metabolize INH, they have higher serum concentrations of the drug and may develop peripheral neuropathies and systemic lupus, whereas rapid acetylators are thought to be more susceptible to INH-induced hepatotoxicity (Weber, 1984).

Cigarette Smoking and Bladder Cancer

Although cigarette smoke contains arylamine compounds, cigarette smoking does not appear to be as strong a factor in the association between NAT phenotype and bladder cancer as occupational exposures. Two studies (Cartwright et al., 1982; Hanssen et al., 1985) found a slight but nonsignificant excess of slow acetylators among smokers, whereas a third study (Miller and Cosgriff, 1983) found no excess of either slow or fast acetylators among smokers. Mommsen and Aagaard (1986) noted no statistically significant differences in the distribution of smokers and nonsmokers between slow and fast acetylators with bladder cancer.

Table 10-2 Human Studies—Association Between Bladder Cancer and Acetylator Phenotype

Reference	Subjects	Test Substrate and Assay Method	Results	Comments
Lower et al., 1979 Sweden	*Cases*—115 histologically confirmed bladder cancer cases *Controls*—118 healthy individuals, hospital personnel, hospital patients admitted for nonmalignant diseases	Sulfamethazine (spectrophotometry)	No statistically significant difference between cases and controls with respect to acetylator phenotype; 69.6% slow acetylators among cases; 66.9% among controls (p < .7) OR = 1.1	Subjects were from a rural population
Wolf et al., 1980 Copenhagen	*Cases*—71 histologically confirmed bladder cancer cases *Controls*—74 healthy individuals, hospital personnel, hospital patients admitted for nonmalignant urological disease	Sulfamethazine (spectrophotometry)	Statistically significant excess of slow acetylators among cases vs. controls; 65% slow acelylators among cases, 51% slow acetylators among controls (p < .06) OR = 1.7	Exposure was presumably to carcinogenic arylamines from occupational or urban exposures and smoking; 95% of subjects smoked
Cartwright et al., 1982 London	*Cases*—111 carcinomas of the bladder *Controls*—95 urological or surgery patients	Dapsone (HPTLC)	Slight but nonsignificant excess of slow acetylators among cases (67%) vs. controls (57%); (p < .15) OR = 1.5 Slight but nonsignificant excess of slow acetylators among former and current cigarette smokers vs. nonsmokers Among bladder cancer cases who were chemical workers,	

			22/23 (96%) were slow acetylators vs. 59% of other cases (p < .01)	
Woodhouse et al., 1982 England	*Cases*—30 histologically confirmed bladder cancer cases *Controls*—27 geriatric patients without malignant disease	Isoniazid (spectrophotometry)	No statistically significant difference in acetylator phenotype between cases and controls, although there were more slow acetylators among cases (70%) vs. controls (59%) (p < .3) OR = 1.6	No patients were known to have industrial exposures to bladder carcinogens. Patients were from an urban population
Miller and Cosgriff, 1983 N.Y. State	*Cases*—26 histologically confirmed bladder cancer cases *Controls*—26 controls, spouses, unrelated friends, or hospital employees	Sulfamethazine (spectrophotometry)	No significant difference in proportion of acetylator phenotypes among cases and controls, although more slow acetylators among controls (69%) than among bladder cancer cases (46%) (p < .1) OR = 0.4 No significant excess of slow acetylators among cases occupationally exposed to chemical carcinogens or cigarette smoking	
Evans et al., 1983 England	*Cases*—100 bladder cancer cases (97 smoked) *Controls*—852 pooled controls from various studies	Sulfadimidine (spectrophotometry)	No statistically significant difference in proportion of acetylator phenotypes between cases and controls; 66/100 (66%) slow acetylators among cases (510/852), 60% slow acetylators among controls OR = 1.3	

(*continued*)

Table 10-2 (*Continued*)

Reference	Subjects	Test Substrate and Assay Method	Results	Comments
Hanssen et al., 1985 Germany	*Cases*—105 histologically confirmed bladder cancer cases *Controls*—42 healthy subjects	Sulfadimidine (spectrophotometry)	Statistically significant excess of slow acetylatos among cases (61.9%) vs. controls (42.9%) (p < .05) OR = 2.2 Greater percentage of slow acetylators among patients who were dye workers (70.4%) as compared to the whole group of patients (61.9%) Slight but nonsignificant excess of slow acetylators among smokers vs. nonsmokers	
Ladero et al., 1985 Spain	*Cases*—130 histologically confirmed transitional cell carcinoma *Controls*—157 normal subjects	Sulfamethazine (spectrophotometry)	No significant excess of slow acetylators among all cases (63.8%) vs. controls (57%) OR = 1.3 Significant excess of slow acetylators among men thought to be occupationally exposed to aromatic amines 41/55 (74.5%) (p < .05)	55 subjects held jobs in which they were thought to be exposed to carcinogenic amines
Mommsen et al., 1985 Denmark	*Cases*—228 histologically confirmed bladder cancer cases *Controls*—100 urologic patients without cancer, matched on age	Sulfamethazine (spectrophotometry)	No statistically significant excess of slow acetylators among cases (63.6%) vs. controls (54.0%) (p < .10) OR = 1.5	Patients were from a rural population
Karakaya et al., 1986 Turkey	*Cases*—23 transitional cell bladder cancer cases *Controls*—109 healthy volunteers	Sulfamethazine (spectrophotometry)	No statistically significant excess of slow acetylators among controls (62%) vs. cases (39%) (p ≃ .05) OR = 0.4	None of the subjects were known to be exposed to chemical carcinogens

Ethical Issues

How will the knowledge of susceptibility status be used? Will the study participants be informed of their status?

The study of susceptibility markers raises many ethical questions for epidemiologists. One key question is how the data will be used. Although screening for potential susceptibility factors can help prevent susceptible people from being exposed to harmful agents, the results of such tests may be used to exclude workers from lucrative employment (Kolata, 1980). Because many susceptibility factors are genetically determined, exclusion from employment could lead to sexual, racial, and ethnic discrimination from certain types of jobs. For example, ethnic groups with a high proportion of slow acetylators could be barred from working in the chemical industry. There is also the fear that insurance companies will use the tests to raise their rates for "cancer prone" individuals (Kolata, 1980). Instead of leading to a cleanup of the workplace and general environment, susceptibility tests may contribute to a "blame the victim" mentality, that is, the persons got sick because of their genetic makeup or life-style (Culliton and Waterfall, 1980). For these reasons, investigators must guarantee the confidentiality of study results.

Another ethical question is whether the subjects themselves should be notified of their susceptibility status. On the one hand, knowledge may allow them to prevent exposure to harmful substances. On the other, unless the association is well established, they may be alarmed unnecessarily. Then again, knowledge of a potential increase in susceptibility may help people make choices they might not otherwise make.

Most occupational susceptibility factors are not well characterized. More is known about acetylator status than about most other occupational susceptibilities, yet no report has recommended routine testing of workers for employment screening. (The magnitude of the risk of bladder cancer between acetylator phenotypes is still unknown.) In fact, no report has recommended routine screening for any occupational susceptibility.

SUMMARY AND CONCLUSIONS

This chapter has discussed the potential significance of markers of susceptibility to epidemiologic research and presented criteria for evaluating potentially useful markers. Given that the goal of epidemiologic research is prevention of disease, markers of susceptibility may aid this effort by identifying population subgroups at particularly high risk of disease after exposure to exogenous agents. Susceptibility markers may also strengthen our understanding of disease by focusing attention on possible pathways of disease causation. Because there is considerable heterogeneity in disease risk within populations, markers of susceptibility may also help to clarify associations between exposures and diseases within population subgroups.

NAT, the example discussed in the chapter, is a promising marker of susceptibility to bladder cancer associated with occupational exposures to N-substituted arylamines. Its metabolic function and genetic inheritance are fairly well understood. The prevalence of each NAT phenotype (fast and slow) among most U.S. caucasians and blacks is about 50 percent, a prevalence that is optimal in terms of its use in epidemiologic studies. Laboratory methods can identify acetylator phenotypes reliably (Weber and Hein, 1985), and the measurement techniques are safe, relatively easy to perform, and fairly noninvasive. Furthermore, they are applicable to large human populations, although some consideration is necessary before one subjects young children, the elderly, or the sick to the test. Because NAT phenotyping is not a routine clinical laboratory test, special arrangements must be made with a laboratory that does the testing.

Epidemiologic studies of the association between acetylator status and risk of bladder cancer suggest that acetylator status is probably not an independent risk factor for bladder carcinogenesis. As would be expected from what is known of NAT function, it is likely that acetylator status modifies the risk of bladder cancer that results from exposure to N-substituted aryl compounds. Slow acetylators are likely to be at increased risk of bladder cancer because they do not detoxify carcinogenic arylamines as well as do fast acetylators. More studies that take the role of acetylator status into consideration are needed, however, to quantify the strength of the association between risk of bladder cancer and exposure to arylamine compounds.

It may be that a simple dichotomy of fast and slow acetylator status is insufficient to explain the relationship with risk of bladder cancer. It is likely that a spectrum of NAT activity lies within these two designations (Iselius and Evans, 1983). The level of NAT activity within each category may be important in terms of future risk of disease. Or, future studies may identify other factors that affect the association between acetylator status and risk of bladder cancer. Such studies should be conducted in industrial settings where it is possible to determine levels of exposure to bladder carcinogens. Given the rarity of bladder cancer, the case-control design is likely to be the most feasible, but future studies should collect incident cases. Because past studies have used prevalent cases, it is not clear whether slow acetylation is associated with the incidence of bladder cancer or survival with bladder cancer (Vineis and Caporaso, 1988).

One final precaution, epidemiologists need to be aware of the ethical implications of their research before they use markers of susceptibility. They need to give some consideration to how the data may be used or misused, and must employ safeguards to keep the test results confidential.

REFERENCES

Ahmad RA, Rogers HJ: Plasma and salivary pharmacokinetics of dapsone estimated by a thin layer chromatographic method. *Eur J Clin Pharmacol* 1980;17:129–133.

Albertini RJ, Castle KL, Borcherding WR: T-cell cloning to detect the mutant 6-thioguanine-resistant lymphocytes present in human peripheral blood. *Proc Nat Acad Sci* (USA) 1982;79:6617– 6621.

Armstrong AR, Peart HE: A comparison between the behavior of Eskimos and non-Eskimos to the administration of isoniazid. *Am Rev Respir Dis* 1960;81:588–594.

Ayesh R, Idle JR, Ritchie JC, Crothers MJ, Hetzel MR: Metabolic oxidation phenotypes as markers for susceptibility to lung cancer. *Nature* 1984;312:169–170.

Cartwright RA, Glashan RW, Rogers HJ, Ahmad RA, Barnham-Hall D, Higgins E, Kahn MA:

Role of N-acetyltransferase phenotypes in bladder carcinogenesis: A pharmokinetic epi-demiological approach to bladder cancer. *Lancet* 1982;ii:842–846.

Cartwright RA: Epidemiological studies on N-acetylation and C-center ring oxidation in neo-plasia: Banbury report No. 16. In: Omenn GS, Gelboin HV, eds.: *Genetic Variability in Responses to Chemical Exposure.* Cold Spring Harbor, NY, Cold Spring Harbor Labora-tory, 1984, pp. 359–368.

Case RAM, Hosker ME, McDonald DB, Pearson JT: Tumors of the urinary bladder in workman engaged in the manufacture and use of certain dyestuff intermediates in the British chemical industry. Role of aniline, benzidine, alpha-naphthylamine, and beta-naphthylamine. *Br J Ind Med* 1954;11:75–104.

Chapron DJ, Kramer PA, Mercik SA: Kinetic discrimination of three sulphamethazine acetyla-tion phenotypes. *Clin Pharmacol Ther* 1980;27:104–113.

Chudley AE: Genetic contributions to human malformations. In: Persaud TVN, Chudley AE, Skalko RG, eds.: *Basic Concepts In Teratology.* New York, Alan R. Liss, Inc., 1985, pp. 31–68.

Cleaver JE: Defective repair replication of DNA in xeroderma pigmentosum. *Nature* 1968;218:652–656.

Colditz GA, Stampfer MJ, Willett WC: Diet and lung cancer: A review of the epidemiologic evidence in humans. *Arch Intern Med* 1987;147:157–160.

Culliton BJ, Waterfall WK: Hazards at work. *Br Med J* August 2, 1980:376–377.

Davies JM: Bladder tumors in the electric-cable industry. *Lancet* 1965;ii:143–146.

Drayer DE, Reidenberg MM: Clinical consequences of polymorphic acetylation of basic drugs. *Clin Pharmacol Ther* 1977;22:251–258.

Evans DAP, Eze LC, Whibley EJ: The association of the slow acetylator phenotype with bladder cancer. *J Med Genet* 1983;20:330–333.

Fontana RS: Screening for lung cancer: Recent experience in the United States. In: Hansen HH, ed.: *Lung Cancer: Basic and Clinical Aspects.* Boston, Martinus Nijhoff Publishers, 1986, pp. 91–111.

Grant DM, Tang BK, Kalow W: A simple test for acetylator phenotype using caffeine. *Br J Clin Pharmacol* 1984;17:459–464.

Hanssen HP, Agarwal DP, Goedde HW, Bucher H, Huland H, Brachmann W, Ovenbeck R: Association of N-acetyltransferase polymorphism and environmental factors with bladder carcinogenesis. *Eur Urol* 1985;11:263–266.

Harnden DG: The nature of inherited susceptibility to cancer. *Carcinogenesis* 1984;5:1535–1537.

Hein DW, Hirata M, Weber WW: An enzyme marker to ensure reliable determinations of human isoniazid acetylator phenotype in vitro. *Pharmacology* 1981;23:203–210.

Hueper WC, Wiley FH, Wolfe HD: Experimental production of bladder tumors in dogs by administration of β-naphthylamine. *J Ind Hyg Toxicol* 1938;20:46–84.

Idle JR, Mahgoub A, Sloan TP, Smith RL, Mbanefo CO, Bababunmi EA: Some observations on the oxidation phenotype status of Nigerian patients presenting with cancer. *Cancer Lett* 1981;11:331–338.

Iselius L, Evans DAP: Formal genetics of isoniazid metabolism in man. *Clin Pharmacokinet* 1983;8:541–544.

Karakaya AE, Cok I, Sardas S, Gögüs O, Sardas OS: N-acetyltransferase phenotype of patients with bladder cancer. *Hum Toxicol* 1986;5:333–335.

Karim AKMB, Elfellah MS, Evans DAP: Human acetylator polymorphism: Estimate of al-lele frequency in Lybia and details of global distribution. *J Med Genet* 1981;18:325–330.

Kellermann G, Shaw CR, Luyten-Kellermann M: Aryl hydrocarbon hydroxylase inducibility and bronchogenic carcinoma. *N Engl J Med* 1973;298:934–937.

Khoury MJ, Stewart W, Beaty TH: The effect of genetic susceptibility on causal inference in epidemiologic studies. *Am J Epidemiol* 1987;126:561–567.

Kolata GB: Testing for cancer risk. *Science* 1980;207:967–969.

Kukongviriyapan V, Lulitanond V, Areejitranusorn C, Kongyingyose B, Laupattarakasem P: *N*-acetyltransferase polymorphism in Thailand. *Hum Hered* 1984;34:246–249.

Ladero JM, Kwok CK, Jara C, Fernandez L, Silma AM, Tapia D, Uson AC: Hepatic acetylator phenotype in bladder cancer patients. *Ann Clin Res* 1985;17:96–99.

Lang NP, Chu DZJ, Hunter CF, Kendall DC, Flammang TJ, Kadlubar FF: Role of aromatic amine acetyltransferase in human colorectal cancer. *Arch Surg* 1986;121:1259–1261.

La Du BN: Isoniazid and pseudocholinesterase polymorphisms. *Fed Proc* 1972;31:1276–1285.

Lee EJD and Lee LKH: A simple pharmacokinetic method for separating the three acetylation phenotypes: A preliminary report. *Br J Clin Pharmacol* 1982;13:375–378.

Littlefield JW: Genes, chromosomes and cancer. *J Pediatr* 1984;104:489–494.

Lower GM, Nilsson T, Nelson CE, Wolf H, Gamsky TE, Bryan GT: N-acetyltransferase phenotype and risk in urinary bladder cancer: Approaches in molecular epidemiology. Preliminary results in Sweden and Denmark. *Environ Health Perspect* 1979;29:71–79.

Lower GM: Concepts in causality: Chemically induced human urinary bladder cancer. *Cancer* 1982;49:1056–1066.

Manchester D, Jacoby E: Decreased placental monooxygenase activities associated with birth defects. *Teratology* 1984;30:31–37.

Miller ME, Cosgriff JM: Acetylator phenotype in human bladder cancer. *J Urol* 1983;130:65–66.

Mommsen S, Barfod NM, Aagaard J: *N*-acetyltransferase phenotypes in the urinary bladder carcinogenesis of a low-risk population. *Carcinogenesis* 1985;6:199–201.

Mommsen S, Aagaard J: Susceptibility in urinary bladder cancer: acetyltransferase phenotypes and related risk factors. *Cancer Lett* 1986;32:199–205.

Murray RF: Tests of so-called susceptibility. *J Occup Med* 1986;28:1103–1107.

Omenn GS: Predictive identification of hypersusceptible individuals. *J Occup Med* 1982;24:369–374.

Omenn GS: Advances in genetics and immunology: The importance of basic research to prevention of occupational diseases. *Arch Environ Health* 1984;39:173–182.

Petersen GM, Scott EM, Rotter JI, Silimpori DR, Hall DB, Ward JI: Uridine monophosphate kinase 3: A genetic marker for susceptibility to Haemophilus influenzae type B disease. *Lancet* 1985;ii:417–419.

Rao DC, Elston RC, Kuller LH, Feinleib M, Carter C, Hawlik R, eds.: *Genetic Epidemiology of Coronary Heart Disease: Past, Present and Future.* New York, Alan R. Liss, Inc., 1984.

Rehn L: Blasengeschwltse bei fuchsin-arbeitern. *Arch Klin Chir* 1895;50:588.

Schmidt W, Popham RE: The role of drinking and smoking in mortality from cancer and other causes in male alcoholics. *Cancer* 1981;47:1031–1041.

Swift M, Sholman L, Perry M, Chase C: Malignant neoplasms in the families of patients with ataxia-telangiectasia. *Cancer Res* 1976;36:209–215.

Thompson JS, Thompson MW: *Genetics in Medicine,* ed. 4. Philadelphia, WB Saunders Co., 1986, pp. 93–94, 130.

USDHEW: *The Health Consequences of Smoking: Cancer—a report of the Surgeon General.* Government Printing Office, 1982, Washington, D.C.

Vineis P, Caporaso N: Applications of biochemical epidemiology in the study of human carcinogenesis. *Tumori* 1988;74:19–26.

Walpole AL, Williams MHC, Roberts DC: Tumors of the urinary bladder in dogs after ingestion of 4-aminodiphenyl. *Br J Ind Med* 1954;11:105–109.

Weber WW, Brenner W: A filter paper method for determining isoniazid acetylator phenotype. *Am J Hum Genet* 1974;26:467–473.

Weber WW, Hein DW: Clinical pharmacokinetics of Isoniazid. *Clin Pharmacokinet* 1979;4:401–422.

Weber WW: Acetylation pharmacogenetics: Experimental models of human toxicity. *Fed Proc* 1984;43:2332–2337.

Weber WW, Hein DW: *N*-acetylation pharmacogenetics. *Pharmacol Rev* 1985;37:25–79.

Wolf H, Lower GM, Bryan GT: Role of *N*-acetyltransferase phenotype in human susceptibility to bladder carcinogenic arylamines. *Scand J Urol Nephrol* 1980;14:161–165.

Woodhouse KW, Adams PC, Clothier A, Mucklow JC, Rawlins MD: *N*-acetylation phenotype in bladder cancer. *Hum Toxicol* 1982;1:443–445.

11

METHODOLOGIC ISSUES
IN MOLECULAR EPIDEMIOLOGY

BARBARA S. HULKA

INTRODUCTION

Most epidemiologic research is designed to identify cause-and-effect relationships. Ideally, epidemiologists like to quantify the disease risk that results from a particular exposure. Exposure and disease relationships form the framework of our thinking. But molecular epidemiology in its current state of development frequently does not fit this construct. Existing molecular epidemiologic studies do not often focus on clinically defined health or disease outcomes. Instead, they often incorporate a substitute outcome that is an internal documentation of external exposure or a postulated step in the natural history of disease. The reasons for this shift in focus lie partly in the early stage of development and partly in the disciplines and sciences from which molecular epidemiology is developing.

Molecular biology and toxicology, disciplines whose primary tools are biological markers, are pushing epidemiology toward the use of biomarkers. Advances in molecular biology and laboratory technology provide the capability for doing molecular epidemiologic studies. And toxicologic studies, although generally performed in animals or in vitro systems, are often used for extrapolating their results to human health and disease.

Biological monitoring in occupational settings offers a prime example of using a biological marker, often an internal dose marker, as the dependent variable in an epidemiologic study. Investigators monitor body fluids for a specific chemical (or its metabolites) known to be in the ambient environment. The internal marker may be on the pathway between exposure and disease outcome, and may be part of a postulated mechanism of disease occurrence. More often, however, the study marker is only a correlate for a marker of disease pathogenesis. In some cases, it may have no documented relationship to a recognized disease entity.

Although the significance of these markers for human health effects are uncertain, they may be used in ways that presume such effects. For example, there are a number of risk assessment strategies that mathematically model postulated adverse health effects (NRC, 1983). A related strategy is the parallelogram approach that extrapolates data from animal models and from in vitro systems, using bacterial, animal, and human cells, to human health effects (Waters et al., 1986). Neither modeling approach is as convincing in its impact or likely validity as empirically derived data from humans.

Epidemiologic research using biological markers must continually strive to establish methods that identify clinical disease or well-established precursors of disease as the outcome variable of interest. This change in focus, using markers as predictor variables of disease outcomes, may be molecular epidemiology's most important contribution to scientific knowledge about human health. This advance opens the door to informed disease prevention and population-based monitoring that uses biological markers as risk factors for disease. Firm data on the relationship between an external exposure and a marker, plus data on a quantitative relationship between the marker and the disease occurrence, offers clear opportunities for effective prevention.

In the rest of this chapter, we discuss reasons why biomarkers may be of use in some studies, but not in others, and we review some of the special considerations for using these markers in epidemiologic research.

CHOICE OF BIOLOGICAL MARKER

Whether it is appropriate to use a biological marker in any given study depends, first, on the goals of the study and, second, on the availability of an assay. A biological marker may or may not contribute useful information to a study.

Consider the use of urinary or salivary cotinine as an indicator of active cigarette smoking. What more do we learn from an assay on a biological sample than from a traditional, well-designed questionnaire? A questionnaire will elicit about 5 percent false-negative and rare false-positive results (NRC, 1986, Chapter 6). In a laboratory experienced in cotinine assays, there will be rare false-positive results at the low end of the distribution of cotinine values because of difficulty in distinguishing between active smoking of occasional cigarettes and heavy exposure to environmental tobacco smoke (ETS). False-negative results for active smoking should be nonexistent.

If one is trying to monitor population-based smoking patterns, the extra degree of accuracy achieved by cotinine assay will probably not be worth the cost and effort. If, however, the goal of the study is to evaluate the effectiveness of a smoking cessation strategy in an intervention trial, the decision to use cotinine is likely to be positive. If the study's goal is to identify recent exposure to ETS among nonsmokers, urinary cotinine levels can integrate that exposure over multiple microenvironments (NRC, 1986, Chapter 8).

In breast cancer studies, steroid hormone receptor levels in the tumor tissue have been used as biological correlates of traditional epidemiologic risk factors. These studies seek to increase knowledge about breast cancer risk factors and to improve the sensitivity of our prognostic abilities. Epidemiologic studies relating estrogen receptor (ER) presence and amount to other breast cancer risk factors have shown that ER-rich tumors are more frequent in older women and in white women (Hulka et al., 1984). These demographic characteristics are also associated with a favorable patient prognosis and longer survival. The ERs have achieved clinical application in patient treatment decisions and as indicators of cellular differentiation independent of clinical stage, histologic grade, and cell type.

The availability of an assay defines in an operational sense the existence of a particular biomarker. Furthermore, availability of the assay can determine its feasibility for epidemiologic research. One can estimate availability by noting the number of different laboratories doing the assay and by the cost. An assay that is done routinely in a hospital's clinical laboratory will have very different properties and availability than one done only by a few research groups. Assay availability, however, can change rapidly. In 1975, for example, the original Southern blot technique for probing specific genomic sequences was published (Southern, 1975). The technique was rapidly applied to the study of different viral genomes in human cells, including human papillomavirus (HPV) DNA in neoplastic cervical cells. Today, the Southern blot technique is used in many laboratories, and commercial kits are available for screening for HPV DNA (Med News and Perspectives, 1988). The rationale for commercial development is the idea that screening for HPV DNA will supplement cervical cytology in identifying carcinoma precursors. The scientific justification is a presumed causal link between HPV and cervical cancer. Recent evidence showing a high frequency of HPV DNA types 16/18/31 in cytologically normal cervices somewhat dampens the enthusiasm for this link (Reeves et al., 1987; Muñoz et al., 1988). Whatever future research may show, however, the rapid development of the Southern blot, Dot blot, and related technologies has made the study of this viral/cancer association possible.

MARKER STABILITY

In choosing a biological marker, the investigators also need to evaluate the marker's stability. Marker stability has a number of components. Some of these involve the pharmacokinetics of a xenobiotic after it enters the body, as well as the persistence of any resulting biological modification formed in the body. Another aspect of stability arises when tissues or other biological media are removed from the body. It is necessary to have transport and storage conditions that ensure marker retention outside the body. The importance of each of these issues, which are reviewed in Chapter 3, varies depending on the character of the exposure and effect under study. For chronic diseases with long latencies, the ability to retain markers in stored biological media will improve opportunities for retrospective cohort or nested case-control studies. If the topic of interest is an acute illness, a physiologic response, or an internal dose marker, the conditions of specimen storage may be of less concern than the pharmacokinetics of a xenobiotic.

Most markers, other than genetically determined susceptibility markers, are transient, either because of the pharmacokinetics of the chemical or because of cell turnover, repair, and death of the tissue in which the marker is found. Even with recent exposures, the timing for collection of the biological medium can be crucial to identifying the marker of interest. After cigarette smoking, for instance, the half-life for cotinine is about 16 hours in plasma and slightly longer in urine (Jarvis et al., 1988). After 3 days of abstinence from cigarettes, the level of cotinine in urine falls below the sensitivity of the assay (Sepkovic et al., 1985). For active smokers, any of the media—

saliva, plasma, or urine—is suitable for cotinine assay, as all exhibit high cotinine values. For identification of ETS exposure, urine is the preferred medium, as it integrates ETS exposure over several hours (Jarvis et al., 1984). Thus, knowledge of the pharmacokinetics of the substance under study aids in the selection of the most appropriate type of specimen and in the timing of specimen collection.

Some chemicals, such as chlorinated hydrocarbons and heavy metals have long storage times in the body. Chlorinated hydrocarbons, found in some pesticides, remain in body fat indefinitely. Equilibration occurs with high levels in adipose tissue compared with blood levels and urinary excretion. For example, residents of Triana, Alabama who were exposed to dichlorodiphenyltrichloroethane (DDT), primarily through consumption of contaminated fish, had high fat levels and significant blood levels of dichlorodiphenyldichloroethylene (DDE) many years after DDT exposure ceased (Kreiss et al., 1981). Although no acute toxicity was observed, the possibility of long-term health effects still exists.

A somewhat different consideration in marker persistence relates to a marker's stability after its removal from the body. Markers that deteriorate rapidly or autolyze must be handled more expeditiously than those that degrade slowly. A study of androgen receptors in prostatic tissue—both cancer and benign prostatic hyperplasia— suffered from a loss of study specimens because of this problem (Hulka et al., 1987). Protein receptors are extremely liable to degradation when tissue is removed from the body. During a transurethral resection, prostatic tissue may fall into the urinary bladder and not be removed promptly. As little as half an hour in this environment makes the tissue useless for receptor assay.

DNA adducts, on the other hand, appear to persist at least 18 hours postmortem, and probably longer (E. Randerath and K. Randerath, personal communication). DNA itself can be retrieved from paraffin-embedded tissue after many years of preservation (Shibata et al., 1988).

The most feasible means for dealing with the problems of transient markers and autolysis is to establish repositories. Serum banks, established in connection with many of the major cardiovascular disease cohort studies, are a recognized epidemiologic resource. They are particularly useful for nested case-control studies in which the biological marker is the independent variable.

Tissue repositories of frozen specimens also exist, and can be useful, if they are adequately documented and available to persons other than the original investigators. If demographic and epidemiologic descriptions of the subjects whose tissues are in these repositories are limited, this reduces their utility for epidemiologic investigation.

Recent interest in oncogenes has provided an impetus for increased tissue storage, and specifically for DNA banks. DNA banks may be extremely valuable for epidemiologic enterprises if other relevant data are collected when the DNA is extracted.

If fixed specimens can be employed, use of biomarkers in cancer epidemiology will be rapidly expanded. This will allow investigators to use tissue blocks and slides that have been conserved in hospital pathology departments from surgical, autopsy, and biopsy specimens. Although common fixatives are problematic in their effects on possible markers, the genetic material persists and can be restored for molecular analyses. The development of techniques for using fixed tissue blocks and slides to identify biomarkers will boost molecular epidemiologic research tremendously. Such techniques are already being developed for the polymerase chain reaction (PCR) to amplify DNA fragments for identification of oncogenes and other genetic markers (Shibata et al., 1988).

BIOLOGICAL VARIABILITY

Epidemiologists are trained to quantify information and to apply statistical methods to determine whether their findings are a chance phenomenon. If statistical procedures show that the subject groups differ in the study factor, the next step is to rule out error as the cause of the differences. The search for error generally concentrates on possible biases in study design and mishaps in measurement. Rarely do we explicitly consider biological variability as the explanation for the results. The possibility that variibility within and between individuals with respect to unmeasured or inadequately measured biological phenomena may bear on the findings deserves more attention. This is especially true because the ability of most epidemiologic questionnaires to tap intrinsic biological phenomena is distinctly limited. The intensive effort to link high dietary fat to breast cancer risk illustrates this point. Dietary intake data obtained by questionnaires are not accurate, although they may be adequate to demonstrate group differences in intake of some micronutrients and macronutrients. Furthermore, questionnaire data tell us nothing about interactions among nutrients, their metabolic pathways, and their ultimate biological effects in the body. For these and other reasons, we have not been able to substantiate a link between dietary fat and breast cancer risk in humans through analytic epidemiologic studies (Hulka, 1989). In this case, a search for biochemical or molecular markers of dietary fat constituents is a promising avenue of research. Biological markers may serve both as a vehicle to refine the concept of biological variability and as an operational means to measure some part of it.

Interindividual variability is a component of random error and can be dealt with analytically if it falls within an expected range and a known distribution. In developmental studies, both individual values for a marker and the distribution of these values may form the outcome of interest. Deviant values may lead to a better understanding of the marker and its relationship to disease. One study identified a subject who had levels of micronucleated red blood cells (RBCs) that were 10-fold higher than the next highest value in a group of 20 individuals (Everson et al., 1988). When folate was administered to this individual, there was a drop in micronucleated RBCs. This example illustrates the importance of recognizing deviant values and using the information to increase knowledge about disease pathogenesis and treatment.

If differential susceptibilities are of interest, interindividual variability may be the object of the study. Many reports have noted significant interindividual variability in enzyme activity, such as aryl hydrocarbon hydroxylase activity. In the absence of environmental exposures, which alter enzymatic activity, such variability reflects allelic polymorphism. It also suggests a potentially important difference in genetic susceptibility to carcinogens because people will have different levels of enzymatic activity to metabolize precarcinogens to electrophilic metabolites (Harris et al., 1985).

DNA adducts illustrate the importance of both tissue type and individual characteristics in contributing to variability. Tissues from the same organ but from different individuals have been found to vary more than 100-fold in their adduct levels. Furthermore, the amount of variability differs from one tissue type to the next. One study found that benzo(a)pyrene adducts in samples of cultured cells from human colon varied 197-fold from one individual to the next compared with threefold in peripheral lung cells (Harris et al., 1985). Although this variation is partially a function of differing numbers of assays per tissue type, much of it stems from a combination of intertissue and interindividual variation.

For a given individual, adduct levels in vivo vary among different organs and tissues. We might expect that carcinogens inhaled through tobacco smoke would produce more DNA adducts in bronchial cells, the tissue of direct contact, than in the more remote sites like heart or brain. Instead, one study done on smokers found the opposite: more adducts in heart and brain (E. and E. Randerath, personal communication). It is not intuitively obvious how we should interpret these findings. One explanation might invoke the differential capacity of cells to multiply and repair. Bronchial epithelial cells, which continually regenerate, may repair the adducted portion of DNA. Because neural and cardiac muscle cells do not divide, the adducts may persist.

Another study found smoking-specific DNA adducts in human placental tissue, but not in WBCs from the same individuals (Everson et al., 1988). Characteristics of the assay itself, however, may determine whether or not the assay detects adducts in a particular tissue, as assays other than the ^{32}P-postlabeling assay have found smoking-related adducts in WBCs (Perera et al., 1987; Shamsuddin et al., 1985).

Intertissue variability can further complicate the design of epidemiologic studies. Consider the prospect of a case-control study of lung cancer with DNA adducts as the exposure variable under investigation. What tissue should be sampled for adduct presence? Would the cancer tissue or the adjacent normal lung tissue be the more likely source? Consider the following points: Adducts involved in tumor initiation would not be present at the time the patient (or subject) is diagnosed with cancer. Because of rapid cell replication and dilution of adduct-containing cells, adducts formed in response to carcinogens in cigarette smoke may rarely be evident in tumor tissue. As a result, phenotypical normal tissue next to the cancerous tissue may yield the best information. Although adducts have been found in both the cancer tissue and the adjacent normal lung tissue, they have not appeared consistently and seem to have little association with smoking status (Perera et al., 1982).

Circulating steroid hormone levels, which have diurnal variation superimposed on pulsatile release patterns, also illustrate intraindividual variability (Wilcox et al., 1987). Two strategies can minimize this variability: one is the choice of specimen (urine integrates the pulsatile release) and the other involves fixing the time of day for specimen collection. The latter helps to control for diurnal variation, which is characteristic of steroid hormones.

The assays that identify biological markers introduce some distinctive new sources of error. Consider the example of DNA adducts for which there are several different laboratory assay methods that use different physicochemical principles. Among these are ^{32}P-postlabeling, ultrasensitive enzymatic radioimmunoassay (USERIA), and synchronous fluorescence spectrophotometry (SFS) (Harris et al., 1985). Because the techniques are new, and still developing, each assay method is likely to differ in some aspect of technique from laboratory to laboratory. The assays vary in their sensitivity to detect adducts and in specificity of the structures they detect (see Chapter 3 for a laboratory definition of sensitivity and specificity). Assay sensitivity and specificity, as epidemiologically defined, are undetermined as the existence of an adduct is only known as a function of the assay. That is, there is no objective standard for "truth" as required for an epidemiologic definition of these terms. Furthermore, results from any one assay technique may not be well reproduced in another, although there is some evidence that different assay methods may identify persons with high levels of specific chemical adducts (Harris et al., 1985).

SAMPLE SIZE AND CONFOUNDING

One feature of developmental studies that use biomarkers is that sample sizes are likely to be small. Feasibility and cost will limit the number of subjects for study. These studies may have more characteristics of clinical research than of traditional population-based epidemiology. Take the example of a study designed to identify smoking-related adducts in sperm through the ^{32}P-postlabeling assay (M. Vine, personal communication). This assay is performed in only a few research laboratories and the methodology is continually being revised. Thus, the investigation must maximize the information gained from each subject.

In addition to problems that stem from a small sample size, developmental studies are also subject to confounding. Potential confounders include endogenous and exogenous factors. In any study of smoking-related adducts, age is a possible confounder. In rats, age has been positively associated with tissue-specific adducts (I compounds) unrelated to known exposures (Randerath et al., 1986). Examples of exogenous confounding factors include both caffeine intake and occupational exposures. Caffeine has been related to adducts in human placentas (Everson et al., 1988). Adducts in WBCs have been found in occupationally exposed individuals (Haugen et al., 1986). Additional exposures and susceptibility factors about which we have no information may produce adducts and could be differentially distributed between cigarette smokers and nonsmokers.

What are the best design and analysis strategies to deal with these problems? To answer these questions we continue using the example of a study of smoking-related adducts in sperm. In this study, the first goal is simply to identify adduct presence. Currently, the literature contains no reports of adducts in human sperm. Assuming adducts are found, the primary question is whether or not there is a significant difference in adduct frequency and type between smoking and nonsmoking men. For this purpose, an unexposed comparison group, concurrent in time with the smoking group, is essential. A study with small numbers of subjects should maximize exposure differences between groups, and thus require heavy smokers of at least one pack of cigarettes per day in the exposed group. A subsequent goal would be the identification of a dose–response relationship between amount smoked and intensity of specific types of adducts. Meeting this goal requires testing a third group of subjects who smoke less than a pack per day. Although sampling of subjects is based on the subjects' stated smoking status, the group designation may be determined more accurately after serum or semen cotinine values, or both, are obtained. These provide information on the internal dose of tobacco constituents.

Some investigators recommend matching exposed and unexposed subjects on potential confounders to increase the precision of the measure of association between exposure and outcome (Hook, 1982). A matched design allows for a simple analysis

cells further highlights the need for standardized quantitative analyses. The SCEs are generally reported as the mean number per cell for each person, and the group value is the mean of the individual means. There is no consensus in the literature, however, on the number of persons to study or the number of cells to score per person. The numbers of each should depend on the amount of variability in SCEs among cells and among persons. One paper provided good evidence that the larger component of variability is interindividual and that counting 50 mitoses per individual provides adequate accuracy and stability of mean SCE levels (Hirsch et al., 1984).

A study may also report the proportion of WBCs with a high frequency of SCEs from each individual (Archer, 1984). The cut point for a high value is determined by the data and the investigator. Although this pragmatic approach may not be ideal, the rationale for a high frequency index is reasonable. The SCEs in a given individual's cells are often not normally distributed. Subjects with a disproportionate number of WBCs that show a high frequency of SCEs may have a particular susceptibility to a known or unknown exposure. The affected cells may also represent a magnified sub-population from the total WBC population.

If each subject's distribution of scored cells by frequency of SCEs were reported, it would be possible to glean more information from SCE scoring. Margolin and Shelby have discussed the use of a heterogeneity index (variance/mean) for scoring an individual's SCEs (Margolin and Shelby, 1985). This index relies on a Poisson distribution of SCEs and a dispersion test to identify deviations from the Poisson (Margolin, 1988). The work of these authors represents an advance in the application of quantitative methods to assays for biological markers.

INTERPRETATION OF MARKERS

Marker interpretation is an issue that goes well beyond the results of any particular study. It focuses on the inferences that can be drawn from a particular marker for human health and disease. Interpretation may be particularly uncertain at the inter-mediate points in the marker spectrum. On the other hand, interpretation of an internal dose marker, near the exposure end of the spectrum, may be reasonably clear. Tri-chloroethanol in the expired air of employees of a dry cleaning establishment is good evidence of recent exposure to trichloroethene (Monster, 1986).

At the disease end of the spectrum, screening with cervical cytology allows us to make clear interpretations about disease. When the cytologic reading is severe dys-plasia, we do not hesitate to recommend treatment, because this morphologic entity has a high probability of progressing to invasive cervical cancer. By itself, however, severe dysplasia has no clinical manifestations.

Moving back from the disease end of the spectrum, we might consider oncogenes as tumor specific markers. What, for instance, are the implications of HER-2/neu oncogene amplification in a series of breast carcinoma cell lines (Slamon et al., 1987)? Slamon and colleagues provided evidence that oncogene amplification has prognostic significance; carcinomas with multiple copies of the oncogene had a poorer prognosis. But data on the causes of amplification and how to identify it before the clinical manifestations of cancer occur are not available.

In animals and in vitro systems, there are various steps by which oncogenes or their protein products lead to tumor development. In humans, there is growing evidence that mutational events or chromosomal translocations activate protooncogenes so that they exhibit oncogenic activity. Exactly how or when this occurs is uncertain. A major hope for the future is the ability to identify oncogenes specific to benign lesions, such as colonic polyps, that are destined to become cancers (Gordon, 1985). This ability would significantly enhance our early detection and cancer prevention strategies.

The significance of DNA adducts, or proxy protein adducts, is much more debatable. In theory, DNA adduct formation could be a first step in mutagenesis or carcinogenesis. Adducted DNA can give rise to a mutation that is replicated in subsequent cell progeny (if the cell divides). The adduct can also be excised or repaired, or the cell may not divide. The actual likelihood that a given adduct will result in an adverse reproductive outcome or cancer must be immeasurably small.

CONCLUSIONS

Biological markers will play a prominent role in epidemiologic research of the 1990s. Growth in the use of biomarkers may be as important to epidemiologic research as the development of quantitative methods was during the 1970s and 1980s. Our first chapter mentions some of the forces responsible for this trend: these include the pervasiveness of molecular biology in scientific inquiry and expanding laboratory technology. Although these developments are taking place outside of epidemiology, the opportunities that they provide are causing them to be drawn inexorably into the fabric of epidemiologic research.

Adding biological markers to epidemiology's set of research tools is particularly timely because it is taking place as the demands on epidemiologic research are increasing. We have entered an era in which many of our studies produce data exhibiting weak associations, with less than twofold relative risk estimates. Fortunately, from the standpoint of human health, epidemiology is unlikely to identify many more associations of the magnitude of cigarette smoking and lung cancer, or estrogens and endometrial cancer. Not many associations of this magnitude are likely to exist. Studies of these exposures and health effects produced large relative risk estimates that were quite consistent in spite of possible flaws in study design or lack of analytic sophistication. Because current research will more frequently identify only weak associations, frailties in study design and analysis may invalidate any substantive conclusions. Because there are limits to our ability to refine and improve conventional epidemiologic strategies, it is necessary to garner all the tools available to strengthen epidemiologic research strategies.

This can occur within the framework of strong biological models for epidemiologic research. To the extent that knowledge permits, the biological rationale can be interwoven with epidemiologic concepts and statistical models. We need to understand exposure factors in terms of their biological behaviors in humans, disease processes as the actual health effects. Biological markers may serve to increase the biological specificity of exposures, diseases, intervening variables, effect modifiers, or confounders. They may reduce bias in study design and create more interpretable data.

REFERENCES

Archer PG: Some statistical and methodologic issues in cytogenetic testing. *Banbury Report 16: Genetic Variability in Responses to Chemical Exposure.* Cold Spring Harbor, Cold Spring Harbor Laboratory, 1984, pp. 369–376.

Everson RB, Randerath E, Santella RM, Cefalo RC, et al.: Detection of smoking-related covalent DNA adducts in human placenta. *Science* 1986;231:54–57.

Everson RB, Wehr CM, Erexson GL, MacGregor JT: Association of marginal folate depletion with increased human chromosomal damage *in vivo:* Demonstration by analysis of micronucleated erythrocytes. *JNCI* 1988;80:525–529.

Everson RB, Randerath E, Santella RM, Avitts TA, et al.: Quantitative associations between DNA damage in human placenta and maternal smoking and birth weight. *JNCI* 1988;80:567–576.

Fleiss JL: *Statistical Methods for Rates and Proportions.* New York, John Wiley & Sons, 1981.

Gordon H: Oncogenes. *Mayo Clin Proc* 1985;60:697–713.

Harris CC, Vahakangas K, Autrup H, Glennwood E, et al.: Biochemical and molecular epidemiology of human cancer risk. In: Scarpelli DG, Craighead JE, Kaufman N, eds.: Chapter 7, *The Pathologist and the Environment.* Baltimore, International Academy of Pathology Monograph No. 26. Williams & Wilkins, 1985.

Haugen A, Becher G, Benestad C, Vahakangas K, et al.: Determination of polycyclic aromatic hydrocarbons in the urine, benzo(a)pyrene diol epoxide-DNA adducts in lymphocyte DNA, and antibodies to the adducts in sera from coke oven workers exposed to measured amounts of polycyclic aromatic hydrocarbons in the work atmosphere. *Cancer Res* 1986;46:4178–4183.

Hirsch B, McGue M, Cervenka J: Characterization of the distribution of sister chromatid exchange frequencies: Implications for research design. *Hum Genet* 1984;65:280–286.

Hook EB: ECPEMC working paper 5/2: Perspectives in mutation epidemiology: 2. Epidemiologic and design aspects of studies of somatic chromosome breakage and sister-chromatid exchange. *Mutat Res* 1982;99:373–382.

Hulka BS, Beckman WC, Checkoway H, DiFerdinando G, et al.: Androgen receptors detected by autoradiography in prostatic carcinoma and benign prostatic hyperplastic tissue. *The Prostate* 1987;10:223–233.

Hulka BS, Chambless LE, Wilkinson WE, Deubner DC, et al.: Hormonal and personal effects on estrogen receptors in breast cancer. *Am J Epidemiol* 1984;119:692–704.

Hulka BS: Dietary fat and breast cancer: Case control and cohort studies. *Prev Med* 1989;18:180–193.

Jarvis MJ, Russell MAH, Benowitz NL, Feyerabend C: Elimination of cotinine from body fluids: Implications for noninvasive measurement of tobacco smoke exposure. *AJPH* 1988;78:696–698.

Jarvis M, Tunstall-Pedoe H, Feyerabend C, Vesey C, et al.: Biochemical markers of smoke absorption and self reported exposure to passive smoking. *J Epidemiol Community Health* 1984;38:335–339.

Kreiss K, Zack MM, Kimbrough RD, Needham LL: Cross-sectional study of a community with exceptional exposure to DDT. *JAMA* 1981;245:1926–1930.

Margolin BH: Statistical aspects of using biological markers. *Stat Science* 1988;3:351–357.

Margolin BH, Shelby MD: Sister chromatid exchanges: A reexamination of the evidence for sex and race differences in humans. *Environ Mutagen* 1985;7(Suppl 4):63–72.

Medical News & Perspectives: DNA probes for papillomavirus strains readied for cervical cancer screening. *JAMA* 1988;260:2777.

Mertz B: DNA probes for papillomavirus strains readied for cervical cancer screening. Medical News & Perspectives. *JAMA* 1988;260:2777.

Monster AC: Biological monitoring of chlorinated hydrocarbon solvents. *J Occup Med* 1986;28:583–588.

Muñoz N, Bosch X. Kaldor JM: Does human papillomavirus cause cervical cancer? The state of the epidemiological evidence. *Br J Cancer* 1988;57:1–5.

National Research Council: Committee on the Institutional Means for Assessment of Risks to Public Health, Commission on Life Sciences: *Risk Assessment in the Federal Government: Managing the Process.* Washington, D.C., National Academy Press, 1983.

National Research Council: Committee on Passive Smoking, Board on Environmental Studies and Toxicology: *Environmental Tobacco Smoke: Measuring Exposures and Assessing Health Effects.* Washington, D.C., National Academy Press, 1986.

Perera FP, Poirier MC, Yuspa SH, Nakayama J, et al.: A pilot project in molecular cancer epidemiology: Determination of benzo(a)pyrene-DNA adducts in animal and human tissues by immunoassays. *Carcinogenesis* 1982;3:1405–1410.

Perera FP, Santella RM, Brenner D, Poirier MC, et al.: DNA adducts, protein adducts, and sister chromatid exchange in cigarette smokers and nonsmokers. *JNCI* 1987;79:449–456.

Randerath K, Reddy MV, Disher RM: Age- and tissue-related DNA modifications in untreated rats: Detection by ^{32}P-postlabeling assay and possible significance for spontaneous tumor induction and aging. *Carcinogenesis* 1986;7:1615–1617.

Reeves WC, Caussy D, Brinton LA, Brenes MM, et al.: Case-control study of human papillomaviruses and cervical cancer in Latin America. *Int J Cancer* 1987;40:450–454.

Schiffman MH. Epidemiology of fecal mutagenicity. *Epidemiol Rev* 1986;8:92–105.

Schlesselman JJ: Sample size. In: Chapter 6, *Case-Control Studies: Design, Conduct, Analysis.* New York, Oxford University Press, 1982.

Schull WJ, Otake M, Neel JV: Genetic effects of the atomic bombs: A reappraisal. *Science* 1981;213:1220–1227.

Sepkovic DW, Haley NJ: Biomedical applications of cotinine quantitation in smoking related research. *Am J Public Health* 1985;75:663–665.

Shamsuddin AKM, Sinopoli NT, Hemminki K, Boesch RR, et al.: Detection of benzo(a)pyrene:DNA adducts in human white blood cells. *Cancer Res* 1985;45:66–68.

Shibata D, Martin WJ, Arnheim N: Analysis of DNA sequences in forty-year-old paraffin-embedded thin-tissue sections: A bridge between molecular biology and classical histology. *Cancer Res* 1988;48:4564–4566.

Slamon DJ, Clark GM, Wong SG, Levin WJ, et al.: Human breast cancer: Correlation of relapse and survival with amplification of the HER-2/Neu oncogene. *Science* 1987;235:177–182.

Southern EM: Detection of specific sequences among DNA fragments separated by gel electrophoresis. *J Mol Biol* 1975;98:503–517.

Waters M, Allen J, Doerr C, Erexson G, et al.: A preliminary investigation of the parallelogram concept in genetic monitoring and risk estimation. In: *Monitoring of Occupational Genotoxicants.* New York, Alan R. Liss, Inc., 1986, pp. 203–215.

Wilcox AJ, Baird DD, Weinberg CR, Armstrong EG, et al.: The use of biochemical assays in epidemiologic studies of reproduction. *Environ Health Perspect* 1987;75:29–35.

GLOSSARY

Aberrations (chromosomal): an irregularity in the number or structure of chromosomes, usually in the form of a gain (duplication), loss (deletion), exchange (translocation), or alteration in sequence (inversion) of genetic material.

Acetyl: an acetic acid molecule from which the hydroxyl group has been removed. It has the molecular formula: CH_3CO^-.

Acetylation: the introduction of an acetyl radical into an organic compound. By the process of acetylation, aryl-amine compounds are detoxified, possibly removing their carcinogenic potential.

Acetylcholinesterase: an enzyme, present in many tissues, that hydrolyzes acetylcholine into choline and acetic acid.

Adipose tissue: tissue that stores fat.

Adduct: stable complexes of reactive chemicals and cellular macromolecules that contain one or more covalent bonds between the two components.

Aflatoxins: toxic metabolites, some of which are carcinogenic, produced by some strains of the fungus *Aspergillus flavus*.

Alkyl: a hydrocarbon radical with the general formula, C_nH_{2n+1}.

Alkylation: the addition of alkyl groups to an organic compound.

Allele: one of several forms of a gene at a given locus on a chromosome.

Alpha$_1$-antitrypsin (ATT): an enzyme that protects connective tissue from damage by elastases and collagenases. Persons with low ATT levels are at higher risk for the development of pulmonary diseases.

Alpha-fetoprotein: a plasma protein produced in utero. Levels decline markedly by the age of 1 year. They are, however, elevated in malignant and benign neoplasms. Alpha-fetoprotein can be used as a marker for monitoring some diseases.

Amino acids: Twenty-one molecules that are the building blocks of proteins.

Aminobiphenyl: a carcinogenic compound found in cigarette smoke that forms hemoglobin adducts. This compound was formerly used as an antioxidant in the rubber industry.

Antibody: immunoglobulins (proteins) that bind to proteins and foreign chemicals enabling the immune system to recognize them (see immunoassays).

Antigen: any molecule that can provoke synthesis of an antibody.

Aryl: an organic radical resulting from the removal of a hydrogen atom from an aromatic hydrocarbon.

Autosomes: paired chromosomes that are alike in men and women, as distinguished from sex chromosomes; 22 of the 23 chromosome pairs in humans are autosomes.

Banding: a staining technique that produces alternating light and dark horizontal zones along the length of the chromosome.

Benzo(a)pyrene (BaP): a carcinogenic chemical found widely in the environment as a by-product of combustion. The genotoxic metabolite of BaP is thought to be benzo(a)pyrene-7,8-dihydrodiol-9,10-epoxide (BPDE-I) (see polyaromatic hydrocarbons).

Biological markers (biomarkers): cellular, biochemical, or molecular alterations measurable in biological media.

Biological monitoring (biomonitoring): the estimation of chemical or physical exposures as measured in biological materials.

Biologically effective dose: the amount of absorbed chemicals that have interacted with subcellular targets.

Bromodeoxyuridine (BrdUrd): a pyrimidine analog that competes with thymidine during DNA synthesis. When used with certain staining procedures, BrdUrd substitution can be used to visualize sister chromatid exchanges and to identify cells with newly synthesized DNA.

Carboxyhemoglobin: hemoglobin combined with carbon monoxide (CO). Carbon monoxide binds strongly to the hemoglobin molecule and occupies sites normally bound to oxygen.

Carcinoembryonic antigen: a glycoprotein in serum originally thought to be a specific marker for adenocarcinoma of the colon. It is now known to appear with a diverse group of neoplastic and nonneoplastic conditions.

Chromatid: one of the two identical longitudinal halves of a chromosome produced during replication.

Chromatin: the DNA and protein complex comprising the nucleus of the interphase cell.

Chromatography: the separation of individual chemical components of a mixture based on their physiochemical properties.

Clastogen: an agent that produces chromosomal breakage (e.g., x-rays, UV light, or certain chemical agents).

Colchicine: a chemical that binds to the tubulin of the spindle fibers. It is used in cytogenetic assays to arrest cellular mitosis at metaphase.

Conjugation: the covalent binding of an exogenous or endogenous compound with a readily available endogenous compound, such as glutathione or glucuronide.

Cotinine: a metabolite of nicotine (see nicotine).

Cytochrome P$_{450}$: a group of enzymes occurring in the liver and other organs that serves as an intermediate electron carrier in the detoxification of many chemicals. They are a component of the mixed funtion oxidase system.

Cytogenetics: the branch of genetics devoted to the study of chromosomes.

Cytology: the examination of cells that have been smeared, fixed, and stained on a slide.

Cytotoxic: poisonous to cells.

Deletions: a type of chromosomal aberration in which a portion of the chromosome is lost. Also refers to a type of DNA mutation in which DNA bases are lost.

Dimethyl sulfoxide (DMSO): a solvent that has the ability to penetrate plant and animal tissues and to preserve living cells during freezing.

DNA (deoxyribonucleic acid): the genetic material. DNA consists of four bases (guanine, thymine, cytosine, and thymine) attached to ribose. The base-ribose complexes are known as nucleosides. The nucleosides are attached by phosphate bonds between the ribose molecules; nucleoside-phosphate complexes are nucleotides. The sequence of bases determines the genetic makeup of the organism.

Dose: (see internal dose).

Dosimeters: methods for measuring dose.

Epithelium: the avascular cellular layer of tissue covering the free surfaces, cutaneous, mucus, and serous structures.

Exfoliated cells: cells sloughed from an epithelium or from any tissue surface.

External exposure: the concentration of a chemical substance in an individual's immediate environment.

Fixed specimens: tissue samples that have been prepared for permanent storage, such as those preserved in paraffin, formalin, or mounted on slides to prevent the denaturization and cross-linking of proteins to maintain cellular morphology.

Free radical: an atom or atoms possessing unpaired electrons. Radicals are usually extremely reactive intermediates in chemical reactions.

Genome: the total gene complement in a set of chromosomes.

Genotoxin: an agent that causes genetic damage.

Genotype: the genetic constitution of an organism.

Glucose: a monosaccharide that is the primary energy source for many organisms.

Heparin: an anticoagulant often added to blood samples to prevent clotting.

Heterozygous: different allelic genes at a locus in homologous chromosomes.

Homozygous: identical allelic genes at a locus in homologous chromosomes.

Hypoxanthine-guanine phosphoribosyl transferase (HGPRT): an enzyme that plays a role in the regulation of purine synthesis. This enzyme can be used to assay for somatic cell mutations.

Immunoassays: various methods for detecting small amounts of a particular compound using antigen-antibody binding. The most common type of enzyme-linked immunosorbent assay (ELISA) requires the use of a primary antibody against the chemical of interest, an enzyme linked to a secondary antibody against the primary antibody, and a colorless substrate that can be converted to a colored compound by the enzyme. Other methods, such as radioimmunoassays (RIA) and ultrasensitive enzymatic radioimmunoassays (USERIA), require radioactive labeling.

Induction (enzyme): the synthesis of a particular enzyme secondary to the presence of its substrate. By this process, the genes that code for the specific enzyme are expressed only in the presence of the substrate.

Initiation: an early step in the process of carcinogenesis, usually causing a mutational change, which leads to the development of a cancer.

Intercalated: refers to chemicals that "slide" between the DNA strands without becoming covalently bound.

Internal dose: the amount of a substance that enters the body as a consequence of ingestion, inhalation, skin absorption, etc.

Karyotype: the photomicrograph of the chromosomes of a cell arranged in a standard format. Also refers to the chromosome complement of a cell.

Kinetics: the study of forces, rates, and mechanisms involved in chemical reactions.

Leukocytes: white blood cells, including lymphocytes, granulocytes, monocytes, and other types.

Locus: the position on a chromosome of the gene for a particular trait.

Lymphocyte: a type of white blood cell having a large, spherical nucleus surrounded by a thin layer of nongranular cytoplasm. Lymphocytes play a central role in the body's immune response.

Macromolecule: a large molecule, such as DNA or protein, consisting of linked subunits.

Matrix: the intercellular substance of a tissue. Also used more broadly to refer to biological materials.

Metabolic activation: the process by which a biologically inactive compound becomes active. Action by the mixed-function oxidase system often results in metabolic activation of chemical procarcinogens.

Mitogen: any substance or agent that stimulates mitotic cell division (see also phytohemagglutinin).

Mixed-function oxidase (MFO): a group of enzymes that transforms many fat-soluble chemicals into water-soluble metabolites. Sometimes genotoxic intermediates are formed in this process.

Mutagens: chemical or physical agents that cause mutations.

Mutation: any change in the base pair sequence of genomic DNA.

N-acetyltransferase: a liver enzyme that detoxifies aryl-amine compounds by acetylation. Genetically determined variation in rates of this acetylation can be measured.

Nicotine: an alkaloid found in tobacco. Cotinine is a metabolite of nicotine. Both substances can be measured as markers of cigarette smoke exposure.

Nucleosides: (see DNA).

Nucleotides: (see DNA).

Oncogene: a gene associated with cellular transformation or tumorigenesis. Under usual genetic control, genes that become oncogenes are thought to encode for proteins involved in normal cellular growth and development until the mechanisms for genetic control are altered. Oncogenes may produce an abnormal product, an excess of a normal product, or a normal product at an abnormal time.

P_{450}: (see cytochrome P_{450}).

Pharmacokinetic: refers to the fate of drugs and other chemicals in the body over a period of time, including their absorption, distribution, metabolism, and elimination.

Phenotype: the appearance or other characteristics of an organism that result from the interaction of its genetic constitution with the environment.

Phytohemagglutinin: a mitogenic plant protein from the red kidney bean, often used in cytogenetic assays to stimulate lymphocyte proliferation.

Polyaromatic hydrocarbon: (polynuclear aromatic hydrocarbon, PAH): a compound consisting of two or more aromatic rings sharing pairs of carbon atoms. These extremely stable compounds, such as benzo(a)pyrene, may be formed as by-products of combustion; many are genotoxic.

Polymorphism: a genetic trait where the least common allele is found in at least 1 percent of the population. The simultaneous occurrence in the population of genomes showing allelic variations.

^{32}P-postlabeling: a method for detecting DNA adducts. This technique involves hydrolysis of the DNA, labeling the nucleotides with radioactive phosphorus, and chromatographing the nucleotides.

Preclinical: the period of pathogenesis before symptoms of disease appear. Also, studies or experiments in nonhuman systems.

Promotion: the process of enhancing the development of a cancer. Conceptually, it is thought to act only after the initial carcinogenic event (see also initiation).

Protein: essential constituents in structure and metabolism. They are composed of linked amino acids such as histidine, cysteine, valine, and proline. Enzymes are proteins.

Radical: (see free radical).

Sensitivity: the proportion of people with a condition whom are correctly classified by a test as having the condition. Also, the ability of an assay to detect differences in an analyte's concentration among samples. The minimum level of an analyte that a test can detect.

Sister chromatid exchange: the breaking, exchange, and rejoining of segments of DNA between sister chromatids. It is analogous to crossing-over between homologous chromosomes.

Somatic: refers to any cell in a multicellular organism other than a germ cell.

Specificity: the proportion of people without a condition who are correctly classified by a test as not having the condition. Also, the degree to which more than one condition can cause a positive test.

Susceptibility marker: a measurable indicator of genetic or acquired factors, existing before and independent of exposure, that influences the probability that disease will result from external exposure.

Thymidine kinase (TK): an enzyme that plays a role in the regulation of pyrimidine synthesis. This enzyme can be used as a marker for somatic cell mutations.

Transformation: the conversion of cells to a state of incompletely restrained growth. In vitro transformation is used as a model for in vivo carcinogenesis. Also used more broadly to refer to a change to another phenotype of a cell.

Translocations: the transposition of two chromosomal segments between nonhomologous chromosomes.

Unscheduled DNA synthesis: the synthesis of DNA as part of a DNA repair process (not DNA replication) occurring in response to chemical exposures.

Volatile: evaporates quickly.

Xenobiotics: chemical substances that are foreign to an organism.

INDEX

N-acetyltransferase (NAT), 22, 199–209. *See also* Cancer
4-aminobiphenyl, 18, 32, 40, 48, 50, 89–90, 93, 200
Aberration, chromosome. *See* Chromosome aberrations
Acetylcholinesterase, 30, 226
Adducts
  assays for DNA adducts, 87–98
    chromatography and spectrometry, 87–88
    comparison of laboratory techniques, 98
    immunoassays, 91–92
    ^{32}P-postlabeling, 94–96
    solid phase assay, 91–92
    in surrogate tissues, 85–86
  assays for hemoglobin adducts, 88
  carcinogenesis and, 81
  dose-response relationships, 84
  in epidemiology, 82–86
  formation, 78–80
    absorption and transport, 78
    chemotherapeutic agents and, 94
    cigarette smoking and, 92–93
    dietary exposures and, 83, 93–94
    endogenous factors, 83
    metabolic activation, 79–80
  heterogeneity, 82
  human studies, 89, 95–98
  mutation and, 81
  in occupational groups, 93
  persistence, 82–85

  stability, 216–218
  variability, 218–219
Adipose tissue, 18, 33–34, 36, 217
Alpha$_1$-antitrypsin, 22, 30
Alpha-fetoprotein (AFP), 10, 20
Ames test, 60–61, 222
  inter- and intraindividual variability, 61–62
  sensitivity and specificity, 61
Amniotic fluid, 21
Amplification, oncogene. *See* Oncogenes
Arylamines and bladder cancer, 204–205
Ataxia-telangiectasia, 11, 85, 201

Banding. *See* Chromosome structure
Benzene, 23, 35, 167
Biochemical epidemiology. *See* Molecular epidemiology
Biological compartments, 33, 35
Biological markers, 3–4, 228
  assay interpretation, 222–223
  biological relationships, 17
  choice of marker, 215–216
  classification, 28–31
    cellular changes, 31
    endogenously produced molecules, 30
    exogenous agents, 28–30
    molecular changes, 30–31
  confounders, 219–221
  definitions, 7–12
  in epidemiologic research, 6–7, 12–14
  interpretation, 16, 223–224